The Ultimate Hormone Balancing Guidebook

A Complete Natural Hormone Balancing Guidebook for Clinicians and Patients

By Dr. Cobi Slater, PhD, DNM®, RHT, RNCP, ROHP

The Ultimate Hormone Balancing Guidebook
A Complete Natural Hormone Balancing Guidebook for Clinicians and Patients
by Dr. Cobi Slater, PhD, DNM®, RHT, RNCP, ROHP

ISBN: 978-1-990830-54-9

1. Endorsements vii
2. Medical Disclaimer ix
3. Acknowledgements xi
4. Introduction xiii
5. Endocrine Overview—The Symphony 15
6. Epidemics Uncovered—Endocrine Disruptors 26
7. Liver Toxicity 34
8. The Stress Effect 43
9. Nutritional Factors 49
10. Testing Procedures 66
11. Bioidentical Hormone Replacement Therapy (BHRT) vs. Hormone Replacement Therapy (HRT) 75
12. Hormonal Conditions 80
    - Anxiety 80
    - Depression 99
    - Adrenal Fatigue 112
    - Thyroid Disorders 127
    - Estrogen Dominance 138
    - Premenstrual Syndrome (PMS) 147
    - Fibroids 158
    - Endometriosis 166
    - Polycystic Ovarian Syndrome (PCOS) 175
    - Ovarian Cysts 184
    - Menopause 192
    - Andropause 206
    - Weight Gain 218
13. Conclusion 237
14. Bibliography 239
15. Appendix 243

Endorsements

"I've known Dr. Cobi Slater for many years and I would definitely say she is the 'hormone guru'. If you suspect any hormonal issues wreaking havoc on your life you can turn these imbalances around with her expert guidance. In The Ultimate Hormone Balancing Guidebook she generously shares her vast wisdom on the subject of hormones."

Michelle Schoffro Cook, MS, PhD, RNCP, ROHP, DNM

International best-selling author of 60 Seconds to Slim, Weekend Wonder Detox, and The Ultimate pH Solution. DrMichelleCook.com

"Dr. Cobi Slater is a true leader in the field of holistic health care and a master at helping women and men with natural solutions concerning hormonal imbalances.
The information in this book is revolutionary for our times, providing clear and practical natural solutions for those searching for answers."

Ellen Tart-Jensen, Ph.D., D.Sc., author of Health is Your Birthright, How to Create the Health You Deserve

Medical Disclaimer

This book is not intended as a substitute for the medical advice of physicians. The reader should regularly consult a physician in matters relating to his/her health and particularly with respect to any symptoms that may require a diagnosis or medical attention.

Acknowledgements

This book is dedicated to the thousands of patients who birthed in me a passion for a deeper knowledge and understanding of hormonal health and healing. I thank you for entrusting me with your health and for allowing me to be a part of your journey to wellness.

I am filled with eternal gratitude for my Mom, Arlene Kubin. I have been abundantly blessed with a Mom who supports me to the most infinite detail in all that I do. Thank you Mom for sitting with me for hours, days, weeks and months editing this book and encouraging each and every word to be printed. Your endless love and daily encouragement has shaped me into to who I am today. Thank you to my dear Dad whose sparkly eyes can light up a room and melt my heart. All that you do behind the scenes does not go unnoticed. Your loving support lifts me when I need it and sets me in flight to pursue my dreams.

Thank you to my 3 Slater boys, Garry, Dane and Kade whom I love with all of my heart. You are the most treasured loves of my life! My cup runneth over.....

Introduction

The North American culture is currently experiencing alarmingly high rates of hormonal imbalances. These imbalances are setting the stage for a cultural shift toward disorders of the endocrine system becoming seemingly "normal." By the time the average North American woman has completed her morning routine, she has exposed her face, body, and hair to over 126 chemicals from twelve different products. *Our Stolen Future,* co-authored by Theo Colborn summarizes the findings of a gathering of international experts in 1991. It was then that they first warned us about chemicals that have the potential to disrupt the hormone systems of humans and animals. These experts estimated with profound confidence that "unless the environmental load of synthetic hormone disruptors is abated and controlled, large scale dysfunction at the population level is possible."[1]

Exposing the many underlying causes of disparity within the hormonal systems of North American females is the first step toward healing. The incidence of hormonal dysfunction is specific to North American females as the rate of their endocrine imbalances far supersedes that of any other culture on our planet. An obvious conclusion is that many women in North America are exposed to far more endocrine disruptors, experience endless stress, and have poor dietary habits, resulting in liver toxicity. People who are native to some cultures live simplistic lifestyles, relying entirely on nature to feed and house them. These people eat indigenously within their land and are not exposed to as many pollutants in the form of electromagnetic radiation, noise pollution, air pollution, pesticides, herbicides, preservatives, and chemicals. Terms such as "hot flashes," "PMS," and "menopause" simply do not exist in their languages. They are relatively free from hormonal irregularities and imbalances. Hormonal stages in a woman's life such as menstruation, childbirth, and the cessation of the menstrual cycle are celebrated through cultural rituals. Interviews with rural Mayan Indian women further illustrates that menopause, as an example, is far from a uniform experience. Researchers found that the women reported no incidences of hot flashes or any other significant menopausal symptoms. Mayan women tend to look forward to menopause because with it comes a progressive change in status within their communities and, in turn, a feeling of freedom. When women from indigenous cultures cross into menopause, they often become known as "wise women," or spiritual leaders, and hold a place of power in their communities[2]. In stark contrast, in North America, these stages have been medicalized and deemed pathological in nature. Menopause, as an example, is treated very much as a medical condition rather than as a natural phenomenon of a woman's life.

There are many proven holistic treatments that are able to bring balance back into the endocrine systems of women. Depression, anxiety, perimenopause, menopause, premenstrual syndrome, fibroids, ovarian cysts, polycystic ovarian syndrome, endometriosis, adrenal fatigue, thyroid disorders, and obesity are some of the main disorders that can result from hormonal imbalances. Rather than compartmentalize each organ of the body, a holistic approach

---

1 Rick Smith and Bruce Lourie, *Slow Death by Rubber Duck*, V111.

2 http://www.everydayhealth.com/menopause/menopause-and-culture.aspx.

is one that considers all aspects involved, including dietary habits, stress, genetics, thought processes, exposure to toxins, liver toxicity, and lifestyle habits. Uncovering the underlying cause of any hormonal imbalance is the most effective way to bring complete resolution and restoration of health.

Endocrine Overview—The Symphony

Every biological process within the body relies upon the hormones that are produced within the body's endocrine glands. Hormones are sophisticated chemical messengers. They form the body's major communication network system, allowing for different parts of the body to interconnect in a symphony.

There are several hormones secreted by the endocrine system. Each hormone affects only the body cells that have a genetic program that allows the cells to react to those hormones. The endocrine system functions like a lock and key mechanism. Therefore each hormone (a.k.a. "key") can only fit into its genetic receptor (a.k.a. "lock"). Although each key has its own lock, there are circumstances when other keys can fit into a lock. An example of the lock and key function, or dysfunction, is the ability of environmental xenoestrogens (estrogen mimickers) to fit into human estrogen receptor sites which may then cause severe hormonal disturbances.

The endocrine system is regulated by feedback in much the same way that a thermostat regulates the temperature in a room. For the hormones that are regulated by the pituitary gland, a signal is sent from the hypothalamus to the pituitary gland in the form of a "releasing hormone." This stimulates the pituitary to secrete a "stimulating hormone" into the circulation. The stimulating hormone then signals the target gland to secrete its hormone. As the level of this hormone rises in the circulation, the hypothalamus and the pituitary gland shut down secretion of the releasing hormone and the stimulating hormone. In response, the secretion by the target gland is slowed down. This system results in stable blood concentrations of the hormones that are regulated by the pituitary gland. [3]

According to the *The Endocrine System—An Overview* written by Susanne Hiller-Sturmhöfel, Ph.D., and Andrzej Bartke, Ph.D., the term "endocrine" implies that in response to specific stimuli, the products of those glands are released into the bloodstream. The hormones are then carried via the blood to their target cells. Some hormones have only a few specific target cells, whereas other hormones affect numerous cell types throughout the body. The target cells for each hormone are characterized by the presence of certain docking molecules (i.e., receptors) for the hormones that are located either on the cell surface or inside the cells. The interaction between the hormone and its receptor triggers a cascade of biochemical reactions in the target cell that eventually modifies the cell's functions or activities.[4]

The endocrine system is comprised of 8 major glands, namely:

1. Hypothalamus
2. Pituitary gland
3. Parathyroid gland
4. Thyroid gland

---

3 http://www.emedicinehealth.com/anatomy_of_the_endocrine_system/article_em.htm

4 Susanne Hiller-Sturmhöfel, Ph.D., and Andrzej Bartke, Ph.D., *The Endocrine System—An Overview.*

5. Adrenal glands
6. Pancreas
7. Ovaries (in the female body)
8. Testes (in the male body)

The following illustration portrays the glands of the Endocrine System:[5]

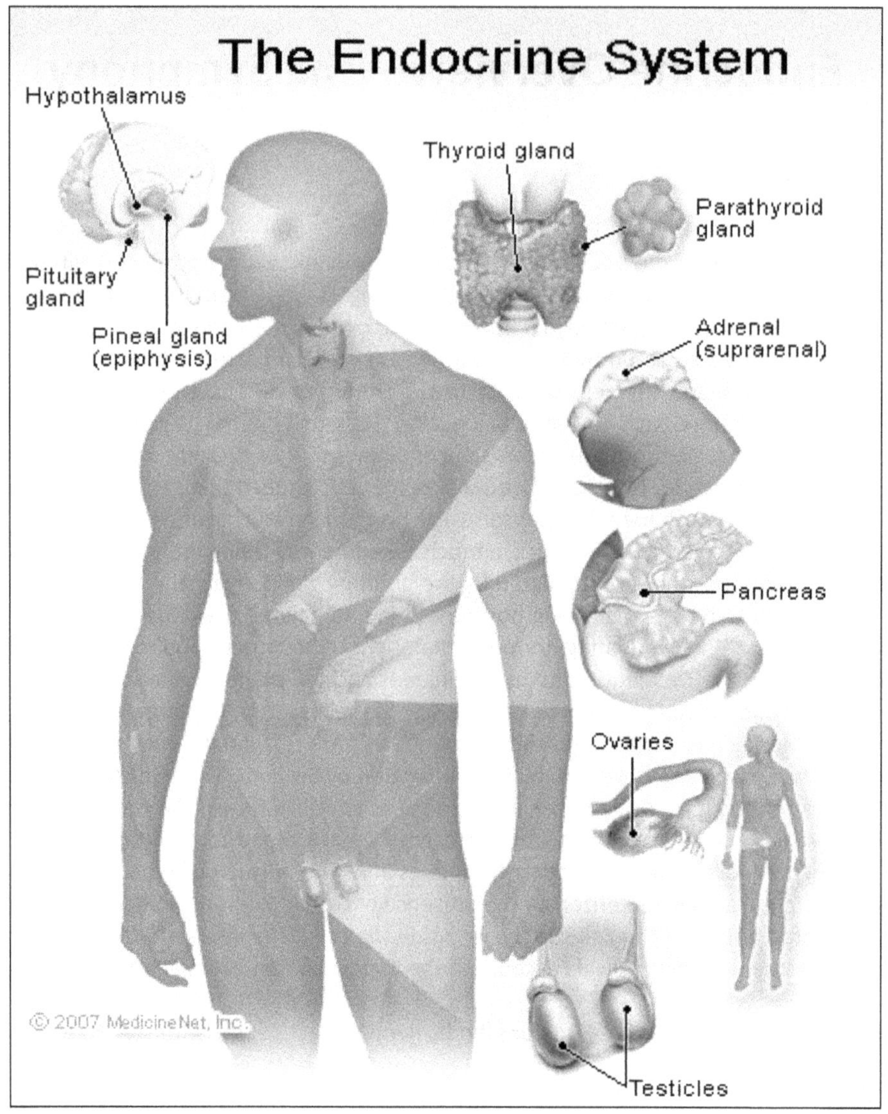

The endocrine system is the body's regulating mechanism. All of the body's functions can be influenced by the endocrine system. This includes metabolism, growth, water and electrolyte balance, sexual function, reproduction, and behavior. The function of the endocrine glands are numerous and specific to each individual gland.

---

[5] http://www.emedicinehealth.com/anatomy_of_the_endocrine_system/article_em.htm.

• **Hypothalamus:** The hypothalamus is the main link between the endocrine system and the nervous system. It is a collection of specialized cells which is located in the lower central part of the brain. The nerve cells of the hypothalamus control the pituitary gland by stimulating or suppressing the hormone secretions.

• **Pituitary Gland:** The pituitary gland is the most important part in the endocrine system. It is often termed the "master gland" and is located at the base of the brain just below the hypothalamus. The pituitary gland secretes hormones on the basis of emotional and seasonal changes. The hypothalamus sends information that is sensed by the brain to the pituitary, triggering production hormones. Endorphins, which act on the nervous system and lower the feelings of pain, are also secreted by the pituitary gland. The pituitary gland is also involved in the production of hormones that signal the reproductive organs to secrete sex hormones and control the menstrual cycle in women.

The pituitary gland is divided into two parts—the anterior lobe and the posterior lobe. The anterior lobe of the pituitary gland regulates the activities of the thyroid, adrenals, and reproductive glands. The anterior lobe also produces hormones such as:

- **Growth Hormone:** To stimulate the growth of the bones and tissues. It also plays a role in the body's absorption of nutrients and minerals.
- **Prolactin:** To activate the production of milk in lactating mothers.
- **Thyrotropin (TSH):** To stimulate the thyroid gland to produce thyroid hormones.
- **Corticotropin:** To stimulate the adrenal glands to produce certain hormones.

The posterior lobe of the pituitary gland produces antidiuretic hormones that help to control the water balance in the body. In addition, oxytocin is produced by the posterior lobe to trigger contractions of the uterus in a woman who is in labor.

• **Thyroid Gland:** The thyroid gland is located in the lower front part of the neck and is shaped like a bowtie or a butterfly. It produces the thyroid hormones thyroxine and triiodothyronine which regulate the metabolism of the body. Triiodothyronine (T3) and thyroxine (T4) look quite similar except for the number of iodine atoms they contain; triiodothyronine has three iodine atoms and thyroxine has four iodine atoms. Very different quantities of these two hormones are produced in the thyroid gland. Approximately 93% of its thyroid hormone production is in the form of T4 and the remainder is in the form of T3.[6] Despite its higher level of production within the thyroid gland, T4 is considered an inactive form of the thyroid hormone. Only T3 or T4 that has been converted into T3 inside the cells can be used to produce energy in our cells. When the body's energy requirements increase, the hypothalamus secretes thyrotropin-releasing hormone (TRH). TRH signals the pituitary gland to secrete thyroid-stimulating hormone (TSH). In turn, TSH stimulates the thyroid gland to produce T4. T4 is secreted by the thyroid gland into the bloodstream and travels to distant cells. After it enters a cell, T4 must be converted into T3, which is the active form of thyroid hormone, so that it can be used to fuel metabolic reactions.[7]

The thyroid gland plays a role in bone growth and development of the brain and nervous system in children. Thyroid hormones also help to maintain normal blood pressure, heart rate, digestion, muscle tone, and reproductive functions.

• **Parathyroid Glands:** These are four tiny glands that are attached to the thyroid gland. They release the parathyroid hormones that help in regulating the levels of calcium and calcitonin, which is produced in the thyroid gland, in the blood.

---

[6] http://www.drhotze.com/Resource-Library/eBooks/eBook-tags.aspx?tagid=1310.

[7] http://www.drhotze.com/Resource-Library/eBooks/eBook-tags.aspx?tagid=1310.

- **Adrenal Glands:** The adrenal glands are triangular-shaped glands located on top of each kidney. The adrenal glands are made up of two parts. The outer part is called the adrenal cortex and the inner part is called the adrenal medulla. The adrenal cortex produces hormones called corticosteroids which regulate the body's metabolism, the balance of salt and water in the body, the immune system, and sexual function. The adrenal medulla, produces hormones called catecholamines, such as adrenaline. These hormones help the body cope with physical and emotional stress by increasing the heart rate and blood pressure.[8]

- **Reproductive Glands or Gonads:** The reproductive glands are the main source of sex hormones. In males, the testes, located in the scrotum, secrete hormones called androgens—the most important of which is testosterone. These hormones affect many male characteristics such as sexual development, growth of facial and pubic hair, and sperm production. In females, the ovaries are located on both sides of the uterus. They produce the hormones estrogen and progesterone as well as producing eggs during ovulation. These hormones control the development of female characteristics such as the breasts and they are also involved in reproductive functions such as menstruation and pregnancy.

- **Pancreas:** The pancreas is an elongated organ located toward the back of the abdomen, behind the stomach. The pancreas has digestive and hormonal functions. One part of the pancreas, the exocrine pancreas, secretes digestive enzymes. The other part of the pancreas, the endocrine pancreas, secretes hormones called insulin and glucagon. These hormones regulate the level of glucose (sugar) in the blood.

- **Pineal:** The pineal gland is located in the center of the brain. This glad secretes melatonin, which regulates the circadian rhythm or the sleep-wake cycle of a person.

The following picture illustrates the main endocrine glands and the hormones they secrete:

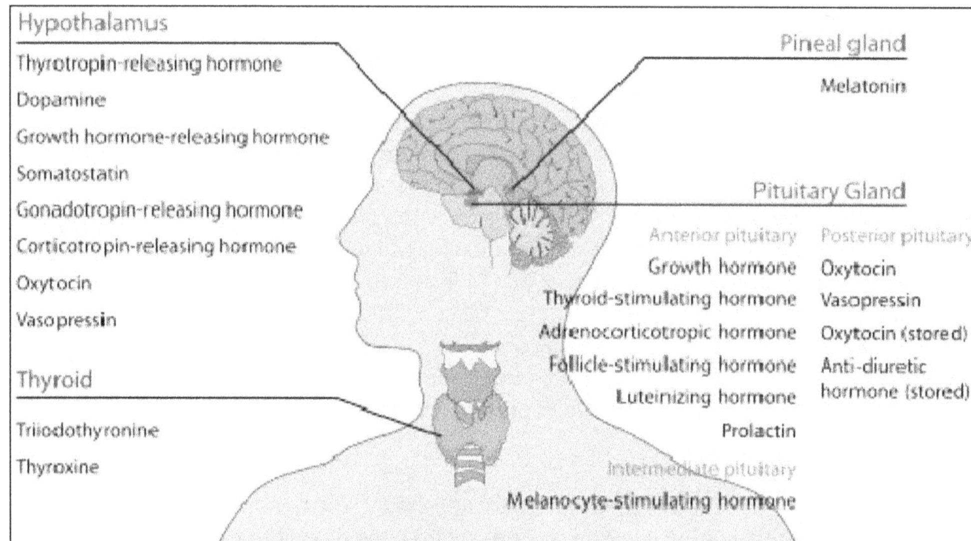

Hormones are molecules that are produced by endocrine glands, including the hypothalamus, pituitary gland, adrenal glands, gonads (i.e., testes and ovaries), thyroid gland, parathyroid glands, and pancreas. Each hormone has a very specific function in the body in order to maintain homeostasis.

---

8 http://www.emedicinehealth.com/anatomy_of_the_endocrine_system/page6_em.htm.

Oxytocin

Oxytocin is a hormone secreted by the pituitary gland. It is one of a group of hormones that control sexual development and processes. The roles of oxytocin are slightly different in males than in females.

The functions of oxytocin hormones in males include:

- Inducing pair bonding
- Playing some role in orgasms
- Facilitating sperm transport in ejaculation

The functions of oxytocin hormones in females include:

- Inducing pair bonding
- Playing some role in orgasms
- Causing contraction of the uterus during labor
- Stimulating milk flow from the breasts by causing the contraction of muscle fibers in the milk ducts
- Inducing maternal behavior

Antidiuretic Hormone (ADH)

Antidiuretic hormone (ADH), also known as vasopressin, is a hormone secreted by the posterior pituitary gland. Antidiuretic hormone increases reabsorption of water by the kidneys, which prevents the body from losing excessive amounts of water.

Prolactin (PRL)

Prolactin (also known as lactogenic hormone, luteotrophic hormone, and luteotrophin) is a hormone secreted by the anterior pituitary gland.

The actions of prolactin in females include:

- Stimulating the production of progesterone in the ovaries
- Stimulating milk production after childbirth

Human Growth Hormone (HGH)

Human growth hormone (HGH), also known as somatotrophin, is a hormone that is synthesized, stored, and secreted by the anterior pituitary gland.

Human growth hormone promotes growth, especially growth of the long bones in the limbs (i.e., the femur, tibia, and fibula in the legs and the humerus, ulna, and radius in the arms). It also increases the synthesis of proteins.

The release of human growth hormone into the bloodstream is controlled by the balancing or opposing effects of the growth-hormone-releasing hormone and somatostatin.

Thyroid Stimulating Hormone (TSH)

Thyroid stimulating hormone (TSH), also known as thyrotrophin, is a hormone that is synthesized and secreted by the anterior pituitary gland.Thyroid stimulating hormone is synthesized and stored in the thyrotroph cells in the anterior lobe of the pituitary gland (which is called the adenohypophysis). Its main function is to stimulate the thyroid gland to release two of its own hormones into the bloodstream. These two hormones are triiodothyronine (T3) and thyroxine (T4).

Synthesis of thyroid stimulating hormone is controlled by thyrotrophin-releasing hormone. The other factor that regulates the amount of thyroid stimulating hormone present in the body is the negative feedback mechanism involving the influence of the thyroid hormones themselves.

Adrenocorticotrophic Hormone (ACTH)

Adrenocorticotrophic hormone (ACTH), also known as adrenocorticotropin, and corticotrophin, is a hormone that is synthesized, stored, and released by the anterior pituitary gland.

Adrenocorticotrophic hormone is released in response to stress and controls the secretion of corticosteroid hormones from the adrenal glands.

These include:

- mineral corticoids
- glucocorticoids
- cortisol (natural anti-inflammatory)
- androgens

Gonadotrophin

The term "gonadotrophin" (or "gonadotropic hormone") may refer to any of several hormones synthesized and released by the anterior pituitary gland. Their function is to promote the production of sex hormones and either sperm or ova by the gonads.

The main gonadotrophins are follicle stimulating hormone and luteinizing hormone.

The production of gonadotrophins by the body is controlled by the gonadotrophin-releasing hormone (GnRH). This is a peptide hormone produced in the hypothalamus and then transported to the pituitary gland via the bloodstream.

Luteinizing Hormone (LH)

Luteinizing hormone (LH) is a glycoprotein gonadotropin hormone secreted by the anterior pituitary gland. It is released by the anterior pituitary in hourly pulses called "circhoral oscillations."

Luteinizing hormone binds to receptors in the testes (in males) and the ovaries (in females). LH also regulates gonadal function by promoting sex steroid production and "gametogenesis," i.e., the processes by which spermatozoa and ova are formed.

The roles of luteinizing hormone are slightly different in males than in females.

The actions of luteinizing hormone in men include:

- Stimulating testosterone production from the interstitial cells of the testes (Leydig cells)
- Playing a role in the maturation of spermatozoa, i.e., mature male sex cells

The actions of luteinizing hormone in females include:

- Stimulating estrogen and progesterone production from the ovaries
- A surge of luteinizing hormone midway through the menstrual cycle leads to ovulation
- Continued secretion of luteinizing hormone stimulates the corpus luteum to produce progesterone, playing a role in controlling the secretion of estrogen from ovarian follicles

Follicle Stimulating Hormone (FSH)

Follicle stimulating hormone (FSH) is a glycoprotein gonadotropin hormone secreted by the anterior pituitary gland.

Follicle stimulating hormone binds to receptors in the testes (in males) and the ovaries (in females). FSH also regulates gonadal function by promoting sex steroid production and "gametogenesis," i.e., the processes by which spermatozoa and ova are formed.

The role of follicle stimulating hormone is slightly different in males than in females.

The actions of follicle stimulating hormone in males include:

- Stimulating testicular growth and enhancing the production of a protein that causes high local concentrations of testosterone near the sperm. This is an essential factor in the development of normal spermatogenesis.
- Playing a role in the maturation of spermatozoa, i.e., mature male sex cells.

The actions of follicle stimulating hormone in females include:

- Controlling the development of ovarian follicles (vessels inside the ovaries in which ova develop).
- Playing a role in controlling the secretion of estrogen from ovarian follicles.

Melatonin

Melatonin is a hormone secreted by the pineal gland. It is important for setting and maintaining the body's biological clock or regulating the day/night rhythm based on periods of light/darkness.

- Melatonin is produced by the pineal gland in darkness but not in bright light
- Melatonin receptors in the brain react to this hormone and synchronize the body to the twenty-four-hour day/night rhythm, informing the brain when it is day and when it is night
- Melatonin is derived from serotonin, which work together to regulate the sleep cycle

Melatonin levels are higher in children than in adults and decline with the aging process.

Thyroxin

Thyroxin (sometimes written "thyroxine") is a hormone secreted by the thyroid gland.

- Thyroxin is important for the regulation of the body's basal metabolic rate (BMR), which is the amount of energy the body uses.
- There are consequences of both excessive quantities of thyroxin in the body (hyperthyroidism), and insufficient quantities of thyroxin in the body (hypothyroidism).

Calcitonin

Calcitonin (also known as "thyrocalcitonin") is a hormone produced by and secreted by the thyroid gland.

- Calcitonin helps to regulate the levels of calcium and phosphate in the blood.
- Calcitonin decreases the amount of calcium in the blood by inhibiting the action of osteoclasts (cells that break down the bone matrix). Hence, calcitonin promotes the movement of calcium ions (Ca^{2+}) into the bone matrix, simultaneously decreasing the quantity of calcium ions (Ca^{2+}) in the blood.

Parathormone

Parathormone is a hormone secreted by the parathyroid glands.

- Parathormone is associated with the growth of muscle and bone.
- Parathormone is responsible for the distribution of calcium and phosphate in the body.

Insulin

Insulin is a protein hormone secreted by the beta cells of the islets of the Langerhans within the pancreas.

Insulin is extremely important for the regulation of the amount of sugar (glucose) in the blood.

The secretion of insulin by the beta cells of the pancreas is stimulated by high concentrations of blood sugar. The insulin secreted prevents the amount of sugar in the blood from rising to a dangerous level by:

- Easing and increasing the rate of diffusion of glucose from the blood into most of the body cells—especially the skeletal muscle fibers.
- Accelerating the conversion of glucose into glycogen and fatty acids.
- Promoting the uptake of amino acids into body cells and increasing the production of proteins within cells.
- Reducing the rate of conversion of liver glycogen into glucose.
- Reducing the rate of formation of glucose by liver cells.

Glucagon

Glucagon is a hormone secreted by the alpha cells of the islets of the Langerhans within the pancreas. Glucagon's presence in the blood causes an increase in the quantity of sugar in the blood (blood sugar level). That is, glucagon in the bloodstream has the opposite effect to that of insulin, which regulates the amount of sugar in the blood.

Glucagon increases blood sugar (or blood glucose) levels when they fall below the "normal" level, i.e., in the range 4-10 mmol/liter, by:

- Accelerating the conversion of glycogen in the liver into glucose.
- Promoting the conversion in the liver of amino acids and lactic acid into glucose.
- Stimulating the release of glucose from the liver into the blood.

Adrenalin

Adrenalin (also known as epinephrine) is a hormone secreted by the adrenal medulla.

Adrenalin prepares the body for "fight or flight" responses and has many effects, including:

- Increasing the action of the heart.
- Increasing the rate and depth of breathing.
- Increasing the metabolic rate.
- Improving the force of muscular contractions.
- Delaying the onset of muscular fatigue.

Noradrenalin

Noradrenalin (also known as norepinephrine) is a hormone secreted by the adrenal medulla.

The effects of noradrenalin are similar to the effects of adrenalin.

The actions of noradrenalin include:

- Constriction of the small blood vessels, leading to increases in blood pressure.
- Increasing the blood flow through the coronary arteries and slowing the heart rate.
- Increasing the rate and depth of breathing.
- Relaxing the smooth muscle in the intestinal walls.

Increased amounts of both adrenalin and noradrenalin are secreted when the body is under stress.

Corticosteroids

Corticosteroids are hormones secreted by the adrenal cortex.

There are two main groups of corticosteroids:

1. The functions of glucocorticoids (e.g., cortisol, cortisone, corticosterone) include:
    - Utilization of carbohydrates, fats, and proteins by the body.
    - Normalizing responses to stress.
    - Anti-inflammatory effects.

2. The functions of mineralocorticoids (e.g., aldosterone) include:
    - Regulation of salt and water balance.
    - Decreasing the potassium levels in the body (via hyper-secretion of aldosterone), affecting nerve impulse transmission and potentially leading to muscular paralysis.

Estrogen

Estrogen is a hormone secreted primarily by the ovaries.

Although estrogen is synthesized mainly by the ovaries, some small quantities of estrogen are also produced by the adrenal cortex, testes, and placenta. Estrogen is present in males but excessive production of estrogen in men can lead to feminization.

The actions of estrogen in women include:

- Controlling female sexual development.
- Promoting growth of female secondary sexual characteristics at puberty.
- Stimulating egg (ovum) production.
- Preparing the lining (endometrium) of the uterus for pregnancy.
- Regulating the growth and functioning of sex organs for sexual reproduction.

Progesterone

Progesterone is a steroid hormone secreted primarily by the ovaries. It is one of a group of steroid hormones that controls female sexual development and processes. Although progesterone is synthesized mainly by the corpus luteum of the ovaries, some small quantities of progesterone are also produced by the adrenal cortex, testes, and placenta.

The actions of progesterone in women include:

- Preparing the inner lining (endometrium) of the uterus for pregnancy.
- Maintaining the uterus after fertilization and then throughout the pregnancy.
- Preventing further release of eggs from the ovaries during pregnancy.
- Regulating the growth and functioning of sex organs for sexual reproduction.

Testosterone

Testosterone is the principal androgen, or male sex hormone, and is secreted primarily by the testes.

Testosterone is important for:

- Development and function of male sex organs.
- Development of secondary sexual characteristics, e.g., body hair, muscle development, voice changes.

SUMMARY—FUNCTIONS OF THE ENDOCRINE SYSTEM[9]

Gland and Hormones	General Function
HYPOTHALAMUS CRF, GnRH, TRH, PIF, GRF, Somatostatin	Controls the secretion of the pituitary gland, body temperature, hunger, thirst, and sexual drive Stimulates the pineal gland to secrete melatonin, which orchestrates body rhythms

[9] Sat Dharam Kaur, ND, *Complete Natural Medicine Guide to Women's Health*, 83-84

PINEAL GLAND Melatonin	Regulates circadian and ultradian rhythms Often called the body's biological clock
PITUITARY GLAND ACTH, TSH, Prolactin, Growth hormone, FSH, LH, Vasopressin, Oxytocin	Controls bone growth and regulates the other glands Often called the master gland
THYROID GLAND T4, T3, Calcitonin	Maintains an optimal metabolic rate in tissues, controlling the rate of fuel use in the body and controlling its sensitivity to heat and cold Supports immune function Protects from bone loss during pregnancy
PARATHYROID GLANDS PTH	Help to regulate the amount of calcium in the blood Stimulate bone building
THYMUS Thymosin	Coordinates white blood cells (especially T cells) and the immune system Destroys viruses, fungi, some bacteria, and cancer cells Shrinks with age
LIVER IGF-1	Regulates growth and blood sugar metabolism Detoxifies body systems
PANCREAS Insulin, Glucagon	Controls blood sugar levels Helps to digest food (non-hormonal function)
OVARIES Estrogen, Progesterone	Controls sexual development, maturation and release of eggs, fertility *Estrogen*: Causes multiplication of breast cells Thickens uterus and uterine lining Maintains vaginal thickness and lubrication Encourages formation of collagen in skin Inhibits breakdown of bone, increasing density *Progesterone*: Prepares uterus for implantation Maintains development of the placenta Develops milk-secreting cells during pregnancy Causes maturation of breast cells during pregnancy Helps prevent breast cysts and cancer Increases libido

ADRENAL GLANDS Cortisol, Aldosterone, DHEA, Testosterone, Adrenaline, Noradrenaline	Control salt and water balance in the body Helps us to adapt to stress Generate "fight or flight" reaction in response to life-threatening situations or unexpected emotional stress Decrease allergies Regulate sleep and mood Increase resistance to viruses, bacteria, fungi, allergies, cancer Stimulate bone formation Prevent osteoporosis, arthritis, Lupus, and autoimmune disease Help to maintain normal sex hormone levels Increase libido and sexual arousal

Epidemics Uncovered—Endocrine Disruptors

Our bodies were created to function in perfect homeostasis. Since the advent of industrialization within the last one hundred years, our once perfect environment became inundated with horrific chemicals that threaten this very homeostasis. Our bodies are now subjected to unprecedented insults from environmental estrogen-like hormones. Our food has changed more in the past fifty years than in the previous one thousand years. We have managed to turn our diets from whole unprocessed foods to a borage of fast and chemically-laden processed foods. Consider cattle that were once raised on grass and natural organic feed and chickens that were allowed to run free and how commercialization has now caged them. To add insult to injury, feeds are now laced with pesticides and hormones. These pesticides and hormones have estrogen-like effects and are passed on to humans as they are consumed. This explains the alarmingly high rate of endocrine disorders in our modern day population.

It has been shown that chronic low dose exposure to pesticides in humans can negatively affect the nervous system and cause immune deficiencies leading to allergies and autoimmune conditions. Exogenous chemicals in the body settle into the organs of high metabolism first. Both the uterus and the ovaries have high metabolic rates.[10] In non-industrialized cultures, women whose diets are indigenous and therefore based on non-processed, whole foods, seldom suffer hormonal imbalances such as those seen in industrialized cultures.

Causes of Hormonal Imbalance

The delicate symphony of hormones that occurs within the endocrine system can be easily disrupted in many different ways. The sheer act of aging can result in upsetting the endocrine system.

As reproductive functions play out over time, hormone levels naturally decline. If the hormones decline too quickly, this can trigger the onset of early menopause and can cause other hormonal imbalances associated with the change of life. Lifestyle habits play a major role in the pace of hormonal decline and premature aging.

Hormone balance is deeply connected to many different factors including nutrition, exercise, detoxification capabilities, obesity, and stress levels. At midlife, the already overstressed adrenal glands must take over much of the hormone production previously handled by the ovaries. Chronic stress that exceeds the body's capabilities causes excess cortisol to flood the system and disrupt the total hormone production. The body sacrifices progesterone in order to make even more cortisol in response to the chronic stress. This depletes the key balancing hormone, progesterone, with obvious implications for estrogen dominance. Prolonged stress deteriorates bones, atrophies muscles, decreases strength and energy, lowers libido, and overwhelms the immune system. This puts women at serious risk

---

[10] "Environmental Illness. COULD CHEMICAL OVERLOAD BE THE CAUSE OF YOUR ILLNESS?" Interview with William J. Rea, M.D., INTERVIEW DATE.

for severe menopausal symptoms as well as chronic illnesses and autoimmune diseases. Many women's ailments are linked to specific hormonal imbalances which can be triggered by any one or a combination of the following:[11]

- Stress and overexertion
- Not enough time for relaxation and play
- Improper breathing
- Improper diet, including excess saturated or hydrogenated fat, sugar, refined carbohydrates, meats, dairy, or toxins from fish
- Nutritional deficiencies, including deficiencies of vitamins B5, B6, and C, zinc, selenium, magnesium, tyrosine, tryptophan, or essential fatty acids
- Food sensitivities
- Environmental allergies
- Infectious organisms and/or imbalances in intestinal flora
- Intestinal toxins, such as yeast toxins
- Impaired liver function or liver stagnation
- Elevated blood sugar
- Excess alcohol consumption
- Smoking
- Exposure to electromagnetic chemicals, including PCBs, dioxin, pesticides, phthalates, Bisphenol A, PVC, fire retardants, or parabens in cosmetics
- Exposure to hormone-disrupting chemicals or hormonal excess *in utero*
- Pharmaceutical drugs, birth control pills, or hormone replacement therapy
- Heavy metals, particularly cadmium, mercury, and lead
- Lack of exercise or excessive exercise
- Exposure to light at night
- Lack of exposure to sunlight
- Shift work
- Insomnia
- Obesity or being underweight
- History of emotional trauma or abuse
- Negative thought patterns and emotions

Xenoestrogens

In 1991, the field of xenoestrogens was first introduced to the world.[12] Xenoestrogens are foreign estrogens, as "xeno" literally means foreign. Not found in nature, man-made toxins are estrogen imposters that make their way into the body on the pretense of being biological estrogen. They mimic the effects of the real hormone but over-stimulate cellular activity to an uncontrollable extent. Xenoestrogens are present in our soil, water, air, and food supply, as well as in personal care and household products. Xenoestrogens accumulate in the fat tissues of our bodies and have the capability of locking into our own estrogen's receptor sites. This deems them to be highly toxic and detrimental to our hormonal environment. Xenoestrogens adversely affect the internal balancing mechanisms of the body, raising the estrogen burden and with it, potential risks for the development of endocrine disorders.

[11] Sat Dharam Kaur, ND, *Complete Natural Medicine Guide to Women's Health,* 85.

[12] "Suite101: List of Xenoestrogens - Chemical Estrogens: How to Avoid Xenoestrogens," http://www.suite101.com/content/list-of-xenoestrogens—chemical-estrogens-a205523#ixzz1lrecjmqZ.

The following is a list of tips for avoiding some of the most common xenoestrogens[13]:

- Avoid organochlorines, one of the largest sources of xenoestrogens. They are used in pesticides, dry cleaning, bleaching of feminine-hygiene products, and the manufacture of plastics.
- Avoid Bisphenol A, a breakdown of polycarbonate, which is used in many plastic bottles. It's found in the lining of many food cans and juice containers.
- Avoid heating plastics, plastic lined-items, and polystyrene foam (e.g., Styrofoam), as the polycarbonates escape during the heating process.
- Use glass, ceramics, or steel to store/consume foods and liquids.
- Choose organic produce, especially when buying thin-skinned fruits and vegetables.
- Buy hormone-free animal products (e.g., eggs, poultry, meats, and dairy) to avoid xenoestrogen injections and bovine growth hormones that are added to non-organic animal products.
- Avoid butylated hydroxyanisole (BHS), which is a common food preservative found in processed food.
- Avoid non-organic coffee and tea.
- Use reverse-osmosis filtered water or purchase your own filter for drinking and bathing.
- Avoid parabens and stearalkonium chloride, which are contained in many creams and cosmetics. Choose natural brands with preservatives made from minerals or grapefruit seed extract.
- Avoid parabens and phenoxyethanol, which are 100% absorbed into the body. They are used in most skin lotions, creams, soaps, shampoos, and cosmetics as preservatives.
- Avoid phthalates, which are commonly found in baby lotions and powders.
- Avoid sunscreen containing benzophenone-3, homosalate, 4-methyl-benzylidene camphor, octal-methoxy-cinnamate, or octal-dimethyl-PABA.
- Avoid artificially-scented perfumes, deodorizers, and air fresheners, which contain phthalates.
- Avoid petrochemical-based perfumes.
- Avoid nail polish and nail polish remover, which contain harsh chemicals.
- The birth control pill contains high concentrations of synthetic estrogen. Choose a condom or diaphragm gels without surfactants. Use a non-spermicidal condom.
- Avoid hormone replacement therapy, which contains synthetic estrogen. Instead, use a as paraben-free progesterone cream.
- Dryer sheets, fabric softeners, and detergents contain petrochemicals that can be absorbed by the skin. Use laundry detergent with fewer chemicals or use white vinegar and baking soda.
- Be aware of noxious gas that comes from copiers and printers, new carpets, and fiberboards.
- Do not inhale and protect your skin from electrical oils, lubricants, adhesive paints, lacquers, solvents, oils, fuel, industrial wastes, packing materials, harsh cleaning products, and fertilizers.
- Avoid pesticides, herbicides, fungicides, parathion, plant and fungal estrogens, industrial chemicals (cad-mium, lead, mercury), conjugated estrogens/medroxyprogesterone (e.g., Prempro®, diethylstilbestrol (DES), Premarin, Cimetidine (e.g., Tagamet®), marijuana, insecticides (e.g., Dieldrin, DDT, Endosulfan, Heptachlor, Lindane/hexachlorocychohexan, and methoxychlor), Erythrosine, FD&C Red No. 3, Nonylphenol, Polychlorinated biphenyls, Phenosulfothizine, Phthalates and Bis(2-ethylhexyl) phthalate (DEHP).[14]

Listed below are the main causes of exposure to endocrine disruptors in North American Women:

1. **Exposure to *In Utero* Xenoestrogens**: When symptoms of anovulation or progesterone deficiency are noted in puberty, exposure to xenoestrogens in utero can be a factor. Five hundred thousand to eight hundred thousand follicles are created in the embryo, each enclosing an immature ovum when a female embryo

---

[13] http://www.suite101.com/content/xenoestrogens-and-your-health-a205476.

[14] http://www.drjudyroth.com/

develops in the womb. Outward changes or symptoms to the pregnant mother may not be obvious when exposed to toxic estrogen-like chemicals. However, the fragile ovarian follicles are extremely sensitive to the environmental pollutants, which can be toxic. The fetus is therefore increasingly affected by the toxins that may damage its ovarian follicles.

2. **Exposure to Petrochemical Compounds**: Petrochemical compounds are found in general consumer products such as creams, lotions, soaps, shampoos, perfumes, hair sprays, and room deodorizers. These compounds have estrogen-like chemical structures and may have estrogen-mimicking effects. Other sources of xenoestrogens include car exhaust, petrochemical-derived pesticides, herbicides, and fungicides, solvents and adhesives such as those found in nail polish, paint removers, and glues, dry-cleaning chemicals, practically all plastics, and industrial waste such as PCBs and dioxins. Synthetic estrogens from urine of women taking HRT and birth control pills are flushed down the toilet and eventually find their way into the food chain and back into the body. They are fat-soluble and non-biodegradable.[15]
3. **Exposure to Industrial solvents**: Industrial solvents are a family of chemicals that are often overlooked as a common source of xenoestrogens. These chemicals enter the body through the skin and accumulate quickly the lipid-rich tissues such as myelin (nerve sheath) and adipose (fat). Some common organic solvents include alcohols such as methanol, aldehydes such as acetaldehyde, glycols such as ethylene glycol, and ketones such as acetone. They are commonly found in cosmetics, nail polish and nail polish remover, glues, paints, varnishes, and other types of finishes, cleaning products, carpets, fiberboards, and other processed woods. Pesticides and herbicides such as lawn and garden sprays and indoor insect sprays are also sources of minute amounts of xenoestrogens. While the amount may be small in each, the additive effect from years of chronic exposure can lead to estrogen dominance.[16]
4. **Exposure to Hormone Replacement Therapy (HRT):** The hormones used in HRT are chemically different in structure than the hormones naturally found in humans. This differing structure is processed in a lab in order to patent the medication and therefore make an economic profit. One of the most popular HRT drugs is called Premarin® and has been the mainstay choice of doctors who are prescribing HRT. Premarin® contains 48% estrone and only a very small amount of progesterone, which is insufficient to have a significant opposing effect. The excessive estrogen from HRT can lead to an increased chance of DNA damage and can result in endometrial and breast cancer.
5. **Exposure to Xenoestrogens in Commercially Raised Cattle and Poultry:** Twenty-five million pounds per year, or half the antibiotics used in the United States each year, are used in livestock. These antibiotics enter our food supply and result in hormone disruption as we consume them as meat. In poultry farms, it now only takes six weeks to grow a chicken to full size, compared to four months in 1940. Feed containing a cocktail of hormone-disrupting toxins including pesticides, antibiotics, and drugs is used to combat disease and is necessary due to the overcrowded conditions of animal warehouses.
6. **Exposure to Commercially Grown Fruits and Vegetables Containing Pesticides**: Over the past one hundred years, several billion pounds of pesticides have been released into the environment. These pesticides are similar in structure to estrogen and therefore can disrupt our hormonal system. Pesticides that were previously banned make their way back into our food supply illegally. Approximately five billion pounds of chemicals have been added to the world each year in the form of pesticides, herbicides, fungicides, and other biocides. It is estimated that the average person eats seventy-five pounds of illegal pesticides per year just by following the guidelines of eating five servings of fruits and vegetables a day if purchasing them from non-organic sources.[17]

---

[15] http://www.drlam.com/articles/Estrogen_Dominance.asp.

[16] http://www.drlam.com/articles/Estrogen_Dominance.asp.

[17] http://www.drlam.com/articles/Estrogen_Dominance.asp.

The following is information and published studies taken from *Our Stolen Future* by Theo Colborn, Pete Myers, and Dianne Dumanoski, which discuss the widespread influence of toxic chemicals on animal and human life.

DDT

A study published in the *Proceedings of the Society of Experimental Biology and Medicine* in 1950 by two Syracuse University Zoologists, Lindeman and Burlington, described how doses of DDT prevented young roosters from developing normally. They injected DDT into forty young roosters for a period of two to three months. The daily doses of DDT did not kill the roosters or even made them sick; it made them look like hens. The bird's testicles were only 18% of normal size. Their combs and wattles remained stunted and pale. The roosters were chemically castrated.

Michael Fry, a wild life toxicologist at the University of California at Davis, injected eggs from western and California gull colonies with DDT and a breakdown product of DDT, DDE, and methoxychlor (another synthetic pesticide known to bind to estrogen receptors). He found a feminization of the male's reproductive tracts. Typical female cells were found in the testicles, and in cases of higher doses, the presence of an oviduct, the egg-laying canal normally found only in females, was detected. Despite all of this internal disruption, the chicks looked completely normal.

DDT was found to bind to the estrogen receptor sites. It is now considered one of the classic xenoestrogens.

DDT was banned in the United States in the early 1970's. However, worldwide production of DDT has never been higher. DDT is metabolized to DDE in the human body within a few months. DDE then may last in the human body for several decades. However, some medical doctors occasionally find DDT in the serum routinely following intensive sauna. So where is this new exposure to DDT coming from? The United States ships DDT to third world countries that spray it on vegetables and fruits. This agricultural produce is shipped to United States supermarkets where Americans consume it. In 1991, the United States exported ninety-six tons of DDT.

Another source of DDT exposure may come from your living area. DDT persists in the soil for several centuries, so you may be exposed if your house is built on or near old agricultural land.

Plastics, Spermicides, Detergents, and Personal Care Products

At Tufts Medical School in Boston in 1987, Soto and Sonnenschein serendipitously discovered that plastic test tubes thought to be inert contained a chemical that stimulated breast cancer cells to grow and proliferate wildly. They were experimenting with malignant breast cancer cells that were sensitive to estrogen. When exposed to estrogen, the cells would grow and multiply, and when isolated from estrogen, the cells would stop multiplying.

During the course of their experiments, they found that the test tube manufacturer changed the formulation of the plastic test tubes that they were using. The manufacturer had used p-nonylphenol, one of the family of synthetic chemicals called alkylphenols, to make these plastics more stable and less breakable. Manufacturers routinely add nonlyphenols to polystyrene and polyvinyl chloride (PVC). These new plastic test tubes caused their estrogen-sensitive breast cancer cells to multiply and grow. Thus, they concluded that p-nonylphenol acts like an estrogen.

Plastic Drinking Bottles and Plastics Used with Food

In 1993 at Stanford University School of Medicine, Dave Feldman, professor of medicine, was experimenting with a yeast protein that binds to estrogen. He used polycarbonate lab flasks, made of a plastic that is routinely used in the giant jugs in which water is shipped, to sterilize the water for his experiments. He found that the polycarbonate bottles used to hold drinking water contained Bisphenol A, due to the fact that Bisphenol A nicely bound to the estrogen protein found in the yeast.

The manufacturer was aware that the bottles would leach, particularly if exposed to high temperatures and caustic cleaners, and so developed a washing regimen to solve the problem. However, the researchers discovered that the manufacturer could not detect samples sent from their lab that were causing proliferation of estrogen-responsive breast cancer cells. This proved to be due to the detection limit of the manufacturer's lab equipment. The Stanford team found that two to five parts per billion of Bisphenol A were enough to cause the breast cancer cells to proliferate.

Professor Feldman noted that though Bisphenol A is two thousand times less potent than estrogen, it still has activity in the parts per billion range.

One Dartmouth University Study showed that plastic wrap heated in a microwave oven with vegetable oil had five hundred thousand times the minimum amount of xenoestrogens needed to stimulate breast cancer cells to grow in the test tube.

Detergent Breakdown Products

From 1978 to 1998, John Sumpter, a biologist from Brunel University in Uxbridge, began to study sexually confused fish reported from anglers fishing in English rivers. Many fish caught in the lagoons and pools just below the discharge from sewage plants looked quite bizarre; even experienced fisherman could not tell if a fish was male or female. The fish showed male and female characteristics at the same time. They were perfect examples of intersex, where an individual is stranded between both sexes.

Sumpter used a marker that helped identify female fish. Normally in females, vitellogenin, a special egg protein, is produced in response to estrogen from the ovaries. On the estrogen signal from the ovaries, the liver produces vitellogenin and the protein is incorporated into the eggs. Since the response is dependent on estrogen, vitellogenin levels found in male fish are a good indication of estrogen exposure.

Caged fish raised in captivity and then kept in the contaminated pools made one thousand times to one hundred thousand times more vitellogenin than control trout kept in clean water.

Nationally, fifteen sites that were sampled had soaring vitellogenin levels. Alkylphenol levels from detergent breakdown products are high on the suspect list. However, Sumpter suspects that the culprit is the synergistic qualities of several xenoestrogens acting together.

Canned Foods

Two Spanish scientists at the University of Granada in 1985 decided to investigate the plastic coatings that manufacturers use to line metal cans to avoid a metallic taste in canned food. These linings are present in about 85% of the cans. Fatima Olea and Nicolas Olea, M.D., specializing in endocrine cancers, worked with Soto and Sonnenschein. In a study analyzing twenty brands of canned foods purchased in the United States and in Spain, they discovered Bisphenol A, the same chemical that the Stanford researchers discovered, in about half of the canned food up to levels of eighty parts per billion. This is a twenty-seven times greater concentration of Bisphenol A than that which was needed to cause the breast cancer cells to proliferate in the Stanford Study.

Commercially Raised Beef, Chicken, and Pork

Commercially raised livestock are routinely given xenoestrogens to fatten them up, help them grow quickly, and cause them to retain water.. Xenoestrogens are an effective, cheap, and quick way to fatten them up. In the 1970s and 1980s there was an epidemic in Puerto Rico of early puberty in girls as young as a year old and even young boys who developed breasts caused by meat and dairy products containing high levels of estrogen. In the United States, the use of estrogen compounds is now slightly better regulated, but it is still very much used and abused.

DES (diethylstilbestrol), a type of synthetic estrogen, was the first hormone to be used by the meat industry to fatten up livestock, until it was discovered that it causes cancer even in extremely minute amounts and was formally banned in North America in the early 1970's.

Birth Control Pills

Birth control pills contain a synthetic estrogen and/or a synthetic progestin to force the body to cycle in a normal manner. Many times it takes one year or more for a woman's period to become normal after stopping birth control pills. This is because the synthetic estrogens and progestins in the birth control pills are oil soluble and difficult for the body to eliminate.

Preservative Methyl Paraben in Skin Lotions and Gels

For many years, parabens were considered among those preservatives with low systemic toxicity, primarily causing allergic reactions. However, as we have become aware that some synthetic chemicals mimic estrogen, our understanding of the toxic effects of both synthetic and natural substances has changed. John Sumpter from the Department of Biology & Biochemistry, Brunel University, Uxbridge, Middlesex, has found that alkyl hydroxy benzoate preservatives (namely methyl-, ethyl-, propyl-, and butylparaben) are weakly estrogenic. In an estrogen receptor-binding assay, butylparaben was able to compete with the female hormone estradiol for binding to estrogen receptors with an affinity approximately five orders of magnitude lower than that of diethylstilbestrol (a highly carcinogenic synthetic estrogen), and between one and two orders of magnitude less than nonylphenol (an estrogenic synthetic industrial chemical).

Although it is reassuring to note that when administered orally, the parabens were inactive, subcutaneous administration of butylparaben produced a positive estrogenic response on uterine tissues. Although approximately one hundred thousand times less potent than 17 beta-estradiol, greater exposure to the parabens may compensate for their lower potency. The researchers concluded that the safety in use of these chemicals should be reassessed. The European Union has asked the European Cosmetics and Toiletry industry about these new findings and the implication for breast cancer. These preservatives are found in the vast majority of skin and body lotions, even in natural progesterone creams. Generally, when taken orally, the sterol hormones are 90% first-pass-metabolized by the liver. Thus, taken orally, only 10% reaches the body. In contrast, anything absorbed by the skin is directly absorbed. In other words, anything absorbed through the skin may be as high as ten times the concentration of an oral dose.

Unfortunately, some natural progesterone creams were found to contain methyl and propyl parabens as a preservative. It is important to use natural progesterone creams that are paraben free.

Shampoos that Purposely Contain Very High Amounts of Estrogen

African Americans have historically favored shampoos with clinically active high doses of estrogen, both for use on adults and on children. In 1998, Chandra Tiwary, former chief of pediatric endocrinology at Brooke Army Medical Center in Texas, published a study of four girls—including a 14-month-old—who developed breasts or pubic hair months after beginning to use such products. The symptoms started to disappear when they stopped using them. The year before, he published a study showing that some of the products used by his patients contained up to one milligram (1 mg) of estradiol per one ounce of shampoo. By comparison, a normal adult topical skin dose for estradiol is 0.02-0.05 mg/day. This means that one ounce of shampoo contains fifty times the daily ADULT dose of estradiol. A small handful of this shampoo on your child every day may give her OR HIM breasts!

Herbicide

Tyrone B. Hayes of the University of California at Berkeley found that atrazine, the most commonly used weed killer in North America, affected frogs at doses as small as 0.1 parts per billion. As the amount of atrazine increased, as many as 20% of frogs exposed during their early development produced multiple sex organs or had both male and female organs. Many had small, feminized larynxes.

Plastic IV Bags

The United States FDA warns that prolonged exposure to fluid from IV bags may affect testicle development in young boys. The chemical DEHP can leach from the plastic into certain liquids, especially fat-containing ones, like blood. Studies of young animals show that this chemical can affect testicle development and production of normal sperm. Some companies already label that their products contain phthalates (DHEP), and the FDA soon will issue a recommendation—not a requirement—that more companies do so.

"FDA's public health notification falls far short of what is needed to protect patients," said Charlotte Brody of Health Care Without Harm, a group working to reduce the amount of phthalates—the family of chemicals that includes DEHP—in a variety of products, from plastic toys to cosmetics.

Five Out of Six Chemicals Used to block UV in Sunscreen are Estrogenic

Margaret Schlumpf and her colleagues from the Institute of Pharmacology and Toxicology, University of Zurich, Switzerland have found that many widely-used sunscreen chemicals mimic the effects of estrogen and trigger developmental abnormalities in rats.[18] Her group tested six common chemicals that are used in sunscreens, lip-sticks, and facial cosmetics. Five of the six tested chemicals (benzophenone-3, homosalate, 4-methyl-benzylidene camphor (4-MBC), octyl-methoxycinnamate, and octyl-dimethyl-PABA) behaved like strong estrogen in lab tests and caused cancer cells to grow rapidly. Only one chemical—a UVA protector called butyl-methoxydibenzoylmethane (B-MDM)—showed no activity.

One very common sunscreen chemical, 4-MBC, was mixed with olive oil and applied to rat skin. This caused a doubling of the rate of uterine growth well before puberty. "That was scary, because we used concentrations that are in the range allowed in sunscreens," said Schlumpf. Three of the six chemicals caused developmental abnormalities in animals. The major cause of sterility in women in the USA is endometriosis, a condition afflicting 5.5% of American women. Exposure to excessive estrogen that may have come from such sunscreens is felt to be the primary cause of endometriosis. Perhaps a sunscreen using zinc oxide is a better choice.

Common Chemicals in Personal Care Products, Fragrances, Paints, Plastics, and Cosmetics May Cause Testicular Defects in Boys

For the first time, scientists have shown that pregnant mothers exposed to high but common levels of a widely used ingredient in cosmetics, fragrances, plastics, and paints can produce baby boys with smaller genitals and incomplete testicular descent. Previous work had shown that prenatal phthalate exposure in rodents can critically affect male hormones, resulting in impaired testicular descent and smaller genital size. The Swan study is the first to look at effects in humans. While none of the boys showed clear malformation or disease, in the 25% of mothers with the highest levels of phthalate exposure, the odds were ten times higher that their sons would have a shorter than expected distance between the anus and the base of the penis. This so-called AGD measurement is a sensitive indicator of impacts on the reproductive system.

The human body is inundated with these harmful chemicals on a daily basis. This creates an overburdened liver and a weakened immune system, and thus the delicate hormonal balance is disrupted, causing effects such as those identified by Swan.

---

[18] Margaret Schlumpf, Beata Cotton, Marianne Conscience, Vreni Haller, Beate Steinmann, Walter Lichtensteiger. *In vitro and in vivo estrogenicity of UV screens.* "Environmental Health Perspectives" Vol. 109 (March 2001). 239-244.

Liver Toxicity

The liver is a complex and unique organ, serving many functions crucial to sustaining life. From circulation to digestion, it is constantly processing blood for use by the rest of the body.

The liver is the largest internal organ in the human body, weighing three to four pounds. The rich supply of blood flowing through it gives it its dark red color and glossy appearance. Sometimes called "The Great Chemical Factory" the liver neutralizes harmful toxins and wastes, stores glycogen (a blood-sugar regulator), amino acids, protein, and fat.

Environmental toxins and over-processed foods which are infused with many unnatural chemicals leave the liver at great risk for contamination. If the liver is not functioning well, a hazardous buildup of toxins may occur.

From its sheltered position in the abdominal cavity, the liver filters blood and performs many functions vital to health including:

1. **Circulation:** The liver stores and regulates the blood in the body and is responsible for nourishing every cell. The liver transfers blood from the portal vein to the systemic circulation.
2. **Excretion:** The liver is responsible for the formation and secretion of bile for digestion and cleansing of blood. It removes ammonia from the blood and excretes substances filtered from the blood, such as heavy metals or dyes.
3. **Metabolism:** Manufacture and storage of many nutrients such as glucose and vitamins occurs in the liver. The metabolism of carbohydrates, proteins, lipids (fat), minerals, and vitamins is also a part of the liver's contribution to metabolism.
4. **Protection and detoxification:** The removal of foreign bodies from the blood (phagocytosis) and detoxification by conjugation, methylation, oxidation, and reduction are some of the liver's main functions.
5. **Production:** The formation of urea, serum albumin, glycogen, and blood coagulating proteins such as prothrombin, fibrinogen, and heparin occurs in the liver. The destruction of erythrocyte (red blood cells) also occurs in the liver. The liver regulates blood sugar levels and stores the balanced amount of sugar as glycogen for future energy usage.
6. **Regulation of hormones:** The process of rendering hormones inactive and causing them to be eliminated through the bile or urine occurs via the liver. Since estrogens and androgens are both growth hormones which stimulate cell division, elevation of their levels in the blood due to the liver's failure to remove them efficiently can cause their accumulation in tissue. This in turn may lead to abnormal growths such as uterine fibroids, ovarian cysts, endometriosis, breast cysts and breast cancer, prostate enlargement, or prostate cancer.
7. **Regulates cholesterol levels:** The liver rids the body of excess cholesterol, subsequently lowering the levels of low-density lipoproteins (LDL) cholesterol and triglycerides.

The body functions which are affected by emotional and mental activities are regulated by the liver. When the liver's blood storage and regulatory functions are affected and bleeding or clots result, the liver is usually in a diseased condition. The joints can become stiff and muscles can become spasmodic and numb when the liver blood is deficient as nourishment to the tendons and blood vessels is decreased. Conditions such as stroke, dizziness, headaches, tinnitus, deafness, fainting, or convulsion can result due to severe liver blood deficiency. When the liver blood is so deficient that it cannot nourish the eyes, night blindness or blurring may result. Stress and negative or unhappy feelings can greatly affect the liver and cause a noticeable decline in liver vitality which can result in hiccups, hernia, and pain surrounding the liver. The bowels may then also become constipated and sleep may become disturbed as nightmares or insomnia can occur.

Symptoms of a poorly functioning liver may include:

- Low energy
- Indigestion, bloating, constipation, gas, or diarrhea
- Foggy thinking
- Weight gain
- Stiff, aching, weak muscles—especially lower back and shoulders
- Altered cholesterol levels
- Blood sugar abnormalities
- Sleep disturbances
- Easy bruising
- Brittle bones
- Fluid retention
- Kidney problems
- Slow wound healing

The liver plays a major role in the detoxification of numerous substances in the body, whether they come from the environment, food, or within the body (from hormones and other substances). In order to metabolize and eliminate these potentially harmful toxins, the liver has developed an intricate, two-step detoxification system. Together, these two phases convert toxins into water-soluble molecules that can be excreted from the body in the stool and urine.

Phase I System:

The Phase I detoxification system, composed mainly of the cytochrome P450 supergene family of enzymes, is generally the first enzymatic defense against foreign compounds. Most pharmaceuticals are metabolized through Phase I biotransformation. In a typical Phase I reaction, a cytochrome P450 enzyme (CypP450) uses oxygen and, as a cofactor, NADH, to add a reactive group, such as a hydroxyl radical. As a consequence of this step in detoxification, reactive molecules, which may be more toxic than the parent molecule, are produced. If these reactive molecules are not further metabolized by Phase II conjugation, they may cause damage to proteins, RNA, and DNA within the cells. Several studies have shown evidence of associations between induced Phase I and/or decreased Phase II activities and an increased risk of disease, such as cancer, systemic lupus erythematous, and Parkinson's disease. Compromised Phase I and/or Phase II activity has also been implicated in adverse drug responses. This process is often referred to as bioactivation. In order to prevent bioactivation from occurring, there must be an orchestrated balance between Phase I and Phase II detoxification. Enhancements of both phases can be achieved through natural medicinal agents. Prior to this process, simple testing can be done in order to reveal the state of detoxification phases. For example, a quantity of caffeine is ingested and saliva samples are taken twice at specified intervals. The efficiency of caffeine clearance is directly related to the efficiency of Phase I detoxification. Rapid clearance shows enzyme induction either from xenobiotic exposure or toxins within the body. Slower rates indicate that CypP450 activity in the liver is abnormal. Patients with slower caffeine clearance will have more difficulty eliminating xenobiotics and other toxins.[19]

The primary nutrients required during phase I detoxification include B vitamins, vitamin C, folic acid, copper, magnesium, and zinc, antioxidants including glutathione, N-acetyl cysteine, and lipoic acid, and the branched-chain amino acids leucine, isoleucine, and valine. Phase I detoxification is further enhanced by indole-3-carbinol, which is found in cruciferous vegetables such as broccoli, Brussels sprouts, cabbage, and cauliflower. It is also enhanced by flavonoids, including Silymarin from milk thistle, curcumin from the spice turmeric, and polyphenol antioxidants from grape seeds and green tea. Nutrients required to support phase II detoxification include vitamins B5, B6, B12, and C, folic acid, selenium, zinc, molybdenum, glutathione, and the amino acids glycine, cysteine, methionine, taurine, and glutamine.

Phase II System:

One of the consequences of Phase I activation is that the product, called the reactive intermediate, is quite often more reactive—and potentially more toxic—than the parent molecule. Therefore, it is important that this molecule be converted to a non-toxic, water-soluble molecule as soon as possible. Conjugation of the reactive intermediate to a water-soluble molecule is accomplished by the Phase II conjugation reactions which include glucuronidation, sulfation, glutathione conjugation, amino acid conjugation, methylation, and acetylation. These reactions not only require the water-soluble molecule that will be attached to the toxicant—such as sulfate in the case of sulfation or glucuronic acid in the case of glucuronidation—but also use a large amount of energy in the form of adenosine triphosphate (ATP). In addition to energy repletion, Phase II reactions require an adequate, continually replenished amount of cofactors since these cofactors are attached to the toxins and then excreted. Several nutrients and phytonutrients support Phase II reactions,[20] including antioxidants, vitamins, amino acids, and other substances the liver needs to have in ample supply to detoxify efficiently.

---

[19] Jacqueline Krohn and Frances Taylor, *Natural Detoxification: A Practical Encyclopedia*, revised edition, Hartley & Marks Publishers, 2000-01.

[20] Deann J. Liska, Ph.D. *ANSR–APPLIED NUTRITIONAL SCIENCE REPORTS,* 650 8/02 Rev. 8/05, "The Role of Detoxification in the Prevention of Chronic Degenerative Diseases "

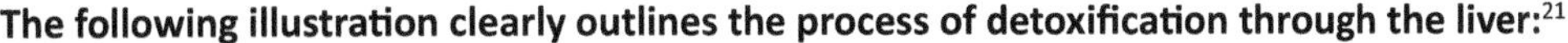

The following illustration clearly outlines the process of detoxification through the liver:[21]

DETOXIFICATION
Toxins enter the body.
Step 2:
(Unhealthy Function)
In Phase I toxins are not completely detoxified in the unhealthy liver.
Step 3:
(Unhealthy Function)
In Phase II toxins are not completely detoxified in the unhealthy liver.
Step 5:
(Unhealthy Function)
Stored toxins recirculate in the blood and may contribute to long term poor health.
Liver Function Phase I
Liver Function Phase II
Fat
Step 1:
(Unhealthy Function)
Toxins and other poisons formed internally leak through the unhealthy intestine and flow to the liver.
Step 4:
(Unhealthy Function)
Unchanged toxins leave the liver and store in tissues such as fat, the brain and nervous system.
Brain
Unhealthy Liver
Unhealthy Intestine
Healthy Liver
Healthy Intestine
Kidney
Step 1:
(Healthy Function)
In the healthy intestine, fewer internal poisons are formed and most of the toxins are excreted, with only a small amount naturally transported to the liver.
Liver Function Phase I
Liver Function Phase II
Some toxins exit the body via the feces.
Step 2:
(Healthy Function)
In the healthy liver toxins are transformed in Phase I to an intermediate substance.
OX-H2O
Step 3:
(Healthy Function)
In the healthy liver the intermediate substance is transformed in Phase II to a more water soluble substance and released to the kidney.
Step 4:
(Healthy Function)
The water soluble substance is excreted via the urine.
Step 2-A:
(Healthy Function)
Harmful free radicals (OX•) are formed as a result of Phase I activity, but are transformed to harmless water (H2O) by antioxidant nutrients.

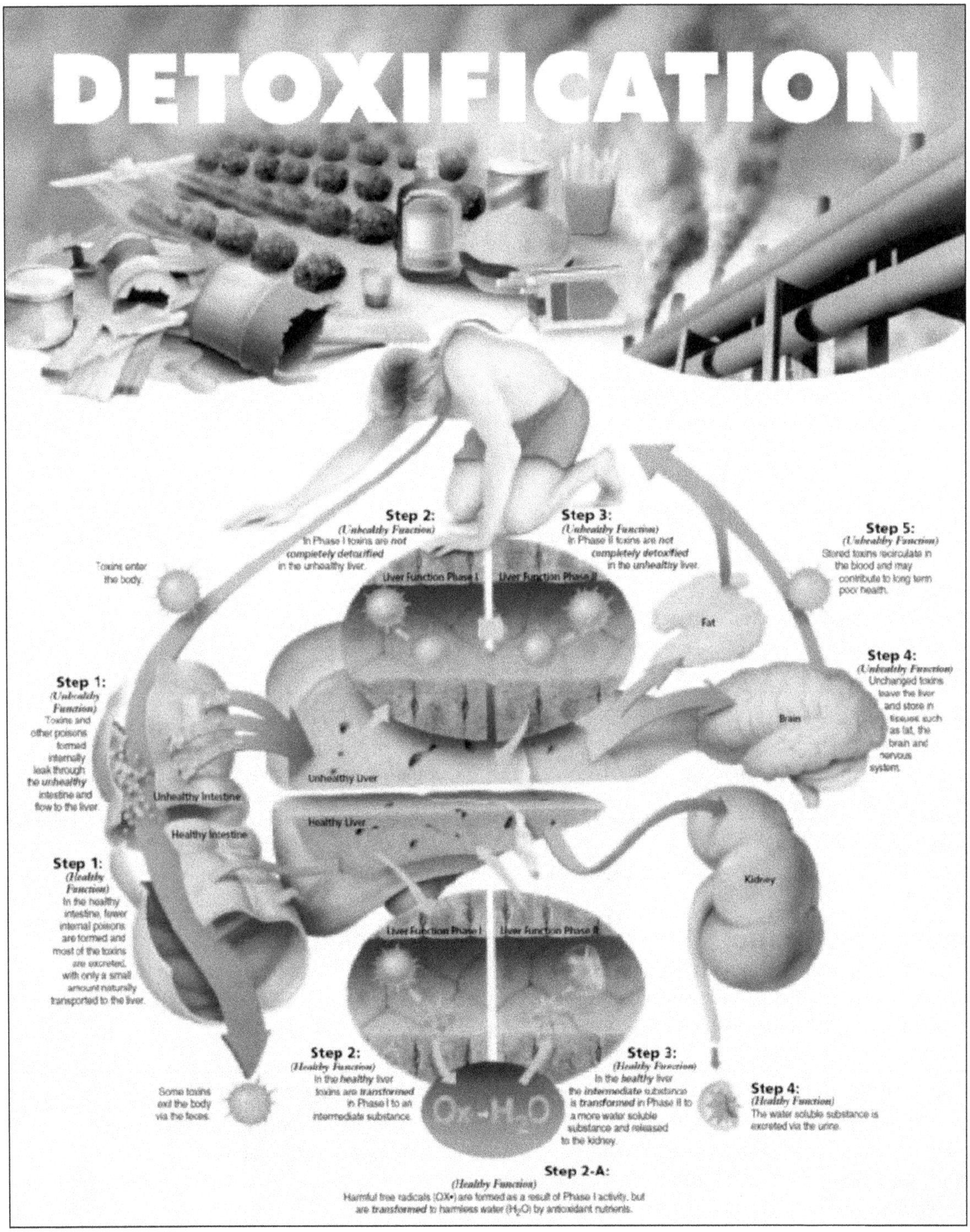

[21] *1994 Advanced Nutrition Publications, Inc.* 010 9/96 Rev 5/04, "Detoxification."

Liver Detoxifiers

Foods to Detoxify the Liver

FOODS TO INCLUDE	FOODS TO AVOID
FRUIT TO INCLUDE strawberries, citrus (except grapefruit), pineapple, apples, apricot, avocado, banana, blueberries, cherries, grapes, kiwi, mango, melons, nectarine, papaya, pear, peach, plums, prunes, and raspberries Organically grown is always preferred.	**FRUIT TO AVOID** grapefruit (grapefruit can alter detoxification enzyme function for up to 72 hours), all sweetened fruits (either canned or frozen) and sweetened fruit juice
VEGETABLES TO INCLUDE arugula, asparagus, artichokes, bean sprouts, bell peppers, bok choy, broccoli, Brussels sprouts, cauliflower, celery, cucumber, cabbage, eggplant, endive, escarole, all types of greens and lettuce, green beans, jicama, mushrooms, okra, green peas, radishes, spinach, squash (summer and winter), sweet potatoes, taro, turnips, yams, and zucchini all fresh, raw, steamed, grilled, sautéed, roasted, or juiced Organically grown is always preferred.	**VEGETABLES TO AVOID** corn, tomatoes, tomato sauce, and any creamed vegetables
GRAINS TO INCLUDE rice (white, brown, sushi, wild), potatoes, oats (gluten-free), quinoa, millet, tapioca, amaranth, and buckwheat	**GRAINS TO AVOID** corn and all gluten-containing products including wheat, spelt, kamut, barley, and rye
LEGUMES TO INCLUDE all legumes including peas and lentils (except soybeans)	**LEGUMES TO AVOID** soybeans, tofu, tempeh, soy milk, soy sauce, and any product containing soy proteins
NUTS/SEEDS TO INCLUDE all nuts except peanuts – almonds, cashews, macadamia, walnuts, pumpkin seeds, brazil nuts, and sunflower seeds—whole or as a nut butter	**NUTS/SEEDS TO AVOID** peanuts, peanut butter, and peanut oil
MEAT AND FISH TO INCLUDE all fresh or frozen wild fish (except shellfish) such as salmon, halibut, sole, mahi mahi, cod, and snapper. Organic, hormone-free chicken, turkey, lamb and wild game (venison, buffalo, elk, etc.),	**MEAT AND FISH TO AVOID** tuna, swordfish, shellfish, beef, pork, cold cuts, hot dogs, sausage, and canned meats

DAIRY AND EGGS TO INCLUDE	DAIRY AND EGGS TO AVOID
milk substitutes such as rice milk, oat milk, hemp milk, and almond or other nut milk and egg substitutes	milk, cheese, cottage cheese, cream, butter, yogurt, ice cream, non-dairy creamers, soy milk, and eggs
FATS TO INCLUDE cold pressed oils such as olive, flaxseed, canola (non-GMO), safflower, sunflower, sesame, walnut, hazelnut, pumpkin seed, and coconut	**FATS TO AVOID** margarine, butter, shortening, any processed or hydrogenated oils, peanut oil, mayonnaise, and fried foods
BEVERAGES TO INCLUDE filtered or distilled water, green tea, herbal tea, pure fruit juices, mineral water, and roasted grain coffee substitutes	**BEVERAGES TO AVOID** sodas and soft drinks (including sugar-free), alcoholic beverages, coffee, tea, or any other caffeinated beverages, and sweetened fruit juice
SWEETENERS TO INCLUDE brown rice syrup (gluten-free), chicory syrup, stevia, blackstrap molasses, fruit sweeteners such as Luo Han fruit, pure maple syrup, agave nectar, and yacon syrup	**SWEETENERS TO AVOID** white or brown sugar, high fructose corn syrup, honey, corn syrup, sucrose, dextrose, turbinado, nutritive corn sweetener, and any artificial sweeteners, colors or flavors
HERBS/SPICES/CONDIMENTS TO INCLUDE vinegars (except grain source), wasabi, mustard, horseradish, pesto (cheese-free), and all spices	**HERBS/SPICES/CONDIMENTS TO AVOID** high salt intake, chocolate, ketchup, relish, soy sauce, BBQ sauce, chutney, MSG, BHA, BHT, nitrates, nitrites, and any other chemical additive or preservatives

Herbs to Detoxify the Liver

Milk thistle *(Carduus marianus)*

Silymarin, a flavanolignan, is the main active compound that gives milk thistle its well-researched liver protecting effects. Silymarin protects the liver from damage by inhibiting damaging substances in the liver. Silymarin has the added ability to increase glutathione, one of the most critical nutrients for liver detoxification, in the liver, intestine and stomach.[22] There are hundreds of studies that involve the ability of milk thistle to protect and regenerate the liver. Milk thistle is proved to be useful in all liver conditions such as hepatitis, cirrhosis, liver damage, cholestasis, and fatty liver. Silymarin's ability to promote the regeneration of damaged hepatocytes renders it as one of the most potent liver detoxifiers.

Turmeric *(Curcuma longa)*

Curcumin, one of the active compounds in turmeric, is a potent liver detoxifier and anti-inflammatory agent. Curcumin is of exponential use in Phase 2 detoxification pathways in the liver as it increases the levels of the enzymes needed to facilitate the action of Phase 2 detoxification. Curcumin also increases the production of bile from the liver, which helps to expel toxins and reduce liver inflammation.

Burdock Root *(Arctium lappa)*

Burdock root is one of the foremost cleansing herbs, providing nourishing support for the blood, liver, and natural defense system. It is rich in vitamins B1, B6, B-2, and E, plus manganese, copper, iron, zinc, and sulfur. Burdock root contains inulin along with bitter compounds and mucilage which provides its ability to control liver damage and

[22] Julieta Criollo, DNM, CHT, *Medicinal Herbs Quick Reference Guide,* 109.

protection from further burdens to the liver. Burdock root also promotes the flow and release of bile, which not only helps in cleansing the liver, but also aids in the digestive process. [23]

Dandelion Root *(Taraxacum officinalis)*
The root of the dandelion plant is effective as a detoxifying agent, acting especially on the liver and gallbladder to remove toxins and waste products. It stimulates and tonifies the digestive system. Its cholagogue, or bile secreting effect, creates a mild laxative effect which allows for expulsion of toxins. Dandelion root is therefore useful in the treatment of liver conditions such as jaundice, metabolic toxicity, hepatitis, and cholelithiasis (gallstones), as seen in two studies cited in *The Australian Journal of Medicinal Herbalism.*[24] Dandelion root has also been proven useful in the treatment of chronic conditions of the digestive system, conditions of the skin such as acne and eczema, and joint problems such as arthritis.

Globe Artichoke *(Cynara scolymus)*
Globe artichoke contains a powerful compound called cynaropicrin, which is a sesquiterpene lactone that stimulates the flow of bile from the liver and makes it a useful liver detoxifier and protector. Due to its ability to promote detoxification and improve bile flow, globe artichoke is useful in all cases of insufficient liver production and digestive insufficiency.

Blue Flag *(Iris versicolor)*
Blue flag has the ability to detoxify almost all channels of elimination. It stimulates the flow and release of bile from the liver, purges the intestines, and promotes secretions from the pancreas. Blue flag also cleanses the blood of impurities and stimulates the lymphatic system, which enhances whole body cleansing effects.

Yellow Dock *(Rumex crispus)*
The major plant chemicals in yellow dock are tannins, oxalates, and anthraquinone glycosides (about 3-4%). Yellow dock also includes nepodin, as well as other chemicals based on chrysophanol, physcion and emodin. These constituents produce alterative, gentle purgative, mild laxative, and mild astringent tonic effects. The iron content of yellow dock makes it useful in treating anemia symptoms. Chrysarobin in yellow dock is found to relieve a congested liver.

The anthraquinone glycosides contained in yellow dock have a laxative effect on the bowels, as well as on the liver and blood, making it beneficial in all detoxification strategies. The release of toxins from the tissues can create an increasingly symptomatic effect on the body if the channels of elimination are not working efficiently.

Barberry *(Berberis vulgaris)*
Barberry is a bark known for containing berberine, the powerful agent which has numerous actions including potent anti-microbial, hepato-protectant, bile secreting, and liver detoxifying benefits. The bark contains a large number of alkaloids (berberine, berbamine, and oxyacantha) and tannins. Barberry is also effective in reducing nausea and vomiting, toning and strengthening the body, and stimulating bowel action.

Nutrients to Detoxify the Liver

Alpha Lipoic Acid (ALA)
ALA is the remarkable "universal antioxidant" as it is both water- and fat-soluble, proving to have antioxidant effects on the inside and outside of the cells. ALA helps to neutralize the effects of all free radicals and enhances the antioxidant functions of vitamins C and E and glutathione.

---

[23] The 4-Week Ultimate Body Detox Plan Michelle Schoffro Cook, DNM, DAc, CNC pg. 237

[24] The 4-Week Ultimate Body Detox Plan Michelle Schoffro Cook, DNM, DAc, CNC pg. 237

Research shows that ALA is effective in neutralizing toxins from over-the-counter and prescription drugs before they can cause liver damage.

Calcium D-Glucarate

Calcium D-glucarate is a substance produced naturally in small amounts by humans. Supplementation of calcium D-glucarate has been shown to prevent recycling of hormones and environmental toxins, promoting liver detoxification and excretion of these potentially detrimental substances.

Glucuronidation is the normal process in the liver of attaching a glucuronic acid molecule to substances for detoxification and elimination from the body.* During phase II liver detoxification, toxic chemicals, steroid hormones, and other fat-soluble toxins undergo glucuronidation and are then excreted through the bile or urine* Calcium D-glucarate helps assure this elimination process occurs uninterrupted

Glutathione

Glutathione is one of the molecules used in Phase 2 detoxification and is produced in the body by the liver. Levels of glutathione naturally decrease with the aging process. Glutathione is made up of cysteine, glutamic acid, and glycine. The amount of cysteine in the body will determine how much glutathione is produced. Glutathione has tremendous liver protecting effects, which block the effects of environmental pollution, medications, radiation, mercury, and other heavy metals. Glutathione aids in detoxification by removing fungicides, herbicides, carbamate, organophosphates, pesticides, nitrates, notrosamines, flavorings, plastics, steroids, phenolic compounds, and certain medications from the liver.

Vitamin C

Vitamin C is a water-soluble antioxidant vitamin which is not produced within the body and therefore must be replenished through dietary means on a daily basis. Deficiencies in vitamin C have been shown to decrease the metabolism of xenobiotics by lowering the level of cytochrome P450.[25] Vitamin C aids in detoxification by combating all free radicals. Vitamin C also prevents damage from exposure to numerous hepato-toxic agents including pollutants, carbon monoxide, heavy metals, sulfur dioxide, carcinogens, stored lipophilic chemicals, medications, anesthetics, radiation, bacterial toxins, and poisons.

N-Acetyl Cysteine (NAC)

NAC is thought to be an intermediate compound in cysteine metabolism, which makes it a derivative of cysteine. NAC has the ability to boost glutathione levels, which is critical to Phase 2 detoxification. NAC protects the liver from toxic compounds, has tremendous chemo-protectant effects, and protects the body from radiation. NAC is a potent liver vasodilator which increases the blood flow to the liver, thereby enhancing its detoxification abilities.

Methionine

Due to methionine's sulfur content, it is a powerful antioxidant that has the ability to inactivate free radicals, support liver detoxification, protect cell membranes against lipid peroxidation, and protect precious glutathione levels in the body. When levels of methionine in the body are sufficient, it has the added effect of preventing the accumulation of fat in the liver.

Coenzyme Q_{10} (COQ_{10})

COQ_{10} is the most powerful antioxidant in the body. COQ_{10}, also called ubiquinone, is a potent free radical scavenger which protects the cellular membranes against damage caused by toxins and is a crucial co-factor for energy production within the body.

---

[25] Jaqueline Krohn, MD and Frances Taylor, MA, *Natural Detoxification: A Practical Encyclopedia,* 276.

Vitamin B5

Vitamin B5, also known as pantothenic acid, is part of the B-complex family of vitamins. B5 is the main vitamin that is used in times of stress as it stimulates adrenal hormone production and supports adrenal function, preventing adrenal exhaustion during prolonged stress. B5 is a critical nutrient involved in Phase 1 detoxification, aiding the body by protecting against harmful radiation. It also counters the effects and toxicity of antibiotics, aids in the production of hydrochloric acid in the stomach, and stimulates the synthesis of cholesterol.

Vitamin B6

Vitamin B6, also known as pyridoxine, is involved in more bodily processes than any other single nutrient and has an effect on both physical and mental health. B6 is needed for the metabolism of methionine, aids in the transport of amino acids across the cellular membrane, and supports liver detoxification. B6 is also needed for the proper metabolism and use of protein, fats, carbohydrates, and hormones.

Folic acid

Folic acid plays a role in both the Phase 1 and Phase 2 detoxification pathways. It is needed for the utilization of amino acids and is involved in protein metabolism and the production of RNA and DNA. Folic acid is required for the formation of both red and white blood cells.

Selenium

Selenium is an essential trace mineral that is found in glutathione peroxidase, which is necessary for the recycling of glutathione. Considered to be one of the beneficial antioxidants, selenium protects the cellular membranes and prevents the breakdown of DNA. It also neutralizes free radicals and enhances the functions of vitamin C and E.

Zinc

Zinc is a trace mineral that is found in over ninety essential enzymes in the body.[26] Zinc is directly involved in Phase 1 detoxification as it is also found in alcohol dehydrogenase, an enzyme that detoxifies aldehydes. In addition, zinc supports liver detoxification and protects the liver from the toxic effects of chemicals. It is a component of superoxide dismutase and it reduces lipid peroxidation.

[26] Jaqueline Krohn, MD and Frances Taylor, MA, *Natural Detoxification: A Practical Encyclopedia,* 284.

The Stress Effect

Stress can be defined as any perceived physical or psychological change that disrupts an organism's metabolic balance.[27] In modern day society, people are faced with constant exposure to stress. A chain of events is automatically activated in response to the stress. Signals are sent throughout the body through the communication efforts of the neuroendocrine system, resulting in "fight or flight" responses. Some of these signals cause positive changes in order for the body to respond to the immediate or acute stress. Long-term or chronic stress poses too many challenges which overload the circuits and cause the systems of the body to eventually shut down.

Surveys and research reports conducted over the past two decades reveal that 43% of all adults suffer adverse effects due to stress. In fact, 75% to 90% of all visits to primary care physicians are in some way related to the adverse impact of psychosocial stress. Furthermore, an estimated one million workers are absent on an average workday because of stress-related complaints. The market for stress management programs, products, and services has skyrocketed in the past decade and is estimated to currently exceed eleven billion dollars annually.[28] While all age groups are affected by stress, the aging population faces compounded susceptibility to stress-induced disorders because of the accumulation of problems mediated by chronic, long-term stress.[29]

Physiological Response to Stress

The autonomic nervous system (ANS), which is a branch of the nervous system, is automatically activated when the stress response is initiated. The autonomic nervous system activities are involuntary and take place completely beyond our conscious control. The automatic functions of the ANS include digestion, heart rate, blood pressure, and body temperature.

The two branches of the ANS that regulate the "fight or flight" response are the sympathetic and the parasympathetic nervous systems. The sympathetic nervous system is the part of the ANS that is responsible for initiating the "fight or flight" response. With each perceived thought of danger or pain, the sympathetic nervous system automatically initiates the "fight or flight" response so that the body can handle any potential danger or pain.

The parasympathetic nervous system returns the body back to balance. During parasympathetic activity, blood concentrates in the central organs for such processes as digestion and storage of energy reserves. Breathing, heart rate, blood pressure, muscle tension, and body temperature are all decreased back to normal.

---

27 *ANSR–APPLIED NUTRITIONAL SCIENCE REPORTS,* "Nutritional Management of Stress-Induced Dysfunction," YEAR.

28 *The American Institute of Stress,* "America's #1 health problem and job stress," November 2001. http://www.stress.org/problem.htm.

29 W.A. Pedersen, R. Wan, and M.P. Mattson, *Mech Ageing Dev,* "Impact of aging on stress-responsive neuroendocrine systems," 2001;122(9):963-83.

The following illustration depicts the differing functions of the sympathetic and parasympathetic nervous systems:[30]

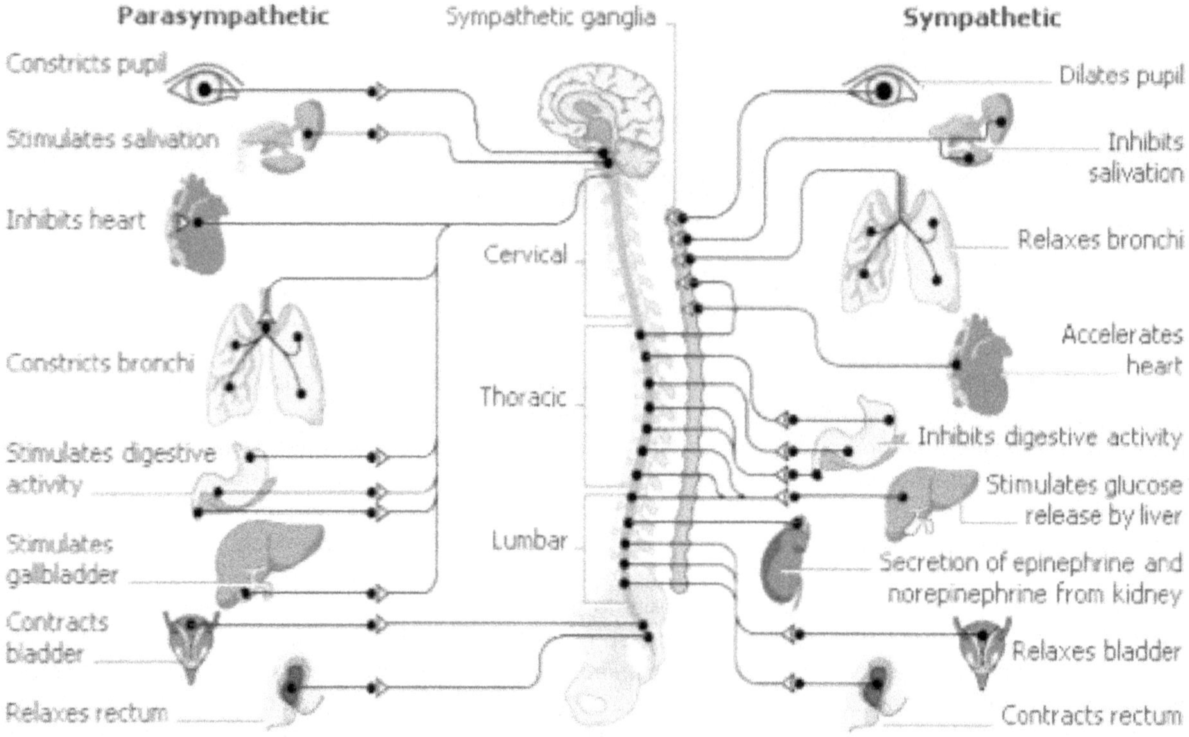

The hypothalamus or "master gland" controls the autonomic nervous system. The hypothalamus receives the message of danger from the higher-order thinking component of the mind. The message is delivered through the nervous system that connects, like a hard-wired neuron system, to every other system of the body. Hormones are secreted upon stimulation of the endocrine system by the hypothalamus. The hormones adrenalin and cortisol are then secreted into the bloodstream and travel throughout the body to deliver information to cells and systems.

Epinephrine (adrenalin) and norepinephrine (noradrenalin) are released into the bloodstream from the adrenal medulla. The adrenal medulla is the part of the adrenal glands positioned on top of the kidneys. Cortisol is the other key hormone released from a portion of the adrenal glands called the adrenal cortex. Together, these hormones flood every cell in the body with the specific message to prepare for fight or flight.

Autonomic Nervous System Responses

Some immediate physiological changes that result from autonomic nervous system activation include:

- Increased central nervous system (CNS) activity
- Increased mental activity
- Increased secretion of adrenaline (epinephrine), noradrenalin (norepinephrine), and cortisol

---

[30] http://medicalterms.info/img/uploads/anatomy/autonomic-nervous-system.gif

- Increased heart rate
- Increased cardiac output
- Increased breathing rate
- Increased metabolism
- Increased oxygen consumption
- Increased oxygen to the brain
- Shunting of blood away from the digestive tract and toward the muscles and limbs
- Increased muscle contraction which leads to increased strength
- Increased blood coagulation (blood clotting ability)
- Increased circulation of free fatty acids
- Increased output of blood cholesterol
- Increased blood sugar released by the liver to nourish the muscles
- Release of endorphins from the pituitary gland
- Dilation of the pupils
- Hair standing on end
- Thinning of the blood
- Increased brainwave activity
- Increased sweat gland secretion
- Increased secretion from apocrine glands resulting in foul body odor
- Constriction of the capillaries under the surface of the skin, consequently increasing blood pressure

There are also several processes in the body that tend to decrease in function when the "fight or flight" response is activated:

- Immune system suppression
- Constriction of blood vessels, except to running and fighting muscles
- Cessation of normal reproductive and sexual system functioning
- Cessation of normal metabolism of food by the digestive system
- Shutdown of the excretory system
- Decreased saliva production
- Decreased perception of pain
- Decreased kidney output
- Closing of the bowel and bladder sphincters

The General Adaptation Syndrome

Dr. Hans Selye, through his research on the physiological effects of chronic stress on rats, developed the General Adaptation Syndrome (GAS). The General Adaptation Syndrome provides a summary of the physiological changes that follow stress. Dr. Selye observed three sets of responses whenever he injected rats with a toxin:

1. Adrenal gland enlargement
2. Lymph node decrease
3. Development of severely bleeding ulcers in the stomach and intestines

Over several years, Dr. Selye theorized that the same physiological changes take place in the human body in reaction to any kind of stress. These patterns had a tendency to result in disease conditions such as ulcers, arthritis, hypertension, arteriosclerosis, and diabetes in humans. Dr. Selye called the pattern the General Adaptation

Syndrome. For decades, researchers have studied the syndrome and Dr. Selye's theories have held up to all levels of scientific scrutiny.

The three stages of the General Adaptation Syndrome include:

1. **Alarm Stage:** In the alarm stage, bursts of the hormones cortisol and adrenaline are released in response to a stressor, resulting in the traditional "fight or flight" responses.
2. **Resistance Stage:** In the resistance stage, the body uses high cortisol levels to free up stored energy to help the body physically resist the stressor. It is now known that a prolonged resistance stage may increase the risk of developing stress-related diseases. If cortisol levels remain elevated, symptoms may include feeling tired but wired, having difficulty sleeping, weight gain around the waist, high blood pressure, hair loss, muscle mass loss, and anxiety. Excess cortisol also interferes with the action of other hormones like progesterone, testosterone, and thyroid hormones, which further creates more imbalances and increases symptoms.
3. **Exhaustion Stage:** At this stage, the adrenals are either depleted from producing too much cortisol or are reacting to the detrimental effects of high cortisol. This reduces the cortisol production significantly. Symptoms of low cortisol include fatigue (especially morning fatigue), increased susceptibility to infections, decreased recovery from exercise, allergies, low blood sugar, a burned out feeling, depression, and low sex drive.

Chronic stress-induced dysfunction can create a significant loss of vitality and can result in serious long-term health problems. While stress is an inevitable consequence of modern life, the devastating damage caused by chronic stress cannot be ignored. A healthy diet, regular exercise, lifestyle changes, relaxation, and holistic therapies can help to normalize the parameters of the stress response.

The Effects of Herbal Adaptogens on Stress

Adaptogens are a group of herbs which have been used for centuries in traditional medicine. There is clear empirical and clinical evidence that adaptogens have the ability to support a healthy response to stress and to normalize HPA activity.[31, 32] Through their complex chemical compositions and broad effects, adaptogens are able to address multiple levels of the stress response, including HPA activation, feedback loops, insulin and glucose homeostasis, energy levels, cognitive function, gastric mucosal strength, blood lipid levels, blood pressure, and immunity.[33]

Some beneficial herbal adaptogens are:

Holy Basil *(Ocimum sanctum)*

Holy basil is an Indian herb which is found to affect multiple aspects of physiology. Research suggests that it has immunomodulatory activities. Holy basil enhances gastric mucosal strength, normalizes blood glucose levels, increases physical endurance, supports healthy blood lipid levels, and modulates adrenal corticosterone levels in animals.[34] Holy basil works directly on stress levels by reducing the harmful effects of elevated cortisol levels and consequently restoring a sense of calm and well-being.

Ashwagandha *(Withania somnifera)*

Also known as Indian ginseng, although it shares no relation to ginseng, ashwagandha traditionally has been used as a tonic for several types of body weaknesses as well as to promote strength and vigor. As an adaptogen, ashwagandha

---

[31] Wagner H, Norr H, Winterhoff H. Plant adaptogens. Phytomedicine 1994;1:63-76.

[32] Panossian A, Wikman G, Wagner H. Plant adaptogens. III. Earlier and more recent aspects and concepts on their mode of action. Phytomedicine 1999;6(4):287-300

[33] 576 1/02 Rev. 11/03 ANSR–APPLIED NUTRITIONAL SCIENCE REPORTS Nutritional Management of Stress-Induced Dysfunction

[34] H. Wagner, H. Norr, and H. Winterhoff, *Phytomedicine,* "Plant adaptogens," 1994, Volume1, 63-76.

has the unique ability to have amphoteric actions on cortisol. Whether cortisol levels are low or high, ashwagandha will restore balance. Known in the Indian system of Ayurveda as a classic rejuvenating herb, ashwagandha has repeatedly proven its adaptogenic potential. While the HPA-modifying mechanisms of ashwagandha are not fully understood, research suggests it may interact with pathways in the CNS that affect HPA activation and catecholamine production. These pathways may include cholinergic, GABAergic, and dopaminergic.[35]

Bacopa *(Bacopa monnieri)*
Bacopa, a nerve tonic from Ayurvedic medicine, has traditionally been used to improve learning, enhance memory, and relieve anxiety and seizures. It has been shown to have neuro-protective and antioxidant properties. The active constituents for cognitive function appear to be saponins called bacosides. Although memory can improve with short-term dosing, it appears chronic (two to three months). Supplementation with bacopa may be necessary for maximum cognitive-enhancing benefits to be demonstrated. Bacopa has been studied in healthy adults and children as well as in children diagnosed with attention deficit/hyperactivity disorder (ADHD). Modern bacopa research confirms its effects on anxiety, which might be mediated by an increase in the brain's level of the inhibitory neurotransmitter GABA (gamma-aminobutyric acid).

Cordyceps *(Cordyceps sinensis)*
Cordyceps is a therapeutic fungus found primarily at high altitudes in China. Research dating back to 1843 states that cordyceps has properties similar to those of ginseng. Cordyceps, like ginseng, is used to strengthen and rebuild the body after exhaustion or long-term illness.[36] Research has also demonstrated immunoregulating activities and cordyceps has been shown to increase adenosine triphosphate (ATP), making it effective in alleviating fatigue and improving physical endurance.[37] In addition, cordyceps is a powerful antioxidant that can defend against oxidative damage occurring within in the cells, including the mitochondria. Studies have shown that cordyceps can help increase lung capacity and lead to easier breathing and better oxygen capacity.

Korean Ginseng *(Panax ginseng)*
Panax ginseng is greatly valued in traditional use as a tonic. It is a substance that acts to normalize the body and aids in creating a state of healthy homeostasis through a variety of pharmacological actions.[38] Panax's main constituent is ginsenoside, which has a corticosteroid-like action and is also hypoglycemic, inhibiting the re-uptake of neurotransmitters and causing a calming balance within the body. It is used to enhance stamina and to provide the capacity to cope with fatigue and physical stress. Although the exact mechanisms of ginseng remain a mystery, animal and human research indicates that ginseng may influence HPA activity by modulating glucocorticoid levels. This influences the positive and negative feedback stress hormone receptors and inhibits cortisone-induced adrenal and thymic atrophy.[39]

Rhodiola *(Rhodiola rosea)*
Rhodiola rosea has been extensively studied in Russia and Scandinavian countries for over 35 years and is categorized as an adaptogen because of its ability to increase resistance to chemical, biological, and physical stressors. Rhodiola

---

[35] H. Wagner, H. Norr, and H. Winterhoff, *Phytomedicine,* "Plant adaptogens," 1994, Volume1, 63-76.

[36] Hobbs C. Medicinal Mushrooms. Loveland, Colorado: Interweave Press Inc.; 1996.

[37] Kiho T, Ookubo K, Usui S, et al. Structural features and hypoglycemic activity of a polysaccharide (CS-F10) from the cultured mycelium of Cordyceps sinensis. Biol Pharm Bull 1999;22(9):966-70

[38] Huang KC. The Pharmacology of Herbs 2nd Ed. New York: CRC Press; 1999

[39] Gaffney BT, Hugel HM, Rich PA. Panax ginseng and Eleutherococcus senticosus may exaggerate an already existing biphasic response to stress via inhibition of enzymes which limit the binding of stress hormones to their receptors. MedbHypotheses 2001; 56(5):567-72.

has been found to inhibit stress-induced depletion of catecholamines and to facilitate the transport of neurotransmitters within the brain. The adaptogenic properties of Rhodiola have been attributed primarily to this ability to influence the levels and activity of neurotransmitters and opioid peptides such as beta-endorphins. Because it is an adaptogen, Rhodiola has the potential to normalize neurotransmitters in the central nervous system without causing drowsiness or fatigue.

Licorice *(Glycyrrhiza glabra)*

Licorice root is one of the most highly regarded herbal adaptogens in terms of treating conditions associated with diminished adrenal function. The adaptogenic activity of licorice is associated with two active components—glycyrrhizin and glycyrrhitinic acid. These components have been reported to bind to both glucocorticoid and mineralocorticoid receptors, possibly displacing endogenous steroids and thus contributing to an increase in availability of cortisol within the body.[40] Licorice is known to have multiple pharmacological actions including adrenocorticoid-like activity. In addition, licorice has anti-inflammatory, antitussive, antiviral, antiulcer, and estrogen- balancing properties.

5-Hydroxytryptophan (5-HTP)

Five-HTP is extracted from the seeds of the African plant Griffonia simplicifolia. It is the intermediate metabolite of the essential amino acid L-tryptophan in the biosynthesis of serotonin. Unlike L-tryptophan, 5-HTP cannot be shunted into niacin or protein production. Therapeutic use of 5-HTP bypasses the conversion of L-tryptophan into 5-HTP by the enzyme tryptophan hydroxylase. This is the rate-limiting step in the synthesis of serotonin but is inhibited by numerous factors which include stress, insulin resistance, vitamin B6 deficiency, magnesium deficiency, and increasing age. It easily crosses the blood-brain barrier and effectively increases central nervous system (CNS) synthesis of serotonin. This makes it an effective treatment in a wide variety of conditions, including depression, fibromyalgia, insomnia, binge eating associated with obesity, and chronic headaches.

Gamma-aminobutyric acid (GABA)

GABA is a major neurotransmitter which is widely distributed throughout the central nervous system. When too much excitation occurs in the CNS, it can lead to irritability, restlessness, insomnia, seizures, and movement disorders and it must be balanced with inhibition. GABA is the most important inhibitory neurotransmitter in the brain. It provides this inhibition and acts like a "brake" during times of runaway stress. Either low GABA levels or decreased GABA function in the brain is associated with several psychiatric and neurological disorders such as anxiety, depression, insomnia, and epilepsy. Studies indicate that GABA can improve relaxation and enhance sleep.

L-theanine

L-theanine is a unique amino acid which is present almost exclusively in the green tea plant (Camellia sinensis) and has been used in Japan for decades. L-theanine has demonstrated the potential to positively modify brain waves and key neurotransmitters involved in mood, focus, and memory. The intensity of brain alpha-wave activity increases within thirty to forty-five minutes of L-theanine supplementation. This results in enhanced relaxation and improved mental focus and acuity. This effect is most pronounced in persons subjectively feeling the highest levels of distress. A small Japanese study of university students showed 200 mg oral L-theanine led to increased brain alpha-waves and a subjective sense of relaxation. Theanine administration caused a dose-dependent relaxed, yet alert, state of mind without sedation, beginning approximately forty minutes after oral dosing. L-theanine enhances production of dopamine and serotonin and appears to play a role in the formation of GABA. L-theanine helps establish balance in the neurotransmitter system, resulting in improvements in the mental, emotional, and physical disturbances resulting from chronic stress.

---

[40] Tamaya T, Sato S, Okada HH. Possible mechanism of steroid action of the plant herb extracts glycyrrhizin, glycyrrhetinic acid, and paeoniflorin: inhibition by plant herb extracts of steroid protein binding in the rabbit. Am J Obstet Gynecol 1986; 155(5):1134-39.

Nutritional Factors

Food production and processing has been greatly changed over the past century. Sporadic eating habits in a fast-paced society have adversely compromised the hormonal health of North Americans.

A study in the journal *Pediatrics* in 2010 that examined 1,238 girls found that nearly 25% of African American girls, 15% of Latin girls, and 10% of Caucasian girls were developing breasts by the age of seven. In the previous decade, only 5% of Caucasian girls were developing breasts that early.

The first genetically engineered product ever brought to market was in 1994 when milk in the United States started coming from cows injected with a genetically engineered growth hormone. At that time, the U.S. Food and Drug Administration (FDA) approved recombinant bovine growth hormone (rBGH) for sale over the objections of consumer and health advocacy groups, such as Consumers Union and the Cancer Prevention Coalition. Recombinant bovine growth hormone, also known as recombinant bovine somatropine (rBST), was not approved for use in both Canada and Europe due to animal welfare and human health concerns.

Although rBGH is manufactured in labs, it actually mimics a naturally occurring hormone that is produced in a cow's pituitary gland. It's injected into cows every two weeks to boost the cow's hormonal activity. This boost allows the cows to produce 10-25% more milk each day which translates into one extra gallon per day. Within four years of its introduction to the market, rBGH was being injected into one third of the US cattle herds.

The label on rBGH's package states that this product is extremely hazardous to the cows. The cited side effects include "increases in cystic ovaries and disorders of the uterus," "decreases in gestation length and birth weight of calves," and "increased risk of clinical mastitis"[41].

Use of rBGH causes as much as a tenfold increase in insulin-like growth factor-1 (IGF-1) in the milk of treated cows. Although IGF-1 naturally occurs in both humans and cows, higher than normal levels of this substance in humans have recently been linked to breast and prostate cancer. There is no definitive proof that drinking milk with high IGF-1 levels will translate to high levels in humans, but IGF-1 can be absorbed into the bloodstream from the digestive tract.[42]

As early as 1998, an article in the *Lancet*, a British medical journal, reported that women with even relatively small increases of a hormone known as insulin-like growth factor 1 (IGF-1) were up to seven times more likely to develop premenopausal breast cancer.[43]

---

41 http://www.allergykids.com/uncategorized/raging-hormones/

42 http://healthychild.org/blog/comments/hormones_in_our_food/

43 http://www.allergykids.com/uncategorized/raging-hormones/

According to a January 1996 report in the *International Journal of Health Services*, rBGH milk has up to ten times the IGF-1 levels of natural milk. More recent studies have put the figure even higher, at approximately twenty-fold.[44]

Non-organic beef is another controversial issue. Farmers use many hormones other than rBGH to raise their animals faster and more efficiently. More than 90% of cows in the U.S. are routinely injected with hormones as the FDA permits six hormones to be given to livestock. Trenbolone acetate, melengestrol acetate, and zeranol are synthetically produced hormones also used on animals. Estradiol, testosterone, and progesterone are the other three hormones that are used, which naturally occur in livestock and humans. Two of these hormones, estradiol—a type of estrogen—and progesterone are considered probable carcinogens by the National Toxicology Program at the National Institutes of Health. Estrogen has been linked to breast cancer in women while progesterone has been found to increase the growth of ovarian, breast and uterine tumors.

Alternatively, organic dairy products come from cows that are not routinely treated with bovine growth hormone (BGH) to increase milk production or with antibiotics and are fed a natural pesticide-free diet. If a cow in an organic herd does need to be treated with antibiotics, she is not returned to the herd for a period of twelve months, at which time testing is done to confirm there are no traces of antibiotic residue. Certified organic beef and dairy producers must comply with stringent production, animal welfare, and processing requirements of an organic standard set by a certifying body. Furthermore, organic beef and dairy production require an audit trail and an annual third-party (independent) verification.

According to the Organic Consumers Association, one benefit of organic milk is that it is higher in vitamins and antioxidants. Some of the vitamins and antioxidants found in greater concentrations in organic milk include vitamin E, beta carotene, omega-3 fatty acids, lutein, and zeaxanthine.

According to a study conducted in Newcastle University by Carlo Leifert and Machteld Huber and published in the *British Journal of Nutrition*, organic milk is associated with 36% lower rates of allergies, asthma, and eczema in children up to age two.

Factory farms are concentrated-animal feeding operations (CAFO's) where non-organic or non-natural beef is raised. According to *Food, Inc.*, the book accompaniment to the documentary film of the same name, tens of thousands of animals are raised in such crowded conditions that normal behavior such as grazing is impossible. Prophylactic antibiotics are routinely administered due to the rampant spread of infections in the overcrowded conditions. Increased use of antibiotics on farm animals leads to antibiotic-resistant strains of bacteria that can be passed to humans.

USDA regulations require that all organic livestock must be fed a diet of agricultural products...that are organically produced and organically handled. Therefore, organic cattle eat grass or organically grown grains that are pesticide-free and not laced with fertilizers or other chemicals. In stark contrast, corn and soybeans are the main staple in the feedlots of conventional cattle. Cattle are naturally inclined to eat grass, but those that eat grains have been found to have more *E. Coli* bacteria in their intestinal tract and feces. During slaughter, this can contaminate meat with these deadly bacteria. Conventionally raised livestock are also fed plastic pellets, formulas containing urea or manure, or slaughter by-products, which are all allowable by the USDA.

Processed Foods

Any food that is canned, frozen, dehydrated, texturized, softened, or chemically laden to increase longevity is a processed food. Research shows that the North American diet consists of 60% processed foods. Researchers have discovered that preservatives are altering our biochemistry and can lead to autoimmune conditions, cancer, obesity, insulin resistance, and accelerated aging.

Butylated hydroxyanisole or BHA, for example, has been "generally recommended as safe" (GRAS) by the FDA but is still considered to be "reasonably anticipated to be a human carcinogen." BHA is a chemical that helps prolong the shelf life of food but it also an endocrine disruptor. BHAs are found in numerous sources such as butter, lard, cereals, baked goods, sweets, beer, vegetable oils, potato chips, snack foods, dehydrated potatoes, flavoring agents,

[44] http://www.allergykids.com/uncategorized/raging-hormones/

sausage, poultry and meat products, dry mixes for beverages and desserts, glazed fruits, chewing gum, active dry yeast, defoaming agents for beet sugar, and yeast and emulsion stabilizers for shortening. BHA is also found in food packaging, lipsticks, lip gloss, mascara, eye shadow, and facial creams. [45]

Hydrogenated Fats

When a regular fat is blasted with a hydrogen ion and the liquid is changed to a solid at room temperature, hydrogenated fats are created. Deemed as one of the worst preserving agents, hydrogenated fats increase cholesterol and triglyceride levels dramatically. Just a 2% increase of trans fatty acids increases the chance of heart disease by 23%. A *New England Journal of Medicine* review of more than eighty studies found that trans fats are more dangerous to health than any food contaminant even when it only makes up 1% to 3% of the total calorie intake.[46]

High Fructose Corn Syrup (HFCS)

In 1967, the US production of HFCS was three thousand tons, compared to 9.3 million tons in 2005. There has been a 350% increase in production since 1980 alone and consumption has increased twenty-fold. Studies conducted at the University of Pennsylvania found that HFCS did not suppress the hormone ghrelin, which is the appetite hormone, in the way that glucose does. The studies showed that when HFCS was consumed, more calories were subsequently taken in than normal in the twenty-four hours following. This translated to an overall weight gain in all of the studies that were performed. HFCS also causes resistance to leptin, which is the hormone that is secreted from the brain to tell the body it is full.

Artificial Sweeteners

Consumption of artificial sweeteners have greatly increased over the past few decades. The consumption rate increased from seventy million in 1987 to 160 million in 2000. There is much research to show that artificial sweeteners such as aspartame and saccharin are not only linked to cancer but also cause increased cravings and weight gain, leading to insulin resistance. Researchers at the University of Texas San Anontio determined that adults aged twenty-five to sixty-four who drank diet soft drinks drastically increased their risk of gaining weight. The study involved examining the weight and soda-drinking habits of more than six hundred subjects of average weight. Eight years later, researchers discovered in subsequent studies that those who consumed one diet soda per day were 65% more likely to be overweight that those who drank none.

When aspartame is broken down in the body, methanol is produced. Methanol is a neurotoxic alcohol which is hundreds of times more potent that the alcohol in alcoholic beverages. Aspartame has thus been shown to cause neurological diseases and symptoms including headaches, muscle spasms, dizziness, twitching, memory loss, migraines, and even seizures.

Refined Grains

When the bran and germ of the grain are removed during the refining of grains to extend shelf life, almost all of the fiber, vitamins, and minerals of the entire grain kernel are also eliminated. In addition, the B vitamins—thiamine, riboflavin, niacin, folic acid, and iron are all stripped away during the processing. Enrichment of the finished product is generally performed to add back synthetic versions of these eliminated nutrients.

Refined grains are easily digestible but cause spikes in blood sugar and insulin, which can result in insulin resistance and diabetes. There is a 30% increased risk of developing diabetes in those people who never eat whole grains or non-refined grains in comparison to those who eat three servings of whole grains per day. A study in the *Journal of Clinical Nutrition* found that people who eat refined grains have a 40% higher level of C Reactive protein, which is an inflammatory marker in the cardiovascular system that can increase the risk of heart attack and stroke.

---

[45] Master Your Metabolism Jillian Michaels pg. 105-106

[46] Master Your Metabolism Jillian Michaels pg. 94

Caffeine

The central nervous system is stimulated when caffeine is consumed, even at doses as small as one third of a cup of coffee. The body is sent into "fight or flight" mode. Once caffeine enters the bloodstream, the adrenals secrete epinephrine and norepinephrine, which sets the stage for a chain of hormonal events that cause weight gain. The liver releases blood sugar and the pancreas subsequently secretes insulin to counteract the sugar, causing the blood to dip. Blood vessels are constricted and sugar cravings then occur which in response to the drop in blood sugar. Cortisol is elevated for up to fourteen hours due to the acid in just one cup of coffee. Over-consumption of caffeine deteriorates the adrenal glands and inflicts the effects of long-term stress on the body. Other effects of caffeine consumption include suppression of the immune system and a decrease in brain oxygenation. Excess cortisol also results in increasing abdominal fat deposits and therefore can lead to insulin resistance.

The phosphoric acid in caffeine-containing beverages blocks calcium absorption, which can lead to a calcium deficiency. This deficiency promotes the loss of bone and contributes to heightened premenstrual syndrome (PMS) symptoms, which include breast tenderness, irritability, and nervousness.

Alcohol

Consumption of even small amounts of alcohol will cause a release of estrogen into the bloodstream, raised cortisol levels, and decreased leptin levels. The extra estrogen in the bloodstream can cause increased fat storage and decreased muscle growth. The raised cortisol levels will cause night waking and disturbed sleep. Decreased leptin levels will result in food cravings.

Influencing Hormone Balance through Nutrition

Organic Foods

Ninety percent of all hormone-disrupting agents are found in everyday food supplies. Consuming organic foods will greatly reduce the toxic exposure accumulated through non-organic foods.

The Environmental Working Group, a non-profit organization dedicated to consumer health and protection, has published a list of the twelve most densely pesticide sprayed fruits and vegetables ("Dirty Dozen") and the fifteen least sprayed fruits and vegetables ("Clean Fifteen").

The Dirty Dozen

1. Peaches
2. Apples
3. Sweet Bell Peppers
4. Celery
5. Nectarines
6. Strawberries
7. Cherries
8. Kale
9. Lettuce
10. Imported Grapes
11. Carrots
12. Pears

The Clean Fifteen

1. Onions
2. Avocado
3. Frozen Sweet Corn
4. Pineapples
5. Mango
6. Asparagus
7. Frozen Sweet Peas
8. Kiwi
9. Cabbage
10. Eggplant
11. Papaya
12. Watermelon
13. Broccoli
14. Tomatoes
15. Sweet Potatoes and Grapefruit tie

Low Glycemic Carbohydrates

The degree to which a carbohydrate raises blood sugar two to three hours after eating is known as its glycemic index. The glycemic index measures how fast an individual food converts to glucose before entering the bloodstream in comparison to the action of glucose itself. On the glycemic index scale, pure glucose is measured at one hundred. Any food that is measured to be above one hundred raises blood sugar faster than pure glucose. Any food that is measured to be below one hundred raises blood sugar that much slower. An example of this would be white rice, corn, and potatoes, which are all high glycemic foods, while pearl barley, legumes and bran all have a low glycemic index. Studies have consistently shown that a diet consisting mainly of high glycemic carbohydrates will cause higher blood levels of insulin and insulin-like-growth factor (IGF-1). Consistently high levels of these hormones in the blood will lead to an increase in fat deposition and the promotion of breast and uterine cell growth, and is linked to the formation of cysts, fibroids and cancer. Combining fiber, protein, or flaxseed oil with the carbohydrates has been shown to lower the glycemic rate.

Consuming a diet consisting of low to medium glycemic foods will restore blood sugar levels and hormonal balance. Complex carbohydrates, such as those found in vegetables and whole grains, are preferred over simple carbohydrates for optimizing estrogen metabolism. Excess consumption of simple carbohydrates raises blood glucose and insulin levels, resulting in adverse influences on sex hormone balance. Conversely, complex carbohydrates attenuate glycemic and insulinemic responses.[47]

[47] Kaaks R. Nutrition, hormones, and breast cancer: Is insulin the missing link? Cancer Causes Control 1996; 7:605 25.

Glycemic Index of Common Foods[48]

Food List	Rating	Food Glycemic Index
Bakery Products		
*Pound cake	Low	54
Danish pastry	Medium	59
Muffin (unsweetened)	Medium	62
Cake, tart	Medium	65
Cake, angel	Medium	67
Croissant	Medium	67
Waffles	High	76
Doughnut	High	76
Beverages		
Soya milk	Low	30
Apple juice	Low	41
Carrot juice	Low	45
Pineapple juice	Low	46
Grapefruit juice	Low	48
Orange juice	Low	52
Biscuits		
Digestives	Medium	58
Shortbread	Medium	64
Water biscuits	Medium	65
Ryvita	Medium	67
Wafer biscuits	High	77
**Rice cakes	High	77
Breads		
Multi grain bread	Low	48
Whole grain	Low	50
Pita bread, white	Medium	57
Pizza, cheese	Medium	60

48 http://www.southbeach-diet-plan.com/glycemicfoodchart.htm

Hamburger bun	Medium	61
Rye-flour bread	Medium	64
Whole meal bread	Medium	69
White bread	High	71
White rolls	High	73
Baguette	High	95
Breakfast Cereals		
All-Bran	Low	42
Porridge, non-instant	Low	49
Oat bran	Medium	55
Muesli	Medium	56
Mini Wheat's (whole meal)	Medium	57
Shredded Wheat	Medium	69
Golden Grahams	High	71
Puffed wheat	High	74
Weetabix	High	77
Rice Krispies	High	82
Cornflakes	High	83
Cereal Grains		
Pearl barley	Low	25
Rye	Low	34
Wheat kernels	Low	41
Rice, instant	Low	46
Rice, parboiled	Low	48
Barley, cracked	Low	50
Rice, brown	Medium	55
Rice, wild	Medium	57
Rice, white	Medium	58
Barley, flakes	Medium	66
Taco Shell	Medium	68
Millet	High	71

Dairy Foods		
Yogurt low- fat (sweetened)	Low	14
Milk, chocolate	Low	24
Milk, whole	Low	27
Milk, Fat-free	Low	32
Milk,skimmed	Low	32
Milk, semi-skimmed	Low	34
*Ice-cream (low- fat)	Low	50
*Ice-cream	Medium	61
Fruits		
Cherries	Low	22
Grapefruit	Low	25
Apricots (dried)	Low	31
Apples	Low	38
Pears	Low	38
Plums	Low	39
Peaches	Low	42
Oranges	Low	44
Grapes	Low	46
Kiwi fruit	Low	53
Bananas	Low	54
Fruit cocktail	Medium	55
Mangoes	Medium	56
Apricots	Medium	57
Apricots (tinned in syrup)	Medium	64
Raisins	Medium	64
Pineapple	Medium	66
**Watermelon	High	72
Pasta		
Spaghetti, protein enriched	Low	27
Fettuccine	Low	32

Vermicelli	Low	35
Spaghetti, whole wheat	Low	37
Ravioli, meat filled	Low	39
Spaghetti, white	Low	41
Macaroni	Low	45
Spaghetti, durum wheat	Medium	55
Macaroni cheese	Medium	64
Rice pasta, brown	High	92
Root Crop		
Carrots, cooked	Low	39
Yam	Low	51
Sweet potato	Low	54
Potato, boiled	Medium	56
Potato, new	Medium	57
Potato, tinned	Medium	61
Beetroot	Medium	64
Potato, steamed	Medium	65
Potato, mashed	Medium	70
Chips	High	75
Potato, micro waved	High	82
Potato, instant	High	83
**Potato, baked	High	85
Parsnips	High	97
Snack Food and Sweets		
Peanuts	Low	15
*M&Ms (peanut)	Low	32
*Snickers bar	Low	40
*Chocolate bar; 30g	Low	49
Jams and marmalades	Low	49
*Crisps	Low	54
Popcorn	Medium	55

Mars bar	Medium	64
*Table sugar (sucrose)	Medium	65
Corn chips	High	74
Jelly beans	High	80
Pretzels	High	81
Dates	High	103
Soups		
Tomato soup, tinned	Low	38
Lentil soup, tinned	Low	44
Black bean soup, tinned	Medium	64
Green pea soup, tinned	Medium	66
Vegetables and Beans		
Artichoke	Low	15
Asparagus	Low	15
Broccoli	Low	15
Cauliflower	Low	15
Celery	Low	15
Cucumber	Low	15
Eggplant	Low	15
Green beans	Low	15
Lettuce, all varieties	Low	15
Low-fat yogurt, artificially sweetened	Low	15
Peppers, all varieties	Low	15
Snow peas	Low	15
Spinach	Low	15
Young summer squash	Low	15
Tomatoes	Low	15
Zucchini	Low	15
Soya beans, boiled	Low	16
Peas, dried	Low	22
Popcorn	Medium	55

Kidney beans, boiled	Low	29
Lentils green, boiled	Low	29
Chickpeas	Low	33
Haricot beans, boiled	Low	38
Black-eyed beans	Low	41
Chickpeas, tinned	Low	42
Baked beans, tinned	Low	48
Kidney beans, tinned	Low	52
Lentils green, tinned	Low	52
Broad beans	High	79

Notes: *high in empty calories **low-calorie and nutritious foods

Whole Grains

Ninety-five percent of grain consumption in North America comes from refined grains.[49] Considering that grains should make up approximately 25% of the daily diet, refined grains are being consumed in excessive amounts. Whole grains are known to be one of the best sources of phytochemicals and antioxidants, even higher than some vegetables. Whole grains contain three specific types of carbohydrates—fiber, resistant starch R,1 and oligosaccharides. These three carbohydrates are fermented in the stomach, giving them prebiotic action which creates short-chain fatty acids such as butyric acid, which feed the healthy cells of the colon. The strengthening of the colon cells enables them to detoxify the body of pharmaceutical and other environmental chemicals, similar to the function of the liver. Grains consumed in their whole form that have not been processed into a flour are filling, as the short-chain fatty acids and fiber stimulate fat cells in the stomach to release leptin, the satiety hormone.

Dietary Fiber

Insoluble dietary fibers such as lignin (found in flaxseeds and the bran layer of grains, beans, and seeds) can interrupt the enterohepatic circulation of estrogens in two ways. This interruption enables the harmful estrogen to be detoxified and not reabsorbed into the system.[50] Dietary fiber, especially lignin, can bind unconjugated estrogens in the digestive tract, which are then excreted in the feces. Dietary fiber can beneficially affect the composition of intestinal bacteria and reduce intestinal b-glucuronidase activity, resulting in a lowered deconjugation of estrogen and reduced reabsorption.[51] Dietary fiber intake also increases serum concentrations of sex hormone binding globulin (SHBG), thus reducing levels of free estradiol.[52]

Forty-five to sixty grams of dietary fiber consumed daily provides the additional benefits of slowing down the aging process, decreasing cancer risks, stabilizing blood sugar, lowering cholesterol, decreasing cardiovascular risks,

---

49 Master Your Metabolism Jillian Michaels pg. 144

50 Shultz TD, Howie BJ. In vitro binding of steroid hormones by natural and purified fibers. Nutr Cancer 1986; 8(2):141-47.

51 Adlercreutz H. Western diet and Western diseases: some hormonal and biochemical mechanisms and associations. Scand J Clin Lab Invest 1990:50(S201):3-23.

52 Adlercreutz H, Hockerstedt K, Bannwart C, et al. Effect of dietary components, including lignans and phytoestrogens, on enterohepatic circulation and liver metabolites of estrogens and in sex hormone binding globulin (SHBG). J Steroid Biochem 1987; 27(4-6):1135-44.

and improving insulin sensitivity. A diet high in fiber has also been shown to modify the bowel floral composition which promotes the growth of beneficial bacteria, resulting in a strengthened immune system. Fiber also improves mineral absorption and decreases osteoporosis risks. Many digestive conditions are greatly improved through increased dietary fiber consumption, which speeds up elimination and decreases toxicity. Valuable fiber sources are found in foods such as beans, raw fruits and vegetables, bran, psyllium, ground flax seeds, and whole grains.

Essential Fatty Acids

Essential Fatty Acids (EFAs) are required in cell membrane formation, are a crucial part of the immune system, and enable the buffering of excessive acids in the body. EFAs protect the membrane of the cell from harmful carcinogens and aid in the oxygen transport of air in the lungs to each cell membrane of the body where the oxygen acts as a barrier to pathogenic microbes. Omega-6 and Omega-3 are EFAs that the body cannot produce. Sixty years ago, the average North American diet consisted of a dietary ratio of one to two of Omega-6 to Omega-3. Currently, the ratio is approximated at twenty-five to one Omega-6 to Omega-3. The optimal ratio has been found to be one to one. Omega-6 fatty acids found in vegetable oils and evening primrose oil consumed in excess without being balanced with at least twice as much Omega-3 fatty acids can be carcinogenic. The most common sources of Omega-6 fatty acids include safflower, corn, and sunflower oils, which are readily used in baked goods and packaged items. Omega-6 fatty acids are now commonly used in replacement of trans fatty acids in trans-fat free products. Omega-3 fatty acids are found primarily in flaxseed oil, purslane, blackcurrant seed oil, and cold water fish oils. Omega-3 fatty acids have been shown to decrease inflammation, pain, and arthritis, improve mental function and memory, decrease cardiovascular risk, prevent diabetes, reduce PMS symptoms, and reduce symptoms of endometriosis.

Legumes

Legumes contain protective phytoestrogens and are one of the richest sources of dietary fiber. Phytoestrogens are weak estrogens that bind to estrogen receptor sites, displacing the body's strong estrogens and environmental estrogens. A constant supply is required in order to prevent the accumulation of excess estrogen, which can cause diseases. The highest sources of protective phytoestrogens are sprouted beans and soy.

Soy is perhaps the most common food source of isoflavones but others include legumes, alfalfa, clover, licorice root, and kudzu root. Higher intakes of soy products and isoflavones, such as those consumed in traditional Japanese diets, are associated with low rates of hormone-dependent cancers.[53] The average daily isoflavone intake of Japanese women is twenty to eighty milligrams, while that of American women is one to three milligrams.[54] In two human studies, women given isoflavone supplements and soy milk for one month experienced longer menstrual cycles and lower serum estradiol levels.[55, 56] Longer menstrual cycles are beneficial because they result in decreased lifetime exposure to estrogen and lowered the risk for breast cancer.

Protein

Protein, when broken down into its subunits, amino acids, is the essential building block of hormones such as serotonin, melatonin, growth hormone, and thyroid hormone. Neurotransmitters such as dopamine, enzymes essential for digestion, and antibodies form the immune system and all come from protein as well. Although protein is essential for tissue healing and repair, an excessive amount of protein can stress the kidneys, exacerbate osteoporosis, and

---

[53] Messina MJ, Persky V, Setchell KD, et al. Soy intake and cancer risk: a review of the in vitro and in vivo data. Nutr Cancer 1994; 21:113-31.

[54] Barnes S, Peterson TG, Coward L. Rationale for the use of genistein-containing soy matrices in chemoprevention Trials for breast and prostate cancer. J Cell Biochem Suppl 1995; 22:181-87.

[55] Cassidy A, Bingham S, Setchell KD. Biological effects of a diet of soy protein rich in isoflavones on the menstrual cycle of premenopausal women. Am J Clin Nutr 1994; 60(3):333-40.

[56] Lu LJ, Anderson KE, Grady JJ, et al. Effects of soya consumption for one month on steroid hormones in premenopausal women: implications for breast cancer risk reduction. Cancer Epidemiol Biomarkers Prev 1996; 5(1):63-70.

negatively affect digestive function. Excessive protein consumed without the balancing effects of carbohydrates can elevate cortisol and lead to adrenal fatigue. Deficiencies of dietary protein can trigger mood disorders, memory loss, increased appetite and cravings, decreased metabolism, sleep disruption, muscle loss, and weight gain. When consumed in the correct portions, protein stimulates the activity of the fat burning and appetite controlling hormones, leptin and glucagon. In addition, protein releases Peptide YY from the digestive system, which causes a suppression of appetite. The average daily intake of protein should make up approximately 30% of the whole diet. This amount can vary depending on gender, activity level, and the amount of lean muscle mass. Optimal protein choices are low in saturated fats and have been shown to increase inflammation in the body and to disrupt hormones. Healthiest sources of vegetarian protein include fermented soy foods (miso, tofu, soy beans, and tempeh), kidney beans, lentils, split peas, chickpeas, almonds, sunflower seeds, pumpkin seeds and sesame seeds. Healthy animal protein sources include non-farmed fish, organic poultry, organic omega-3 eggs, organic lamb, organic grass fed wild game, and organic dairy (plain yogurt, low-fat ricotta cheese, and cottage cheese).

Berries

Berries have extremely high concentrations of anthocyanins, particularly flavonoids, which are responsible for the bright colors of berries. A Japanese researcher discovered that anthocyanins can stop individual fat cells from increasing in size and can also help to secrete adiponectin, which is a hormone that reduces inflammation, lowers blood sugar, and reverses leptin and insulin resistance. Other studies have found that anthocyanins are capable of reducing post-prandial blood sugar levels, preventing insulin spikes, and blocking the digestive enzyme activity of specific starches and fats, thereby reducing their absorption.

Cruciferous Vegetables

Cruciferous vegetables contain phytochemicals known as isothiocyanates, which stimulate our bodies to break down potential carcinogens. They work by preventing the transformation of normal healthy cells into cancerous cells. Some examples of cruciferous vegetables are arugula, bok choy, broccoli, Brussels sprouts, cabbage, cauliflower, Chinese cabbage, collard greens, daikon, kale, kohlrabi mustard greens, radishes, rutabaga, turnips, and watercress. In particular, broccoli contains sulforaphane, which is a natural chemical that stimulate our bodies to produce enzymes and destroy carcinogens. This substance is particularly rich in broccoli sprouts and about twenty to fifty times richer in mature broccoli.

At the Harbor UCLA Medical Center in Torrance, California, a study was conducted to document the effects of eating broccoli among men and women aged fifty to seventy-four. The results showed that those who consumed more broccoli (3.7 half-cup cooked servings weekly on average) were 50% less likely to develop colorectal cancer than those who never ate broccoli.[57]

Many cruciferous vegetables also contain a compound called indole-3-carbinol. This compound is said to reduce the risk of hormone dependent cancers such as prostate, breast, and ovarian cancer.

---

[57] http://www.drlam.com/opinion/cruciferous_vegetables.asp

Phytochemical Sources and Health Values[58]

PHYTOCHEMICAL	EFFECT	FOOD SOURCES
ALLYL SULPHIDES	Increases liver enzymes to detoxify carcinogens	Garlic, onions, and leeks
CAPSAICIN	Prevents carcinogens from binding to DNA	Chili peppers
CAROTENOIDS	Act as antioxidants that neutralize free radicals, enhance immunity High intake is associated with low cancer rates	Parsley, carrots, spinach, kale, winter squash, apricots, cantaloupe, and sweet potatoes
FLAVANOIDS	Prevent the attachment of cancer-causing hormones to cells by blocking receptor site	Most fruits and vegetables, including parsley, carrots, citrus, broccoli, cabbage, cucumber, squash, yams, eggplant, peppers, and berries
CURCUMIN	Decreases inflammation Assists the liver in detoxifying carcinogens and hormones Arrests cell division in cancer cells	Turmeric
ELLAGIC ACID	Neutralizes carcinogens in the liver Antioxidant Inhibits cancer cell divisions	Red raspberries and walnut skin
ISOFLAVONES *(genestein and diadzen)*	Bind to the estrogen receptor so that harmful estrogens can't bind Block the formation of blood vessels to tumors Inhibit enzymes that might cause cancer Inhibit activation of breast cancer genes	Soy beans, tofu, miso, lentils, dried beans, split peas, garbanzo beans, green beans, green peas, mung bean sprouts, and red clover sprouts
INDOLES	Decrease the estrogen that initiates breast cancer	Raw cabbage, broccoli, Brussels sprouts, kale, cauliflower, bok Choy, kohlrabi, mustard, and turnips
ISOTHIOCYANATES	Prevents DNA damage Block the production of tumors induced by environmental chemicals Act as antioxidants Assist liver detoxification	Mustard, horse radish, radishes, turnips, cabbage, broccoli, cauliflower, Brussels sprouts, kale, bok Choy, watercress, and garden sorrel
LIMONOIDS	Induce protective enzymes in liver and intestines that fight cancer	Citrus fruit rind, essential oils of lemon, orange, celery, and lemongrass

[58] Complete Natural Medicine Guide to Women's Health Sat Dharam Kaur, ND pg. 52-54

LINOLENIC ACID	Regulates production of prostaglandins in cells	Flax seeds and flaxseed oil
LYCOPENE	Protects from cell damage	Tomatoes, red grapefruit, and guava
LUTEIN	Protects from cell damage	Spinach, kiwi, tomatoes, and grapes
MONOTERPENES	Antioxidant properties Induce protective enzymes Inhibit cholesterol production in tumors Stimulate the destruction of breast cancer cells Inhibit growth of cancer cells	Cherries, lavender, parsley, yams, carrots, broccoli, cabbage, basil cucumbers, peppers, squash, eggplant, mint, tomatoes, and grapefruit
PHENOLIC ACIDS	Block the effects of free radicals Inhibit the formation of nitrosamine, a carcinogen	Berries, broccoli, grapes, citrus, parsley, peppers, soy, squash, tomatoes, and grains
PLANT STEROLS *(beta-sitosterol)*	Prevent cells from becoming cancerous and lower cholesterol levels in the body	Broccoli, cabbage, soy, peppers, and whole grains
POLYPHENOLS	Act as antioxidants Reduce damaging effects nitrosamines Kill human cancer cells	Broccoli, carrots, green tea, cucumbers, squash, basil, and citrus
PROTEASE INHIBITORS	Block the activity of enzymes involved in the growth of tumors	Beans and soy products
QUERCETIN	Slows down cell division in cancer cells Anti-inflammatory	Onions, apples, and green cabbage
QUINONES	Neutralize carcinogens	Rosemary and Pau d'arco tea
SULPHORAPHANE	Increases the ability of the liver's detoxifying enzymes to remove carcinogens Antioxidant	Broccoli sprouts, broccoli, cauliflower, and Brussels sprouts

Consumption of the following "Super Foods" on a daily basis will prevent inflammation as well as lower cholesterol and balance hormones.

Super Food Health Effects[59]

SUPERFOOD	GOOD HEALTH EFFECTS
FLAX SEED *Two tablespoons freshly ground flax seeds daily*	High fiber for increasing bowel movements and cleansing the colon Contains phytoestrogens to prevent breast cancer and alleviate menopausal hot flashes A complete protein
FLAXSEED OIL OR UNCONTAMINATED FISH OIL *Two tablespoons per day uncooked*	High in Omega-3 EFAs to help prevent cancer, arthritis, heart disease, depression, skin affections, and Alzheimer's disease Keeps the cell membranes strong
TURMERIC *Two teaspoons or more daily*	One of the best anti-inflammatories to alleviate arthritic symptoms Decreases the risk of most cancers and helps prevent Alzheimer's disease Assists in liver detoxification
GARLIC *Two cloves daily*	Natural antibiotic and anti-parasitic Lowers cholesterol and blood pressure, preventing heart disease Helps to prevent many types of cancer Assists in liver detoxification
RAW NUTS AND SEEDS *Two to four tablespoons daily*	High in zinc and magnesium, which are common mineral deficiencies linked to lowered immune function, anxiety, and heart disease Pumpkin seeds are anti-parasitic
SEAWEED *Two tablespoons daily*	Good sources of calcium and iron Nori, dulse, hiziki, arame, and kombu are highly alkaline, rich in minerals, and high in beta carotene Brown seaweed, like kelp, helps to pull radioactive particles out of the body so they can be excreted
ORGANIC SOY (NON-GMO) *Twenty-five grams daily*	Helps to lower cholesterol and blood pressure Helps to prevent breast and uterine cancers Eat with seaweed as a source of iodine Avoid if allergic
RAW BRASSICAS *Half a cup or more daily*	Cabbage, cauliflower, broccoli, and kale assist the liver in detoxification pathways, improve estrogen metabolism, and help to prevent breast and uterine cancer when eaten raw Raw cabbage juice health stomach and duodenal ulcers

[59] Complete Natural Medicine Guide to Women's Health Sat Dharam Kaur, ND pg. 61-61

SHITAKE MUSHROOMS *Half a cup or more daily*	Enhance the immune system and help prevent cancer
BLUEBERRIES, RASPBERRIES, AND STRAWBERRIES *Half a cup or more daily*	High in antioxidants that help to prevent cancer and improve vision
COOKED TOMATOES *Weekly*	High in lycopene, an antioxidant that helps prevent breast, lung, and cervical cancer
EXTRA VIRGIN OLIVE OIL *One to two tablespoons daily*	Moves the bile through the liver and gallbladder, facilitating a removal of toxins
LEGUMES *Half a cup or more daily*	Contain high amounts of potassium and magnesium Low glycemic index Contain phytic acid which helps to prevent the growth of cancer
ROSEMARY AND CORIANDER *Several times per week*	Rosemary facilitates liver detoxification of hormones and chemicals Coriander helps to remove toxic metals such as mercury, cadmium and lead
ORGANIC GREEN TEA *Two or more cups daily*	Stimulates metabolism to assist in weight loss and helps to prevent cancer

Multiple dietary and nutritional factors have the ability to influence the endocrine system into a state of harmony or dysfunction. Incorporating dietary changes with the use of select nutritional supplements can have profound beneficial effects in influencing hormone balance and thus preventing hormone-related diseases and conditions.

Testing Procedures

The Science of Saliva Testing

The amount of hormones delivered to receptors in the body is most accurately represented by hormone levels in saliva samples. Comparatively, serum represents the hormone levels that may or may not be delivered to receptors of the body. Clinically, it is far more relevant to test the amount of hormones delivered to the tissue receptors as this is a reflection of the active hormone levels of the body.

The majority of hormones in the blood exist in two forms: free (5%) or protein-bound (95%). Free bioavailable hormone levels in the body are measured through saliva while blood serum measures only the protein bound non-bioavailable hormone levels. When assessing functional hormone levels, blood serum is a much less accurate measurement than saliva.

When blood is filtered through the salivary glands, the bound hormone components are too large to pass through the cell membranes of the salivary glands. Only the unbound hormones pass through and into the saliva. What is measured in the saliva is considered the "free," or bioavailable hormone, that which will be delivered to the receptors in the tissues of the body.

In order for steroid hormones to be detected in serum, they must be bound to circulating proteins. In this bound state, they are unable to fit into receptors in the body, and therefore will not be delivered to tissues. They are considered inactive, or non-bioavailable.

The discrepancy between free and protein bound hormones becomes especially important when monitoring topical, or transdermal, hormone therapy. Studies show that this method of delivery results in increased tissue hormone levels (thus measurable in saliva), but no parallel increase in blood serum levels. Therefore, blood serum testing cannot be used to monitor topical hormone therapy.

Saliva, Serum, and Urine Testing Comparative Analysis[60]

Saliva Tests	Serum Tests	Urine Tests
Real Life Hormone Function Evaluation		
Multiple salivary specimens throughout the day or month. Can be collected under real life situations, at work, at home, etc. Hormone values reflect real life physiological conditions and responses.	Serum collection requires clinic visit and creates apprehension due to anticipation of venipuncture. Stress causes an artificial increase in cortisol. Only approximates real life conditions.	Twenty-four-hour urine has metabolites of the hormones and is not time specific and does not reflect time sensitive hormonal and stress responses.
Ease of Collection		
Saliva is easily collected by the patient.	Serum tests require clinic staff and disruption of routine schedule of patient.	Twenty-four-hour urine collection is cumbersome and time-consuming, especially for women.
Biohazard		
Patient collects sample with minimal biohazard to clinic staff.	Serum collection is bio-hazardous to clinic staff, especially when handling serum of patients with AIDS and Hepatitis.	Urine collection is minimally bio-hazardous to clinic staff.
Time-Specific		
Multiple saliva samples collected at different times allow evaluation of hormonal stress response and circadian rhythm.	The routine single serum sample does not allow circadian rhythm evaluation, i.e., no real time component.	Twenty-four-hour urine is not time-specific and does not reflect circadian rhythm variation at all.
Bioactive hormonal fraction		
Saliva reflects the unbound bioactive hormone level to which living cells are subjected. This is the hormone level that needs to be evaluated.	Routine serum hormone testing reflects total hormone level, not the bioactive fraction. Total levels are crude estimates of unbound bioactive hormone.	Urine hormones reflect production and catabolism and do not reflect tissue level hormone concentrations to which the living cells are exposed. Urine hormone interpretation is very misleading.
Therapeutic Discrimination		
Because saliva testing can sub-classify hormonal dysfunction into time-related values, the subclasses of dysfunction are discernible. Consequently, therapeutic options are expanded and treatments are very specific.	Serum testing results are reported as high, low, or normal. Hormone values and treatment options are limited and not always synchronized with the natural circadian cycle of the patient. Urine testing results are reported as high, low, or normal.	Hormone values and treatment options are limited and not always synchronized with the natural circadian cycle of the patient.

[60] http://www.diagnostechs.com/ProviderPortal/SalivaSerumandUrineTestingComparison.aspx

Female Hormone Panel

Estradiol (E2)

The correct balance between estrogen and progesterone is one of the critical factors for maintaining hormonal health. Estradiol is needed for the proper function of progesterone receptors. High estradiol levels may compete with T3, a thyroid hormone, at the T3 responsive gene sites and interfere with the tissue activity of T3, leading to hypothyroidism. High estradiol levels may also increase thyroid binding globulin levels, which bind up free T3 and T4 hormone, resulting in decreased tissue action of T3. Low estradiol levels post-menopause may be a consequence of adrenal dysfunction as post-menopausal production of estradiol comes via conversion from the adrenal hormone DHEA.

Progesterone

Progesterone enhances the sensitivity of estrogen receptors. Even with normal E2 levels, progesterone deficiency contributes to, or exacerbates, estrogen deficiency symptoms.

Estradiol and progesterone levels and their ratio are an index of estrogen/progesterone balance. An excess of estradiol, relative to progesterone, can explain many symptoms in reproductive-age women, including endometrial hyperplasia, premenstrual syndrome, fibrocystic breasts, and uterine fibroids.[61] When estrogen supplements are prescribed without the balancing effects of progesterone, a deficiency in progesterone can also result. Symptoms of estrogen dominance, which include weight gain in the hips and thighs, fibrocystic and tender breasts, uterine fibroids, irritability, water retention, and thyroid problems, can occur from this imbalance. Estrogen dominance can lead to cancers of the uterus and breasts and insulin resistance. Low estradiol levels occurring at the onset of menopause can trigger a multitude of symptoms including hot flashes, night sweats, vaginal dryness, sleep disturbances, foggy thinking, more rapid skin aging, and bone loss. Maintaining appropriate levels of estradiol adequately balanced with progesterone at any age is essential for optimal hormonal health. Only endogenous levels of progesterone and estradiol are used in the calculation of the progesterone to estradiol ratios. The most commonly observed range in regularly cycling women in the luteal phase is between eight and thirty days, with fifteen being the median value.

Testosterone

Unbalanced testosterone can lead to hormonal disruption, whether levels are deficient or excessive. Elevated testosterone often caused by ovarian cysts leads to conditions such as polycystic ovarian syndrome (PCOS), excessive facial and body hair, acne, and oily skin and hair. Testosterone deficiency is often caused by excessive stress, medications, contraceptives, and surgical removal of the ovaries.[62] This leads to symptoms of androgen deficiency including loss of libido, thinning skin, vaginal dryness, loss of bone and muscle mass, depression, and memory lapses.

Sex Hormone Binding Globulin

Sex hormone binding globulin (SHBG) is a protein produced by the liver when exposed to any type of estrogen. This exposure can include estrogen produced naturally by the body or consumed as a synthetic oral contraceptive estrogen, estrogen therapy, or as foods or herbs (phytoestrogens). SHBG binds tightly to circulating estradiol and testosterone. This prevents their rapid metabolism and clearance and limits their bioavailability to tissues. SHBG gives a good index of the extent of the body's overall exposure to estrogens. The SHBG level is also used to calculate free (unbound) testosterone levels when blood spot is used to measure sex hormones.[63]

---

[61] Northrup C. Estrogen dominance. Available at: http://www.drnorthrup.com/womenshealth/healthcenter/topic_details.php?topic_id=118. Accessed 9/19/08.

[62] Miller KK. Androgen deficiency in women. J Clin Endocrinol Metab. 2001 Jun; 86(6):2395-401.

[63] Selby C. Sex hormone binding globulin: origin, function and clinical significance. Ann Clin Biochem. 1990 Nov; 27 (Pt 6):532-41.

DHEA sulphate

DHEA sulphate (DHEA-S), which is produced by the adrenal glands, generally reflects adrenal gland function. DHEA is normally present in greater quantities than all the other steroid hormones as it is the precursor for estrogen and testosterone production. DHEA levels peak in the late teens to early twenties and then naturally decline with age. Cortisol and DHEA have opposite effects on immune function and insulin regulation. When cortisol levels are increased, more DHEA is required to be released to balance the effects of the elevated cortisol. Thus, chronically elevated cortisol can result in a deficiency of DHEA. Low DHEA can result in decreased libido and general malaise, while high DHEA can have masculinizing effects on women because it metabolizes into androgens, including testosterone. The ratio of cortisol to DHEA-S increases with age, mostly due to declining DHEA. Low DHEA-S levels may be associated with hypothyroidism and chronic illnesses such as lupus and rheumatoid arthritis.

Cortisol

Cortisol levels portray overall adrenal function and indicate exposure to stressors. Healthy adrenal cortisol production is highest early in the morning, soon after waking, and then falls to lower levels at mid-day and continues to decrease into the evening. Low cortisol levels can indicate adrenal fatigue (a reduced ability to respond to stressors), and can leave the body more vulnerable to poor blood sugar regulation and immune system dysfunction. Chronically high cortisol is a consequence of high, constant exposure to stressors, and this has serious implications for long-term health, including an increased risk of cancer, osteoporosis, and possibly Alzheimer's disease.[64] Elevated cortisol can interfere with the action of progesterone and testosterone at gene regulatory sites. A functional deficiency can result when women with normal progesterone and/or testosterone levels exhibit signs of deficiency when cortisol levels are high. High cortisol can also induce the enzyme aromatase, which speeds the conversion of testosterone to estradiol, resulting in elevated estradiol levels and estrogen dominance. Excess cortisol is also linked to significant bone loss. Elevated cortisol in the evening has been associated with depression and a poorer prognosis in breast cancer survivors. Chronically high cortisol levels may progress to adrenal exhaustion and eventual low cortisol levels as the adrenal glands are no longer able to produce enough cortisol in response to stress.

Luteinizing Hormone (LH)/Follicular Stimulating Hormone (FSH)

LH and FSH tests are included in the female fertility profiles to give information on the possible presence of ovarian insufficiency (elevated FSH) or PCOS (elevated LH/FSH). These hormones are released from the pituitary gland and stimulate the ovaries and testes. High levels are found in cases of menopause, infertility, amenorrhea, and premature ovarian failure. Low levels indicate pituitary gland dysfunction. An excess of LH compared to FSH is a common finding in PCOS.

Thyroid Profile

The thyroid profile (free T4, free T3, TSH, and TPO) can indicate the presence of an imbalance in thyroid function. Some of the associated symptoms of low thyroid include cold intolerance, low stamina, fatigue (particularly in the evening), depression, low sex drive, weight gain, dry brittle nails, coarse hair, hair loss, infertility, constipation, and high cholesterol.

Thyroid Stimulating Hormone (TSH)

TSH is produced by the pituitary gland and acts on the thyroid gland to stimulate production of T4. High levels of TSH can indicate a low functioning thyroid gland, while low TSH can indicate an over-production of T4, which acts as a negative feedback on the pituitary to reduce TSH production. Low TSH can also be caused by problems in the pituitary gland itself which result in insufficient TSH being produced to stimulate the thyroid (secondary hypothyroidism).

---

64 Magri F, Cravello L, Barili L, Sarra S, Cinchetti W, Salmoiraghi F, Micale G, Ferrari E. Stress and dementia: the role of the hypothalamic pituitary-adrenal axis. Aging Clin Exp Res. 2006 Apr; 18(2):167-70.

Free T4 – Thyroxine

T4 is an inactive thyroid hormone that is most predominantly produced by the thyroid gland. T4 converts to T3 within cells. Free T4 is the non-protein-bound fraction of the T4 circulating in the blood, representing about 0.04% of the total circulating T4, which is available to tissues. Low TSH combined with low T4 levels indicates hypothyroidism, while low TSH and high T4 levels indicate hyperthyroidism. High TSH and low T4 indicate a thyroid gland disease such as thyroiditis.

Free T3 – Triiodothyronine

Free T3 is the active thyroid hormone that regulates the metabolic activity of cells. Free T3 is a non-protein-bound fraction circulating in the blood. This represents about 0.4% of the total circulating T3, which is available to tissues. Elevated T3 levels are seen in hyperthyroid patients but levels can be normal or abnormal in hypothyroid patients.

TPO – Thyroid Peroxidase Antibodies

Thyroid peroxidase is an enzyme used by the thyroid gland in the manufacture of T4. The body produces antibodies that attack the thyroid gland in patients with autoimmune thyroiditis (predominantly Hashimoto's disease). Levels of these antibodies in the blood can be used to diagnose this condition and indicate the extent of the disease.

Adrenal Stress Index

Cortisol Rhythm

Analysis of four saliva samples, taken upon waking, before lunch, before dinner, and before bed, reflects accurate salivary cortisol measurement. Results indicate the awake diurnal cortisol rhythm generated in response to everyday normal stress. The test results facilitate the diagnosis of stress maladaptation and adrenal fatigue.

DHEA/DHEA-S

Multiple saliva samples are used to measure the average DHEA/DHEA-S levels for the day. The many facets of stress maladaptation are highlighted by the cortisol to DHEA relationship. The cortisol/DHEA ratio also helps to determine the projected time for recovery from stress maladaptation, as well as the substances, hormones, supplements, and botanicals that will facilitate the recovery.

17-Hydroxyprogesterone (P17-OH)

The Adrenal Stress Index measures P17-OH levels in order to evaluate the efficiency of the conversion of adrenal precursors into cortisol. A small percentage of the population is genetically predisposed to low cortisol production and hence will not benefit from exogenous supplementation of pregnenolone or progesterone.

Insulin

Fasting and non-fasting insulin measurements are used to diagnose insulin resistance-functional insulin deficit (pre-diabetes). These levels are also used to correlate elevated cortisol with insulin and can explain glycemic dys-regulation problems. The combined results of insulin and cortisol can help in designing an effective glycemic control treatment plan that may include lifestyle modifications, nutritional support and botanical supplementation.

Secretory IgA (SIgA)

Mucosal immunity is measured by using SIgA as a stress impact biomarker. SIgA values are sensitive to increased cortisol/DHEA ratio and sympathetic tone. Detection of depressed mucosal immune function allows for a number of therapeutic modalities to be utilized. These can range from botanical supplementation to control of heart rhythm variability.

Gliadin Antibodies

The Adrenal Stress Index provides objective identification of grain-intolerant patients. Measurements of gliadin antibodies detect subclinical grain intolerance even when celiac disease (gluten intolerance) is not present. Positive findings indicate restriction of gluten intake, which will reduce inflammation and adrenal stress.

Hormonal Imbalances in Women[65]

ESTROGENS Elevated estrogen (estrogen dominance)	**Conditions:** early puberty, uterine fibroids, uterine cancer, ovarian cysts, breast fibro adenoma, breast cancer, PMS, endometriosis, hypothyroidism, autoimmune diseases, increased risk of gallbladder disease **Symptoms:** blood clots, impaired blood sugar, water retention, depression, anxiety, headaches
ESTROGENS Estrogen deficiency	**Conditions:** infertility, amenorrhea, osteoporosis, menopausal hot flashes, vaginal dryness **Symptoms:** decreased sexual arousal, poor memory, depression, elevated cholesterol, high LDL, low HDL, elevated blood pressure, poor sleep, aging skin with wrinkles
ESTROGENS Disturbed estrogen quotient	**Conditions:** breast cancer, uterine cancer
PROGESTERONE Progesterone deficiency	**Conditions:** infertility, PMS, prolonged or heavy menstrual bleeding, breast tenderness, breast cysts, breast fibroadenomas, breast cancer, uterine fibroids, uterine cancer, ovarian cysts, polycystic ovarian syndrome, lowered libido, hypothyroidism, adrenal fatigue, miscarriage, increase cardiovascular disease **Symptoms:** fatigue, insomnia, anxiety, coronary artery spasm
ACTH Low ACTH	**Symptoms:** low energy and motivation, poor memory
CORTISOL High cortisol	**Conditions:** PMS, polycystic ovary syndrome, hypothyroidism **Symptoms:** muscle weakness, muscle wasting, thinning skin, elevated glucose, insulin resistance, easy weight gain, diabetes, fat deposition in chest, abdomen and

[65] Complete Natural Medicine Guide to Women's Health Sat Dharam Kaur, ND pg. 92-94

	head; peptic ulcer, slow wound healing, lowered immune function, increased infections, constriction of blood vessels with elevated blood pressure
CORTISOL Low cortisol	**Conditions:** PMS, menopausal hot flashes, nausea in pregnancy, hypothyroidism, lupus, chronic fatigue syndrome, fibromyalgia, low libido, allergies, asthma **Symptoms:** inability to handle stress, crave stimulants—sugar, chocolate, caffeine, cigarettes; mental confusion, poor concentration, low blood pressure, dizziness, rapid heartbeat with exertion, fatigue, joint pain, increased inflammation anywhere, increased skin pigmentation, hypoglycaemia, aching calves, flat feet, weak ankles and knees, increased white blood cell production, inflammation, autoimmune disease susceptibility
ALDOSTERONE High aldosterone	**Conditions:** PMS (water and salt retention), high blood pressure **Symptoms:** increased potassium loss in the urine, slow irregular heartbeat, muscle cramps, fatigue, constipation, insomnia
ALDOSTERONE Low aldosterone	**Symptoms:** low blood pressure, dizziness, fatigue, frequent urination, excessive perspiration, salt craving, muscle twitches, cardiac arrhythmia
DHEA High DHEA	**Conditions**: converted to estrogen in breast cancer cells; may increase tumor growth in estrogen driven cancers
DHEA Low DHEA	**Conditions:** heart disease, fibromyalgia, lupus, osteoporosis **Symptoms:** fatigue, poor memory, decreased libido, anxiety, nervousness, decreased dreaming, elevated blood pressure, high cholesterol, atherosclerosis, increased infections, poor recovery after stress
TESTOSTERONE High testosterone	**Conditions:** PMS, amenorrhea, polycystic ovary syndrome, miscarriage, increased breast cancer risk **Symptoms:** easily angered, increased facial hair, increased muscle mass
TESTOSTERONE Low testosterone	**Symptoms:** low energy, low motivation, poor memory, depression, no sexual orgasms, low libido, elevated blood pressure during or after menopause, loss of muscle mass

INSULIN Elevated insulin	**Conditions:** precocious puberty, amenorrhea, dysmenorrhea, polycystic ovary syndrome, diabetes, hypothyroidism, cardiovascular disease, breast cancer, uterine cancer, ovarian cancer **Symptoms:** high cholesterol, atherosclerosis, elevated testosterone, elevated estrogen
INSULIN Insulin resistance or insensitivity (metabolic syndrome)	**Conditions:** irregular periods, polycystic ovarian syndrome, preeclampsia in pregnancy, cardiovascular disease, adult onset diabetes **Symptoms:** high blood pressure, high cholesterol, elevated LDL, low HDL
INSULIN Low insulin	**Condition:** type 1 diabetes **Symptoms:** low endurance, dizziness, irritability hunger, shakiness, sweating, rapid heartbeat
INSULIN-LIKE GROWTH FACTOR (IGF-1) Elevated IGF-1	**Conditions:** precocious puberty, breast cancer, lung cancer, polycystic ovary syndrome, uterine fibroids, uterine cancer, ovarian cysts, ovarian cancer **Symptoms:** causes increased growth of tissue, promotes growth and invasiveness of malignant cells, decreases production of SHBG which results in more available estrogen, stimulates increased estrogen production in the ovaries
GROWTH HORMONE Elevated growth hormone	**Conditions:** precocious puberty and early breast development, breast cancer, polycystic ovary syndrome, uterine fibroids, uterine cancer, ovarian cysts, ovarian cancer **Symptoms:** increase estradiol long-term, elevated IGF-1, promotes cell multiplication
GROWTH HORMONE Decreased growth hormone	**Conditions:** amenorrhea, osteoporosis **Symptoms:** exhaustion, poor recovery from exertion, high LDL, low HDL, high blood pressure
THYROID HORMONES Underactive thyroid gland	**Conditions:** amenorrhea, PMS, heavy periods, menopausal hot flashes, endometriosis, polycystic ovary syndrome, infertility, miscarriage, breast cysts, breast cancer, breast cancer, fibromyalgia, osteoarthritis, cardiovascular disease

	Symptoms: low energy—especially in the morning, poor memory, slow thinking, anxiety and depression—especially in the morning and better when physically active, elevated cholesterol, high or low blood pressure, slow pulse, numbness in hands and feet, carpal tunnel syndrome, dry skin, decreased perspiration, weight gain with puffy face and eyelids, hair loss, husky voice, intolerance to cold, slow digestion, gas, constipation
THYROID HORMONE Underactive thyroid gland	**Conditions:** menopausal hot flashes **Symptoms:** nervousness, restlessness, irritability, insomnia, palpitation, rapid pulse, bulging eyes, enlarged thyroid, diarrhea, increased hunger, infrequent or scanty periods, weight loss, muscle weakness, tremors, increased perspiration, hair loss, heat intolerance, high blood pressure
PTH Decreased PTH	**Symptoms:** low levels of calcium in the blood, muscle spasms
PTH Elevated PTH	**Symptoms:** high levels of calcium in the blood, possible calcium-containing kidney stones
PROLACTIN Elevated prolactin	**Conditions:** amenorrhea, PMS, polycystic ovary syndrome, infertility, breast cancer, osteoporosis **Symptoms:** increases cell division in breast cells causing increased breast density, can inhibit estrogen, causing amenorrhea or osteoporosis, may cause breast milk secretion in non-breastfeeding women
MELATONIN Low melatonin	**Conditions:** precocious puberty, uterine fibroids, uterine cancer, breast cancer **Symptoms:** low energy in the morning, disturbed body rhythms, insomnia, morning anxiety and agitation, increased effects of estrogen dominance

Bioidentical Hormone Replacement Therapy (BHRT) vs. Hormone Replacement Therapy (HRT)

On January 13, 1964, *Newsweek* published an article titled "No More Menopause" which reported on the work of Dr. Robert A. Wilson, a New York gynecologist who had been studying menopause since 1920. Teaming up with Ayerst Laboratories, Dr. Wilson, along with the financial backing of the pharmaceutical industry, developed the first conjugated estrogen called Premarin. Dr. Wilson subsequently published his infamous book, *Feminine Forever.* This book informed the readers as to how estrogen-only hormone replacement therapy (ERT) could prevent the "curse" of menopause, which was causing women to become shriveled up, old, and decrepit. News of this flooded the media and sales of ERT blossomed into an economic boom for the pharmaceutical industry. At the time, estrogen was very poorly researched. Synthetic estrogen gained approval in the pharmaceutical realm based on a very small and poorly conducted trial in Puerto Rico. The study was based on an insignificant number of women who took a birth control pill containing progestin and a synthetic estrogen. During the trial, three women died and 20% reported negative side effects that were actually disregarded. The evidence was clear that the "pill" caused blood clots and strokes but it was dismissed and suppressed for the supposedly higher good of controlling the population explosion and consequently, synthetic estrogen was approved as a drug.

Although ERT remained controversial over the decades, it was not until 2002, after a long-term government funded study of hormone replacement therapy called the Women's Health Initiative (WHI) was abruptly halted, that the controversy ended for most people. The study was ended three years early as the data had clearly shown that the risks of long-term HRT use clearly outweighed the benefits. The randomized, double-blind study was composed of sixteen thousand healthy menopausal women aged fifty to seventy-nine years. One group was placed on Prempro® (Premarin-equine estrogens, plus Provera-synthetic progestin). Five years into the trial, those using Prempro® had a 29% higher risk of breast cancer, a 26% higher risk of heart disease, and a 41% higher risk of stroke.[66] The National Cancer Institute released a second study on the same day that reported that women who used estrogen-only hormone replacement for longer than ten years doubled their risk for ovarian cancer.[67] In addition, a report from the Harbor-UCLA Research and Education Institute found that the cancers tended to be diagnosed at more advanced stages and resulted in substantial increases in the percentage of women with abnormal mammograms. This increased risk was not reported with the first findings. Although the breast tumors were most likely already present, they were not detected because synthetic hormones caused increased breast density. Therefore, Prempro® taken by women who had tumors in their breasts made it much more difficult to detect them. Consequently, when the

---

[66] Writing Group for the Women's Health Initiative Investigators (2002). Risks and benefits of estrogen plus progestin in healthy postmenopausal women: Principal result from the Women's Health Initiative randomized controlled trial, *JAMA, 228, 327-333*

[67] Lacey, J.V., et al. (2002) Menopausal hormone replacement therapy and risk of ovarian cancer. *JAMA, 228, 334-341.*

tumors were detected, the cancer was much more advanced.[68] Studies published in the last several years continue to provide alarming evidence against the use of HRT. In April 2007 researchers reported that breast cancer rates remained low in 2004 after a substantial decline in 2003. Powerful evidence published in the *New England Journal of Medicine* expressly linked the significant drop in breast cancer to the sharp drop in the synthetic hormones used by menopausal women. In March 2008, the *JAMA* published a study which found that women who stopped taking Prempro® still had a 24% higher risk of developing breast cancer years later.[69]

The word "bioidentical" is derived from the words "bios," meaning "life," and "identical," meaning "the same as." Therefore, "bioidentical" means "the same as life" or identical to what is in the living body, as opposed to synthetic substances such as conjugated hormones. Although bioidentical hormones are created in a lab (not extracted from humans), they have the exact same molecular structure as hormones made in the human body, making them chemically indistinguishable from one another. Bioidentical hormones generate the same physiologic responses in the body as do hormones already produced by the body because their chemical structures are identical.

In 1939, Russell E. Marker devised a method to convert sarsasapogenin, which is a sapogenin found in the sarsaparilla plant, into a progesterone-like compound. Shortly after, he devised methods to convert disogenin from the wild yam (*Dioscorea villosa)* into progesterone. It was quickly discovered that progesterone was a fat-soluble compound and when administered orally it was ineffective due to the first-pass effect of the liver. Efforts to dissolve the progesterone-like compound in vegetable oil and to administer it via injection were quickly aborted due to the difficulty of administration. Progesterone was then given as a suppository in the rectum or vagina to effectively treat conditions such as PMS and ovarian cysts and to prevent miscarriages.

Bioidentical hormones are made from botanical plants such as soy and yams. The human body cannot convert soy or yams directly into natural hormones. Because of this, the natural plants must be pharmaceutically processed to produce natural bioidentical progesterone and estrogen in the form of a transdermal cream. The body responds to the hormones as if they were the naturally produced hormones of the body rather than foreign substances being introduced which occurs with synthetic hormones. This cream may technically be yam-based but its active ingredient is not the wild yam itself but the USP (United Sates Pharmacopeia) progesterone that has been converted from the yam. The USP progesterone used for hormone replacement comes from plant fats and oils via a substance called diosgenin, which is extracted from a very specific type of wild yam that grows in Mexico or from soybeans. In the laboratory, diosgenin is chemically synthesized into real human progesterone. The other human steroid hormones, including estrogen, testosterone, progesterone, and the cortisones are also nearly always synthesized from diosgenin.

In contrast, conventional hormone replacement therapy often involves the use of non-bioidentical hormones which have been modified so that their chemical structure is not the same as endogenous human hormones (hormones the body naturally makes). These conventional hormones can also be extracted from animals which have non-human estrogens (e.g., equine from horses' urine does not occur in humans naturally). Another example is when a molecule is added to progesterone to make medroxyprogesterone acetate. This process makes this form of synthetic progesterone more bioavailable via oral routes and patentable but it also increases the risk of cancer.

Bioidentical hormone replacement therapy (BHRT) is a modification of conventional hormone replacement therapy that involves the use of supplemental doses of hormones with three important criteria:

1. BHRT has the identical chemical structure to the hormones that exist naturally in the human body.
2. BHRT is used to replenish levels to physiologically normal concentrations, never exceeding physiological levels.

---

68 Rowan T. Chlebowski, Susan L. Hendrix, Robert D. Langer, et al., for the WHI Investigators, "Influence of Estrogen Plus Progestin on Breast Cancer and Mammography in Healthy Menopausal Women, *"JAMA 289, no. 24 (2003);* C.L, Dillis and J.S. Schreiman, "Change in Mammographic Breast Density Associated with the Use of Depo-Provera," *Breast Journal, no.4 (2003): 312-15*

69 M. Ravdin, K.A. Cronin, N. Howlander, et al., "The Decrease in Breast Cancer Incidence in 2003 in the United States," *New England Journal of Medicine 356, no. 16 (2007).*

3. BHRT is administered transdermally to avoid metabolic by-products which are produced by first-pass metabolism to the liver upon oral dosing and can have negative side effects such as increased risk of blood clotting.

Many studies and media statements discuss hormones in general terms without making a distinction between bioidentical and non-bioidentical forms of hormones. For example, a clinical study involving medroxyprogesterone (a progestin), a non-bioidentical form of progesterone, may inaccurately refer to the hormone as "progesterone." Yet medroxyprogesterone and progesterone differ in their molecular structure, their derivation, and, most importantly, their effects on the body. Therefore, the results from such a study reflect only those of the particular progestin used and does not involve any other types of progestin, or progesterone itself, which might, in fact, produce different results.

In the late 1800s, laws were passed in the United States that allowed medicines to be patented only if they were not natural substances. If a drug company discovered a naturally occurring medicine, then anyone was also free to capitalize on the discovery. However, if the drug company could isolate an "active ingredient" within a naturally occurring plant medicine and chemically alter the molecular structure by even one molecule, then it could be patented into a drug which no one else could manufacture. When a drug company manufactures a synthetic hormone, they do not alter it by only one molecule. Instead they add whole chains of molecules so that it will behave similarly enough to the natural hormone, yet it is different enough to be patentable. The grave changes to the molecular structure are the very reason that there are so many side effects attached to synthetic hormone replacement therapy. Conversely, pharmaceutical companies have no interest in bioidentical hormone replacement therapy because these forms of hormones are not patentable and therefore useless from an economic standpoint.

Progesterone and Progestin

Progesterone and Progestin are often confused although they are not related. Progestin is defined as any compound able to sustain the human secretory endometrium.[70] Progesterone is the only such hormone that is made by the body and has many significant functions that are not provided by synthetic progestins. One clear example of the differences in function between progesterone and progestin is the fact that progesterone is necessary for the survival and development of the embryo and throughout gestation. Conversely, Provera, the most commonly prescribed progestin, carries the warning that its use in early pregnancy may increase the risk of early abortion or congenital deformities of the fetus. There is only one type of progesterone and it is produced via the ovaries. There are seven commonly prescribed synthetic progestins. Two of these, medroxyprogesterone acetate and megesrol acetate, are synthesized from the 21-carbon nucleus of progesterone. The other five—norgestrel, norethindrone acetate, norethynodrel, lynestrenol, and norethisterone—are from the 19-carbon nucleus of nortestosterone. The basic body of the synthetic hormones remains identical to progesterone or nortestosterone and thus the compounds will likely bind to the same receptor sites as the natural hormones. It is the alteration (e.g., acetate or ethyl groups) linked to the C-17 site that will convey a different "message" to the target cell. This undoubtedly explains the alarming array of listed warnings, contraindications, precautions, and adverse reactions attached to the synthetic progestins.

Potential side effects of medroxyprogesterone acetate (Provera) [71]

Warnings:

- Increased risk of birth defects such as heart and limb defects if taken during the first trimester of pregnancy
- Beagle dogs given this drug developed malignant mammary nodules
- Discontinue this drug if there is sudden or partial loss of vision

[70] Natural Progesterone-The multiple roles of a remarkable hormone John R. Lee MD pg. 17

[71] Natural Progesterone-The multiple roles of a remarkable hormone John R. Lee MD pg. 18

- This drug passes into breast milk; consequences unknown
- May contribute to thrombophlebitis, pulmonary embolism, and cerebral thrombosis

Contraindications:

- Thromboembolic disorders
- Cerebral apoplexy
- Liver dysfunction or disease
- Known or suspected malignancy of genital organs
- Undiagnosed vaginal bleeding
- Known sensitivity to any included ingredient

Precautions:

- May cause fluid retention, epilepsy, migraine, asthma, or cardiac or renal dysfunction
- May cause breakthrough bleeding or menstrual irregularities
- May cause or contribute to depression
- The effects of prolonged use of this drug on pituitary, ovarian, adrenal, hepatic, or uterine function is unknown
- May decrease glucose tolerance; diabetic patients must be carefully monitored
- May increase the thrombotic disorders associated with estrogens

Adverse Reactions:

- May cause breast tenderness and galactorrhea
- May cause sensitivity reactions such as urticaria, pruritus, edema, or rash
- May cause acne, alopecia, and hirsuitism
- Edema, weight changes (increase or decrease)
- Cervical erosions and changes in cervical secretions
- Cholestatic jaundice
- Mental depression, pyrexia, nausea, insomnia, or somnolence
- Anaphylactoid reactions and anaphylaxis (severe, acute allergic reactions)
- Thrombophlebitis and pulmonary embolism
- Breakthrough bleeding, spotting, amenorrhea, or changes in menses

When taken with estrogens, the following have been observed:

- Rise in blood pressure, headache, dizziness, nervousness, fatigue
- Changes in libido, hirsuitism and loss of scalp hair, decrease in T-3 uptake values
- Premenstrual-like syndrome, changes in appetite
- Cystitis-like syndrome
- Erythema multiforme, erythema nodosum, haemorrhagic eruption, itching

The Official Black Box Warning for Premarin Issued by the USDA

Important Safety Information

What is the most important information you should know about PREMARIN (estrogens), Prempro® (a combination of estrogens and a progestin), or PREMARIN Vaginal Cream (a cream of estrogens)?

- Estrogens increase the chances of getting cancer of the uterus. Report any unusual vaginal bleeding right away while you are using these products. Vaginal bleeding after menopause may be a warning sign of cancer of the uterus (womb). Your health care provider should check any unusual vaginal bleeding to find out the cause.
- Do not use estrogens with or without progestins to prevent heart disease, heart attacks, strokes or dementia.
- Using estrogens with or without progestins may increase your chances of getting heart attacks, strokes, breast cancer and blood clots. Using estrogens, with or without progestins, may increase your risk of dementia, based on a study of women 65 years or older. You and your health care provider should talk regularly about whether you still need treatment with estrogens.

Hormonal Conditions

Anxiety

The most common psychiatric disorders in North America re anxiety disorders. Sixty-five percent of North Americans take prescription medications daily; 43% take mood altering prescriptions regularly. Paxil and Zoloft (two of the more popular anti-anxiety medications) ranked seventh and eighth in the top ten prescribed medications in North America. These two medications totaled almost $5 billion in sales in 2002.[72] While anxiety is a symptom that everyone experiences at some point in his or her life, in some individuals it can be more than just occasional nervousness or stress. People with anxiety disorders often have symptoms that go beyond a simple response to stressful situations. The manifestations of an anxiety disorder are extremely debilitating and can prevent the individual from engaging in a fully functional life. The consequences of anxiety encompass all areas of life, including emotional, occupational, and social.

Common anxiety symptoms include:[73]

- Back pain, stiffness, tension, pressure, soreness, spasms, immobility in the back or back muscles
- Blushing, turning red, flushed face
- Body jolts, body zaps, electric jolt feeling in body, intense body tremor or "body shake"
- Burning skin, itchy, "crawly," prickly or other skin sensations, skin sensitivity, numbness of the skin
- Chest pain, chest tightness
- Chronic fatigue, exhaustion, worn out feeling
- Clumsiness, coordination problems with the limbs or body
- Chills, feeling cold
- Craving sugar
- Difficulty speaking
- Dizziness, feeling lightheaded
- Heart palpitations, racing heart
- Hyperactivity, excess energy, nervous energy
- Increased or decreased sex drive
- Mouth or throat clicking or grating sound when you move your mouth or jaw, such as when talking
- Muscle twitching
- Nausea and/or vomiting

---

[72] http://www.anxietycentre.com/anxiety-statistics-information.shtml

[73] http://www.anxietycentre.com/anxiety-symptoms.shtml

- Night sweats
- Startle easily
- Trembling, shaking
- Urgency to urinate, frequent urination
- Weight loss, weight gain
- Find it hard to breathe, feeling smothered, shortness of breath
- Fears (anxiety symptoms commonly associated with fear)
- Heightened self-awareness, or self-consciousness
- Frequent headaches, migraine headaches
- Ringing in the ears
- Difficulty concentrating, short-term memory loss
- Nightmares
- Repetitive thinking or incessant 'mind chatter'
- Short-term learning impairment, have a hard time learning new information
- "Stuck" thoughts, mental images, concepts, songs, or melodies that "stick" in your mind and replay over and over again.
- Depression
- Dramatic mood swings
- Aerophagia (swallowing too much air, stomach distention, belching)
- Difficulty swallowing
- Irritable bowel syndrome (IBS)
- Difficulty falling or staying asleep

In addition to these anxiety symptoms, you may also find yourself worrying compulsively about:

- Having a heart attack
- Having a serious undetected illness
- Dying prematurely
- Going insane or losing your mind
- Suddenly snapping
- Uncontrollably harming yourself or someone you love
- Losing control of your thoughts and actions
- Being embarrassed or making a fool out of yourself
- Fainting in public
- Choking or suffocating
- Being alone

There are several recognized types of anxiety disorders including:

1. **Generalized anxiety disorder (GAD):** This disorder involves excessive, unrealistic worry and tension, even if there is little or nothing to provoke the anxiety. Individuals with GAD have great difficulty trying to control their worries and may have symptoms similar to those of depression.
2. **Panic disorder:** People with this condition have feelings of terror that strike suddenly and repeatedly with no warning. Other symptoms of a panic disorder include sweating, chest pain, palpitations (irregular heartbeats) and a feeling of choking which may make the person feel like he or she is having a heart attack or "going crazy." These symptoms may occur with or without agoraphobia (morbid fear of having a panic attack or panic-like symptoms in a situation that is perceived to be difficult from which to escape).

3. **Obsessive-compulsive disorder (OCD):** Characterized by persistent mental images, thoughts, or ideas with compulsive, repetitive behaviours that are rigid and ritualistic.
4. **Post-traumatic stress disorder (PTSD):** A re-experiencing or flashbacks of symptoms, avoidance and hyper-arousal after exposure to a traumatic event.
5. **Social anxiety disorder:** Also called social phobia, social anxiety disorder involves overwhelming worry and self-consciousness about everyday social situations. The worry often centers on a fear of being judged by others or behaving in a way that might cause embarrassment or lead to ridicule.
6. **Specific phobias:** A specific phobia is an intense fear of a specific object or situation such as snakes, heights, or flying. The level of fear usually is inappropriate to the situation and may cause the person to avoid common, everyday situations.

There are a variety of underlying medical conditions, lifestyles, medications and toxins that can cause anxiety disorders. Some of the main medical conditions are listed below:[74]

Medical Conditions That Can Cause Anxiety

System Involved	Conditions
Cardiovascular	Arrhythmia Congestive heart failure Coronary artery disease Pulmonary embolism
Endocrine/Hormonal	Cushing's syndrome Hyper/hypothyroidism Hypoglycaemia Hormonal Imbalances
Metabolic	Porphyria Vitamin B-12 deficiency B-Vitamin deficiency Amino Acid deficiency Mineral deficiency Essential fatty acid deficiency Cerebral allergies (Foods and food substances) Elevated blood lactate levels
Neurological	Neurotransmitter imbalances Encephalitis Neoplasms Temporal lobe epilepsy
Pulmonary	Asthma COPD Pneumonia

[74] Uphold CR, Graham MV. Anxiety Disorders. Clinical Guidelines in Family Practice. 3rd ed. Gainesville, Fl: Barmarrae Books, 1989:106-13.

Substances That Can Cause Anxiety Symptoms

Category of Substances	Various Types
Medications	Anaesthetics Analgesics Stimulants Anticholinergic Insulin Thyroid preparations Antihistamines Corticosteroids Anti-hypertensive Anti-consultants Anti-psychotics Antidepressants
Dietary Substances	Alcohol Caffeine
Illicit Substances	Cannabis Cocaine Hallucinogens Inhalants
Accidental/Purposeful Exposure to Volatile Substances	Gasoline Paint Insecticides Carbon monoxide
Withdrawal from Substances	Alcohol Cocaine Sedatives Hypnotics Anxiolytics

The underlying causes of anxiety disorders are vast and often numerous. In order to identify the medical diagnosis of an anxiety disorder, the following DASS (Depression, Anxiety and Stress Scale) questionnaire can be used to differentiate between depression, anxiety, and stress so that the appropriate healing protocol can be prescribed. The Depression, Anxiety, and Stress Scale (DASS) was developed by researchers at the University of New South Wales (Australia).[75]

[75] University of New South Wales Depression Anxiety Stress Scales http://www2.psy.unsw.edu.au/groups/dass/

DASS

Name: *Date:*

Please read each statement and circle a number 0, 1, 2 or 3 which indicates how much the statement applied to you *over the past week*. There are no right or wrong answers. Do not spend too much time on any statement.

The rating scale is as follows:

0 Did not apply to me at all
1 Applied to me to some degree, or some of the time
2 Applied to me to a considerable degree, or a good part of time
3 Applied to me very much, or most of the time

1	I found myself getting upset by quite trivial things	0	1	2	3
2	I was aware of dryness of my mouth	0	1	2	3
3	I couldn't seem to experience any positive feeling at all	0	1	2	3
4	I experienced breathing difficulty (eg, excessively rapid breathing, breathlessness in the absence of physical exertion)	0	1	2	3
5	I just couldn't seem to get going	0	1	2	3
6	I tended to over-react to situations	0	1	2	3
7	I had a feeling of shakiness (eg, legs going to give way)	0	1	2	3
8	I found it difficult to relax	0	1	2	3
9	I found myself in situations that made me so anxious I was most relieved when they ended	0	1	2	3
10	I felt that I had nothing to look forward to	0	1	2	3
11	I found myself getting upset rather easily	0	1	2	3
12	I felt that I was using a lot of nervous energy	0	1	2	3
13	I felt sad and depressed	0	1	2	3
14	I found myself getting impatient when I was delayed in any way (eg, lifts, traffic lights, being kept waiting)	0	1	2	3
15	I had a feeling of faintness	0	1	2	3
16	I felt that I had lost interest in just about everything	0	1	2	3
17	I felt I wasn't worth much as a person	0	1	2	3
18	I felt that I was rather touchy	0	1	2	3
19	I perspired noticeably (eg, hands sweaty) in the absence of high temperatures or physical exertion	0	1	2	3
20	I felt scared without any good reason	0	1	2	3
21	I felt that life wasn't worthwhile	0	1	2	3

Reminder of rating scale:

0 Did not apply to me at all
1 Applied to me to some degree, or some of the time
2 Applied to me to a considerable degree, or a good part of time
3 Applied to me very much, or most of the time

22	I found it hard to wind down	0	1	2	3
23	I had difficulty in swallowing	0	1	2	3
24	I couldn't seem to get any enjoyment out of the things I did	0	1	2	3
25	I was aware of the action of my heart in the absence of physical exertion (eg, sense of heart rate increase, heart missing a beat)	0	1	2	3
26	I felt down-hearted and blue	0	1	2	3
27	I found that I was very irritable	0	1	2	3
28	I felt I was close to panic	0	1	2	3
29	I found it hard to calm down after something upset me	0	1	2	3
30	I feared that I would be "thrown" by some trivial but unfamiliar task	0	1	2	3
31	I was unable to become enthusiastic about anything	0	1	2	3
32	I found it difficult to tolerate interruptions to what I was doing	0	1	2	3
33	I was in a state of nervous tension	0	1	2	3
34	I felt I was pretty worthless	0	1	2	3
35	I was intolerant of anything that kept me from getting on with what I was doing	0	1	2	3
36	I felt terrified	0	1	2	3
37	I could see nothing in the future to be hopeful about	0	1	2	3
38	I felt that life was meaningless	0	1	2	3
39	I found myself getting agitated	0	1	2	3
40	I was worried about situations in which I might panic and make a fool of myself	0	1	2	3
41	I experienced trembling (eg, in the hands)	0	1	2	3
42	I found it difficult to work up the initiative to do things	0	1	2	3

DASS 42 SCORE SHEET

Enter each score from the questionnaire into the first two columns.
Add up each row and enter the score into the available box (D, A or S)
Add up the each of the D, A and S columns.
The total for each column is the score for that trait:

D = Depression
A = Anxiety
S = Stress

Use the ratings table below to assess the meaning of each score.

Score Calculation:

Q	Score	Q	Score	All D scores	All A scores	All S scores
1		22				
2		23				
3		24				
4		25				
5		26				
6		27				
7		28				
8		29				
9		30				
10		31				
11		32				
12		33				
13		34				
14		35				
15		36				
16		37				
17		38				
18		39				
19		40				
20		41				
21		42				
				Total for D	Total for A	Total for S

Score Interpretation:

	Depression (D)	Anxiety (A)	Stress (S)
Normal	0 – 9	0 – 7	0 – 14
Mild	10 – 13	8 – 9	15 – 18
Moderate	14 – 20	10 – 14	19 – 25
Severe	21 – 27	15 – 19	26 – 33
Extremely Severe	28+	20+	34 +

In order to further evaluate the underlying causes of anxiety, specific laboratory testing can be implemented. **The following are common lab tests to determine the underlying causes of anxiety:**

Specific Lab Test	Description
ELISA/EIA Food Allergy Testing	This is based on the findings that certain subclasses of IgG have been associated with the *in vitro* degranulation of basophils and mast cells, the activation of the complement cascade (both of which are important mechanisms in allergy and anaphylaxis), and the observation that high circulating serum concentrations of some IgG subtypes have been measured in certain atopic individuals. The premise behind this testing is that high circulating levels of IgG antibodies are correlate with clinical food allergy signs and symptoms. The ELISA/EIA test itself involves coating a ninety-six-well plate with food antigens, adding a patient's sera, and looking for a classic antigen/antibody interaction.
Micronutrient Testing for Nutritional Deficiencies	The micronutrient tests measure how micronutrients are actually functioning within the white blood cells. Micronutrient's patented testing chemically-defined control media contains the minimal amount of each essential micro-nutrient that is needed to support optimal lymphocyte growth or mitogenic response. The functional intracellular status of micronutrients involved in cell metabolism is evaluated by manipulation of the individual micronutrients in the media followed by mitogenic stimulation and measurement of DNA synthesis.
Neurotransmitter Testing	Medical science has discovered that neurotransmitters are at the foundation of many psychiatric and neurological disorders. Imbalances in neurotransmission, due to excessive or deficient neurotransmitter levels at the synaptic cleft, are associated with depression, insomnia, anxiety, behavioural disorders, memory disorders, and a spectrum of other brain-related functions. Because neurotransmitters play an integral role in these disease states, they are prime targets for treating disorders of the nervous system and mental health concerns. Neurotransmitters are recognized as the primary bio-chemical messengers of the central and peripheral nervous systems. Studies have demonstrated that urinary neuro-transmitter measures are reflective of circulating levels, as evidenced by renal neurotransmitter clearance mechanisms. Laboratory methodology for the accurate assessment of urinary neurotransmitter levels has been established. Urinary measures are not recognized as a direct reflection of central activity, however,

	definite associations exist. The ability to measure neurotransmitters has led to the generation of scientific literature that demonstrates that urinary neurotransmitter measurements have clinical value as representative biomarkers of various neurological, immunological, and endocrinological conditions.
Adrenal Stress Index	The panel utilizes four saliva samples. Salivary cortisol measurement reflects the free (bioactive) fraction of serum cortisol. The test report shows the awake diurnal cortisol rhythm generated in response to real-life stress. The cortisol/DHEA relationship highlights the many facets of stress maladaptation. The cortisol/DHEA ratio helps determine the projected time for recovery and the substances (hormones, supplements, and botanicals) that promote this recovery. The cortisol/DHEA ratio regulates a multitude of functions. The panel measures P17-OH levels in order to evaluate the efficiency of the conversion of adrenal precursors into cortisol. Certain adrenal fatigue patients who are genetically predisposed to low production of cortisol will not benefit from exogenous supplementation of pregnenolone or progesterone. The panel includes fasting and non-fasting insulin measurements. The insulin values are used to diagnose insulin resistance-functional insulin deficit (pre-diabetes), as well as to correlate elevated cortisol with insulin to help explain glycemic dysregulation problems.
Complete Female Hormone Panel	Estradiol and progesterone levels and their ratio are an index of estrogen/progesterone balance. An excess of estradiol, relative to progesterone, can explain many symptoms in reproductive age-women. Testosterone levels can also be either too high or too low. Testosterone in excess, often caused by ovarian cysts, leads to conditions such as excessive facial and body hair, acne, and oily skin and hair. Polycystic ovarian syndrome (PCOS) is thought to be caused, in part, by insulin resistance. On the other hand, too little testosterone is often caused by excessive stress, medications, contraceptives, and surgical removal of the ovaries. This leads to symptoms of androgen deficiency including loss of libido, thinning skin, vaginal dryness, loss of bone and muscle mass, depression, and memory lapses. SHBG binds tightly to circulating estradiol and testosterone, preventing their rapid metabolism and clearance and limiting their bioavailability to tissues. SHBG gives a good index of the extent of the body's overall exposure to estrogens.

Thyroid Hormone Testing	A complete thyroid profile includes free T4, free T3, TSH, and TPO and can indicate the presence of an imbalance in thyroid function. Hypothyroidism includes feeling cold all the time, low stamina, fatigue (particularly in the evening), anxiety, depression, low sex drive, weight gain, and high cholesterol. Hyperthyroidism includes heat intolerance, anxiety, palpitations, weight loss, tired but wired visual disturbances, and insomnia.

Conventional Medicine Therapies Commonly Prescribed for Anxiety Disorders

Benzodiazepines

The most commonly prescribed pharmacologic therapy for anxiety is benzodiazepines. Benzodiazepines bind to a macromolecular complex that is found within the central nervous system. This complex is called the Gamma-aminobutyric acid (GABA)-benzodiazepine receptor-chloride ion channel complex. [76]

The somatic symptoms and hypervigilence, which are part of anxiety, are lowered by benzodiazepines. Benzodiazepines are usually prescribed on an as-needed basis due to their short half-life. This short half-life also causes them to be rapidly absorbed and therefore often abused.

Commonly Prescribed Benzodiazepines[77]

Name	Half-Life (hours)	Dosage Range (per day)	Initial Dosage (per day)
Alprazolam (Xanax)	14	1-4mg	0.25-0.5mg 4 times per day (Q.I.D.)
Chlordiazepoxide (Librium)	20	15-40mg	5-10mg 3 times per day (T.I.D.)
Clonazepam (Klonopin)	50	0.5-4.0mg	0.5-1.0mg 2 times per day (B.I. D.)
Chlorazepate (Tranxene)	60	15-60mg	7.5-15mg B.I. D.
Diazepam (Valium)	40	6-40mg	2-5mg T.I.D.
Lorazepam (Ativan)	14	1-6mg	0.5-1.0mg T.I.D.
Oxazepam (Serax)	9	30-90mg	15-30mg T.I.D.

[76] Trevor AJ, Way WL. Sedative-hypnotic drugs. In Katzung BG (Ed). Basic and Clinical Pharmacology, ^the d. Norwalk. CT:Appleton and Lange, 1995; 338-39

[77] Gliatto MF. Generalized Anxiety Disorder. AM Fam Physician 2000; 62:1591-1600, 1602

Side Effects of Benzodiazepines

Chronic use of Benzodiazepines can results in dependence. The dependence is measured by the effects of withdrawal when discontinued. Withdrawal symptoms can include anxiety, irritability, and insomnia for up to seventy-two hours. Following withdrawal, the patient often returns to his or her recurrent anxiety state.[78]

Selective Serotonin Reuptake Inhibitors (SSRIs) and Tricyclic Antidepressants (TCAs)

SSRIs are believed to increase the extracellular level of the neurotransmitter serotonin by inhibiting its reuptake into the presynaptic cell, increasing the level of serotonin in the synaptic cleft available to bind to the postsynaptic receptor. They have varying degrees of selectivity for the other monoamine transporters, with pure SSRIs having only a weak affinity for the noradrenaline and dopamine transporter.[79]

The majority of the TCAs act primarily as serotonin-norepinephrine reuptake inhibitors (SNRIs) by blocking the serotonin transporter (SERT) and the norepinephrine transporter (NET), which results in an elevation of the extracellular concentrations of these neurotransmitters, and therefore an enhancement of neurotransmission. Notably, the TCAs have negligible affinity for the dopamine transporter (DAT), and therefore have no efficacy as dopamine reuptake inhibitors (DRIs).[80]

Commonly Prescribed SSRIs and TCAs for Anxiety Disorders[81]

SSRIs and Newer Agents

Name	Usual Starting Dose	Typical Therapeutic Dose	SSRI Side Effects
Fluoxetine (Prozac)	10mg daily in the a.m.	20-80mg per day	Somnolence, agitation, sweating, nausea, anorexia, and sexual dysfunction
Paroxetine (Paxil)	10mg daily	20-50mg per day	(As above)
Sertraline (Zoloft)	25mg daily	50-200mg per day	(As above)
Fluvoxamine (Luvox)	25mg at bedtime	50-300mg per day	(As above)
Nefazodone (Serzone)	50mg daily	150-300mg per day	(As above)
Venlafaxine (Effexor)	18.75-25mg daily	75-150mg per day	(As above)

78 Schatzberg AF, Cole JO, DeBattista C. Manual of Clinical Physcopharmacology. Third ed. Washington, DC; American Psychiatric Press, Inc., 1997

79 http://en.wikipedia.org/wiki/Selective_serotonin_reuptake_inhibitor

80 Tatsumi M, Groshan K, Blakely RD, Richelson E. (1997). "Pharmacological profile of antidepressants and related compounds at human monoamine transporters." Eur J Pharmacol. 340 (2-3): 249–258. doi: 10.1016/S0014-2999(97)01393-9. PMID 9537821.

81 Uphold CR, Graham MV. Anxiety Disorders. Clinical Guidelines in Family Practice. 3rd ed. Gainesville, Fl: Barmarrae Books, 1989:112

TCAs

Name	Usual Starting Dose	Typical Therapeutic Dose	TCA Side Effects
Imipramine (Tofranil)	10mg at bedtime	100-200mg per day	Anticholinergic; dry mouth, constipation, blurred vision, orthostatic hypotension, weight gain, and somnolence
Desipramine (Norpramin)	10mg at bedtime	100-200mg per day	(As above)
Amitriptyline (Elavil)	10mg at bedtime	100-200mg per day	(As above)
Nortriptyline (Pamelor)	10mg at bedtime	50-100mg per day	(As above)

Nutritional Factors Affecting Anxiety

Clinical anxiety, including panic attacks, can be produced by caffeine, certain other drugs, and the infusion of lactate into the blood. The most significant dietary factors affecting anxiety are elevated blood lactic acid levels and an increased lactic acid to pyruvic acid ratio. Lactate (the soluble form of lactic acid) is the final breakdown product of blood sugar (glucose) when there is a lack of oxygen. This occurs, for example when a person exercises so vigorously that he or she cannot catch his or her breath. Lactic acid is changed into lactate and transported to the liver where it is converted into harmless pyruvic acid. People who tend to suffer panic attacks and anxiety are unable to convert lactate into pyruvic acid and so have elevated blood levels of lactate. If people who get panic attacks are injected with lactate, severe panic attacks are produced. In normal individuals, nothing happens.[82] Reducing the level of lactate is a critical goal in the treatment of anxiety disorders.

Nutrition plays a pivotal role in reducing lactate levels and preventing the conversion of lactic acid back to pyruvic acid. There are six main nutritional factors that may be responsible for elevated lactate levels or lactic acid to pyruvic acid ration:[83]

1. Alcohol
2. Caffeine
3. Sugar
4. Deficiency of the B-vitamins niacin, pyridoxine, and thiamine
5. Deficiency of calcium or magnesium
6. Food allergens

Simple avoidance of alcohol, caffeine, and refined sugar can make remarkable improvements to anxiety disorders. A small study was conducted on the effects of abstaining from caffeine on anxiety symptoms. Four males and two females who had been diagnosed with generalized anxiety disorder or panic attacks decreased their intake of caffeine consumption from an average of one and a half to three and a half cups of coffee per day to none. After one week, there was significant reduction in anxiety symptoms. Follow-up exams six to eighteen months later indicated that five out of the six patients were completely without symptoms and the sixth patient required a very small dose of Valium.[84] Patients with anxiety disorders appear to be more susceptible than healthy individuals to the

[82] Encyclopedia of Natural Medicine Revised 2nd ed. Michael Murray MD Joseph Pizzorno ND pg. 254

[83] M.Werbach, Nutritional Influences on Mental Illness: A Sourcebook of Clinical Research (Tarzana, CA: Third Line Press, 1991)

[84] M. Bruce and M. Lader, Caffeine Abstention in the Management of Anxiety Disorders, Psychol Med 19 (1989):211-4.

anxiety-inducing effects of caffeine. This increased sensitivity may be due in part to slower caffeine metabolism, a higher peak caffeine concentration following caffeine ingestion, or exaggerated response to caffeine.[85]

Food Allergens

Disturbances in brain function can also involve masked or delayed cerebral allergic responses to foods or beverages. These reactions to foods can occur hours or even several days after the ingestion of allergenic foods.[86] The foods most commonly associated with allergies are as follows:

- Dairy products
- Wheat
- Eggs
- Corn
- Chocolate
- Tea
- Coffee
- Sugar
- Yeast
- Soy
- Citrus fruits
- Pork
- Rye
- Beef
- Tomato
- Peanuts
- Barley
- Nuts
- Seafood

Hypoglycemia and Anxiety

Hypoglycemia results when an excessive fall in the blood glucose level leads to a compensatory response by the sympathetic nervous system which includes the release of epinephrine and nor-epinephrine. This type of a response will enable the glucose levels to restore toward normal levels. It will also induce a "fight or flight" response which can result in anxiety, palpitations, sweating, hunger, and irritability. Patients with anxiety caused by reactive hypoglycemia may experience a worsening of symptoms in the late morning or late afternoon (before mealtime) and a significant improvement after eating. This type of patient tends to crave sweets and may note that consumption of refined sugar relieves their symptoms temporarily but will often be followed by an exacerbation of symptoms. In order to stabilize blood sugar levels, certain dietary recommendations should be taken under counsel. A nutritional regime that involves consuming six smaller meals per day rather than the standard three meals per day has been shown to dramatically decrease hypoglycemic tendencies. The hypoglycemic patient's diet should be one that is high in protein and fats and low in carbohydrates. Protein in moderately high amounts will decrease the release of insulin from the pancreas. If the protein-to-carbohydrate ratio is 0.75 or greater, the insulin release from the pancreas will

[85] Levy M Zulber-Katz E. Caffeine metabolism and coffee-attributed sleep disturbances. Clin Pharmacol Ther 1983;33:770-775

[86] Gaby AR. The role of hidden food allergy/intolerance in chronic disease. Altern Med Rev 1998; 90-100.

be slowed down and the subsequent decline in blood glucose following meals will not be as rapid.[87] Macronutrient percentages kept at levels of 40% carbohydrates, 30% protein, and 30% fat have been found to balance blood sugar levels substantially.

Herbal Medicine Indicated for Anxiety Disorders

Passion Flower *(Passiflora incarnata)*

The alkaloids, namely Harman and Harmaline, are responsible for the sedative and muscle relaxant properties of passion flower. Passion flower has been used traditionally in the Americas and later in Europe as a "calming" herb for anxiety, insomnia, seizures, and hysteria. It is believed that passion flower works by increasing the levels of GABA in the brain. GABA lowers the activity of some brain cells, resulting in noticeable relaxation.

Valerian *(Valeriana officinalis)*

The volatile oils, mainly valerianic acid, give valerian its well-known sedative and anti-spasmodic properties. Germany's Commission E approved valerian as an effective mild sedative and the United States Food and Drug Administration listed valerian as "Generally Recognized as Safe" (GRAS). Scientists aren't sure how valerian works, but they believe it increases the amount of GABA in the brain. GABA helps regulate nerve cells and has a calming effect on anxiety.

Kava kava *(Piper methysticum)*

Kava lactones, including kavain, dihydrokavain, methysticum, and dihydromethysticum, have been found to produce effective anxiolytic effects. Germany's Commission E has approved kava for the treatment of conditions of nervous anxiety, stress, and restlessness. In a review of seven scientific studies, researchers concluded that a standardized kava extract was significantly more effective than placebo in treating anxiety. Another study found that kava substantially improved symptoms after only one week of treatment. Another study found that kava may be as effective as some prescription anti-anxiety medications. In fact, according to one study, kava and diazepam (Valium) cause similar changes in brain wave activity, suggesting that they may work in the same ways to calm the mind.[88]

Lemon Balm *(Melissa officinalis)*

Volatile oils, including citral, citronellal, citronellol, geraniol, and caryophyllene, give lemon balm its anti-spasmodic and calming effects on the central nervous system. In a double-blind, placebo-controlled study, eighteen healthy volunteers received two separate single doses of a standardized lemon balm extract (300 mg and 600 mg) or placebo for seven days. The 600 mg dose of lemon balm increased mood and significantly increased calmness and alertness.[89]

Skullcap *(Scutellaria leteriflora)*

It is the flavonoid glycosides and the volatile oils that are responsible for skullcap's calming properties. Skullcap has been used for more than two hundred years as a mild relaxant and as a therapy for anxiety, nervous tension, and convulsions.

---

[87] Westphal SA, Gannon MC, Nuttall FQ. Metabolic response to glucose ingested with various amounts of protein. Am J Clin Nutr 1991;52:267-72

[88] http://www.umm.edu/altmed/articles/kava-kava-000259.htm

[89] http://www.umm.edu/altmed/articles/lemon-balm-000261.htm

Specific Nutrients in the Treatment of Anxiety

5-HTP (5-hydroxytryptophan):

Five-HTP, extracted from the seeds of the African plant *Griffonia simplicifolia,* is the intermediate metabolite of the amino acid L-tryptophan in the serotonin pathway. After tryptophan is converted into 5-HTP, the chemical is then converted into another chemical called serotonin (a neurotransmitter that relays signals between brain cells). Five-HTP acts primarily by increasing levels of serotonin within the central nervous system. Five-HTP dietary supplements help raise serotonin levels in the brain. Since serotonin helps regulate mood and behaviour, 5-HTP may have a positive effect on sleep, mood, anxiety, appetite, and pain sensation. Other neurotransmitters and CNS chemicals such as melatonin, dopamine, norepinephrine, and beta endorphin have also been shown to increase following oral administration of 5-HTP. Dosage: 100-600mg per day

Relora

Relora is a proprietary blend of the plant extracts from *Magnolia officinalis* and *Phellodendron amurense*. Relora has been found to bind to GABA receptor sites, resulting in the immediate relief of anxiety and providing a sense of relaxation. In addition, as relora binds to GABA sites, the signalling from the brain to produce the stress hormone cortisol is ceased, resulting in a calming, non-sedative effect. In central nervous system receptor binding assays, the plant extracts in relora bind to several important targets associated with anxiety. They do not bind to the benzodiazepine receptors that would cause sedation, yet they have the relaxing qualities of the benzodiazepine class of drugs in a validated anxiolytic animal model. In addition, relora normalizes hormone levels associated with stress-induced obesity and eating/drinking behaviour. Dosage: 500-1000mg per day

Gamma-aminobutyric acid (GABA)

GABA is a major neurotransmitter widely distributed throughout the central nervous system. Due to the fact that too much excitation can lead to irritability, restlessness, insomnia, seizures, and movement disorders, it must be balanced with inhibition. GABA is the most important inhibitory neurotransmitter in the brain, acting like a "brake" during times of runaway stress. Medications for anxiety, such as benzodiazepines, stimulate GABA receptors and induce relaxation. Either low GABA levels or decreased GABA function in the brain is associated with several psychiatric and neurological disorders including anxiety, depression, insomnia, and epilepsy. Studies indicate that GABA can improve relaxation and enhance sleep. Clinical studies have shown that natural GABA is produced via a fermentation process that utilizes Lactobacillus hilgardii, which is the bacteria used to ferment vegetables in the preparation of the traditional Korean dish known as kimchi. GABA increases the production of brain alpha-waves, decreases stress-related beta-waves, and creates a profound sense of physical relaxation while maintaining mental focus. In addition to changes in brain waves, GABA has been shown to produce relaxation as evidenced by reduced pupil diameter, heart rate, and markers of stress, namely salivary cortisol and chromogranin A. Dosage: 100-600mg per day

Flaxseed Oil

Patients who suffer from panic attacks and anxiety have been shown to be deficient in alpha-linolenic acid, which is the essential fatty acid found in high concentrations in flaxseed oil. In one study, three out of four patients with a history of agoraphobia over ten or more years improved within two or three months after taking two to six tablespoons daily in divided doses depending upon their response.[90]

Inositol

Inositol, sometimes referred to as vitamin B8, is a water-soluble fatty lipid that is required by the body for the formation of healthy cells. Inositol has been shown to be effective in treating some cases of depression, anxiety,

[90] D.O. Rudin, The Major Psychoses and Neuroses as Omega-3 Essential Fatty Acid Deficiency Syndrome: Substrate Pellagra, Biol Psychiatry 16 (1981): 837-50

OCD, and other psychological disorders that respond to serotonin uptake inhibitors. Inositol is a "second messenger," triggering the release of calcium in cells. It is also involved in the transmission of messages between neural cells and the transport of fats within cells. Its most important role seems to be in the central nervous system, where it serves to help transmit messages along neural pathways. Various studies have shown its efficacy in treating a number of psychological disorders that have a chemical basis, including bulimia, OCD, depression, and bipolar mood disorder. Inositol is present in greater concentration in the cells in and around the central nervous system, including brain cells and retinal cells, and in other specialized cells such as bone marrow and intestinal cells. Dosage: Large doses (12-18g per day) are used in the treatment of anxiety and psychiatric disorders.

Vitamin B3 (Niacinamide)

Niacinamide is involved in over two hundred enzymatic reactions in the body. The mechanisms of action of niacinamide are multifactorial and include the correction of subclinical pellagra, correction of an underlying vitamin B3-dependency disorder, benzodiazepine-like effects, the ability to increase the production of serotonin, and the ability to modify the metabolism of lactic acid.[91] Both benzodiazepines and niacinamide exert similar anxiolytic effects through the modulation of neurotransmitters commonly unbalanced in anxiety. Optimal doses of niacinamide increase the production of serotonin by diverting more tryptophan to become a substrate for serotonin synthesis.[92] Dosage: 500-3000mg per day in divided doses

Vitamin B1 (Thiamine)

Thiamine's effectiveness in the reduction of anxiety symptoms comes from its ability to reduce the production of lactate in the body. Thiamine's anxiolytic functions result from its coenzyme function in the pyruvate dehydrogenase enzyme resulting in a reduction in blood lactate and less anxiety symptoms due to an increased conversion of pyruvate to acetyl-CoA.[93] Dosage: 100mg-1800mg have been observed in the treatment of anxiety

Vitamin B6 (Pyrodoxine)

Pyrodoxine has three critical roles in the treatment of anxiety, the first being its role in the conversion pathways of tryptophan to serotonin. Secondly, pyrodoxine is involved in the production of GABA. Pyrodoxine is a coenzyme for glutamic acid decarboxylase, which facilitates the conversion of glutamic acid to GABA. Finally, pyrodoxine is partly responsible for a reduction in the formation of blood lactate. Dosage: 200mg-600mg per day. Doses higher than 200mg per day should be monitored for the development of neurotoxicity.

Magnesium

Magnesium deficiency can cause both anxiety and decreased stress tolerance. In addition, various types of physical and mental stress can lead to magnesium depletion and an increased requirement for magnesium. Thus, a vicious cycle can occur in which anxiety and stress leads to a magnesium depletion which further exacerbates anxiety and stress. It is also indicated that magnesium depletion is associated with an increased lactate-pyruvate ratio. Dosage: 5mg per kg of body weight

Adjunctive Therapies

Breathing Therapy

Breathing is not a function that is detached from your emotional and mental states but rather just the opposite because the way in which you breathe reflects your state. When asleep, breathing patterns become deep, slow, and

---

[91] Anxiety Orthomolecular Diagnosis and Treatment Dr. Jonathan Prousky BPHE, BSc, ND, FRSH pg. 47

[92] Velling DA, Dodick DW, Muir JJ. Sustained release niacin for prevention of migraine headaches. Mayo clin Proc 2003;78:770-771

[93] Buist RA. Anxiety neurosis The Lactate connection. Int Clin Nutr Rev 1985; 5:1-4

forceful. When under strain, breathing patterns become shallow and rapid. During anger, breathing can be quite irregular. Alternatively, a state of relaxation produces slow breathing as well as rhythmic and quiet breathing patterns.

By having knowledge of breathing exercises, you can control panic or distress. You can also steady yourself and reduce tension, resulting in lowered blood pressure and cholesterol levels. Breathing techniques can be "First Aid" in preventing stress and tension from injuring your body. Regular breathing exercises, especially done early in the morning when the air is fresh, will clear the mind and invigorate the body.

First Aid Breathing

"First Aid" breathing exercises can be used in times of acute stress. The simplest breathing exercise is an exercise to bring calm. Sit comfortably in a chair and allow the shoulders to drop. Move outward to widen the chest. Allow the head to float upward from the shoulders as if it were being lifted from above. Look straight ahead as if gazing at a place on the wall. Practice this initial letting go. Once able to do this easily, the lungs will be free to fill from top to bottom. Next, take a few deep, slow, but gentle breaths. Breathe in freely to the count of three and out again also to the count of three. Let the chest expand and deflate. Try not to exaggerate the movements. This is a way of controlling the stress response, quieting the nervous system, and allowing for balance to be restored.

Breathing Exercises to Aid in Sleep

Breathing exercises can be helpful for those whose minds will not switch off from the events of the day. With the eyes closed, breathe deeply and gently, letting the stomach expand and contract while deepening the breathing. Visualize the breath as exhaling, moving up from the diaphragm through the lungs and out of the mouth. In the mind's eye, watch the air; follow an arc like a rainbow from the mouth back to the abdomen and through an imaginary hole and back to the diaphragm. Then start again with a slow rhythm, breathing and seeing the breath flow through the lungs and over the chest to the mouth, counting to four, then blow it back to the diaphragm while again counting to four. Keep visualizing the circle of air as it moves through the body and around to the diaphragm. Keep the mind fully involved with this process and sleep will gently enfold you.

Breathing Exercises to Reduce Tension

Begin by standing up, stretching the arms above the head and then letting them fall loosely to the sides of the body. Straighten the back, hold in the stomach, and tuck the gluteal muscles under. Allow your head to rise and shoulders to drop. This will encourage blood flow. Take a slow breath in and count to four. Hold it in for four counts and then breathe, again counting to four. This should allow the shoulders to drop further. Next, make a circle with the head: let it drop onto the chest, roll the head over the left shoulder, let it drop behind and roll over the right shoulder, and back onto the chest. Roll the head three times to the left, then three times to the right, breathing easily the whole time. Finally, lift the head and take a deep, steady breath.

EMDR (Eye Movement Desensitization and Reprocessing)

EMDR is an integrative psychotherapy approach that has been extensively researched and proven effective for the treatment of trauma. EMDR is a set of standardized protocols that incorporates elements from many different treatment approaches. To date, EMDR has helped an estimated two million people of all ages relieve many types of psychological stress.

Until recently, psychologists thought that trauma permanently altered brain chemistry. It is now believed that eye movement somehow liberates the natural healing process to reverse such effects. It seems that eye movement stimulates the neurochemical communication between the two hemispheres of the brain, which results in the trauma no longer containing the negative emotional charge that was originally associated with it.

Researchers at the Human Resource Institute's Trauma Center (Brookline, MA) have been using SPECT brain-scan imaging to map changes that occur from EMDR treatments. They found that traumatic material appears to be held in the right parietal region, which is concerned with body states and is mostly nonverbal. Following EMDR, areas of the left frontal regions that have to do with verbal processing and future planning come back online. Although the brain has a natural mechanism for processing disturbing events, when a traumatic experience is overwhelming, the brain may not be able to process it in the same way. This is why severely traumatized people often find themselves struck with disturbing memories long after the traumatic event. Research suggests that an important part of the natural trauma processing happens during rapid eye movement (REM) sleep, which provides alternating stimulation of the right and left hemispheres of the brain. This may help explain why EMDR therapy seems to jump-start the brain's natural healing ability, allowing the traumatic memory to become less and less disturbing.

EMDR is now the most researched treatment for Posttraumatic Stress Disorder (PTSD), and many scientific studies have shown that it is effective and long-lasting. For example, in December 1995, a study by Wilson, Becker, and Tinker was published in the *Journal of Consulting and Clinical Psychology*, where eighty subjects diagnosed with PTSD showed significant improvement after EMDR therapy. Treatment benefits were unchanged at a fifteen-month follow-up.

Exercise for Anxiety Reduction

There is a great deal of recent scientific evidence demonstrating that regular physical activity leads to significant symptom reduction. Consistent findings show that aerobic exercise, such as brisk walking, for at least thirty minutes three to five times a week at 60% to 80% of one's maximum heart rate results in improved mood in people with depression or anxiety disorder.[94]

Exercise can help to relieve stress, tension, and anxiety. By expelling your excess negative emotions and adrenaline through physical activity, you can enter a more relaxed, calm state of being from which to deal with the issues and conflicts that are causing your anxiety. Exercise is one of the most important coping medium to combat anxiety and stress.

Exactly how exercise helps in relaxation and stress management is not clear. The benefits of exercise can come from many factors: the decision to take up exercise, the symbolic meaning of the activity, the distraction from worries, the acquisition of mastery over a sport, the effects on self-image, and the biochemical and physiological changes that accompany the activity.

Exercise increases blood flow to the brain, releases hormones, stimulates the nervous system, and increases levels of morphine-like substances found in the body (such as beta-endorphin) that can have a positive effect on mood. Exercise may trigger a neurophysiological high that produces an antidepressant effect in some, an antianxiety effect in others, and a general sense of "feeling better" in most.[95]

Exercise is only a short-term fix for anxiety. The relaxation induced by the exercise lasts for only four hours or so. So if you are suffering from chronic anxiety, you may have to moderately exercise every day to see an effect. If you become anxious during the day, such as the case if you experience job stress, you may want to exercise first thing in the morning. On the other hand, if you suffer from insomnia, you may want to exercise in the late afternoon. (Note: Exercising too late in the day may make it difficult for you to fall asleep.)

Studies are inconclusive when examining whether you need to exercise vigorously in order to reduce anxiety. Some studies suggest that exercise should be fairly intense, but not exhausting, to best elicit the tranquilizer effect of exercise. Other researchers have found that light exercise such as walking or swimming decreases anxiety just as effectively as vigorous jogging. Exercises such as golf, tennis, handball, biking, and other sports have shown to help people relax. Choose an exercise (the type and the level of exercise) that work best for you.

---

[94] Dunn, A.L., Trivedi, M.H., Kampert, J.B., Clark, C.G., & Chambliss, H.O. (2005). Exercise treatment for depression: Efficacy and dose response. American Journal of Preventive Medicine, 28(1), 1-8.

[95] Michael H. Sacks, M.D.: Exercise For Stress Control

Top 5 Strategies for Anxiety

1. Complete Hormone Panel testing
2. Food Allergy testing
3. Eliminate caffeine
4. Balance blood sugar levels- heal hypoglycemia
5. Supplement with GABA, Relora, Magnesium,
6. B-complex vitamins and Theanine

Louise's Story - Anxiety

Louise is a forty-six-year-old female who presented with severe, progressing, and chronic anxiety. Louise is a mother of two teenage children who works full-time. The anxiety began when Louise was thirty-six years old and suffered a miscarriage at twelve weeks gestation. Shortly after the miscarriage, she underwent a cone biopsy for cervical dysplasia. The stress and grief involved in both of those situations set Louise into a pattern of long-term anxiety.

At first, Louise experienced anxiety as short bursts of overwhelming stress that occurred intermittently. The anxiety continued and grew exponentially into daily anxiety, palpitations, insomnia, severe mood swings, depression, anger, and irritability; all of these symptoms increased the week before her period.

Louise's diet was sporadic. For a short duration, Louise would eat a very well-balanced diet, with long durations of time when she would skip meals and rely on quick carbohydrate-dense convenience snacks to get her through the day. Louise also consumed at least two cups of coffee per day and very little water. One of Louise's goals was also to lose five to ten pounds. Louise then underwent lab testing for her anxiety.

Lab testing results:

- Extremely elevated cortisol, especially between the hours of 4:00 p.m. to midnight
- Hypoglycemia
- Depressed Salivary SIgA
- Depressed progesterone
- Elevated testosterone

Management Plan

Louise was administered the following natural medicine therapies:

- Estrogen detoxification: isoflavones, turmeric, rosemary, resveratrol, B6, B12, folic acid; three times per day
- Adrenal support: vitamins C, B5, and B6, magnesium, citrus bioflavonoids; two times per day
- Adrenal support: licorice root, ashwagandha root; two times per day
- Modified Mediterranean Lifestyle Nutrition Plan to balance hormones and correct hypoglycemia (See "Specific Guidelines for Nutritional Lifestyle Management in Weight Gain" section)

Louise returned three weeks later for a follow-up visit and reported that during the first week of treatment her anxiety was extreme, but over the course of the following two weeks, it had dissipated an incredible amount. Insomnia and PMS were still major issues with which she was dealing. Louise was instructed to add the following forms of therapy to her protocol:

- Exercising with a personal trainer three to five times per week
- Counseling therapy to deal with the past miscarriage and current issues in her life as well as stress management techniques

The following changes were made to Louise's protocol:

- Continue with adrenal support: vitamins C, B5, and B6, magnesium, citrus bioflavonoids; two times per day
- Cortisol management: ashwagandha, L-theanine, phosphatidylserine one capsule at 4:00 p.m. and one capsule before bed
- Chinese stress-reducing formula including: rhemannia root, schisandra fruit, don quai, Chinese asparagus root, scrophularia root, Asian ginseng root and Chinese salvia root two to six tablets per day as needed for stress
- Progesterone-balancing formula including Vitex and Black cohosh
- High potency purified fish oils 1000mg three times per day

Four weeks later, Louise came for a follow-up and reported that her anxiety was completely gone. She was sleeping much better at an average nightly amount of seven hours. She had no PMS symptoms at all during her last cycle and she had lost eight pounds. She reported that she was exercising regularly, eating consistently, and undergoing counseling.

Depression

In affluent countries, depression is the leading cause of disease burden for women.[96] Studies have also shown that depression will become the second leading cause of death and disability worldwide by 2020, second only to ischemic heart disease. The greatest burden of depression occurs in North America and the United Kingdom.[97] The Medical Outcome Study, a four year longitudinal report, corroborates these projections and adds that depression is more debilitating than other chronic medical disorders such as diabetes, arthritis, hypertension, and cardiovascular disease.[98] Over the course of a year, 9.5% of the North American population suffers from depression and depression-related mood disorders. In the course of a lifetime, one out of every four women and one out of every ten men will develop depression.[99]

The official definition of clinical depression (also referred to as major depression or unipolar depression), according to the American Psychiatric Association in its Diagnostic and Statistical Manual of Mental Disorders (DSM-IV), is based on the following eight primary criteria:

1. Poor appetite accompanied by weight loss or increased appetite accompanied by weight gain
2. Insomnia or excessive sleep habits (hypersomnia)
3. Physical hyperactivity or inactivity
4. Loss of interest or pleasure in usual activities or decrease in sexual drive

---

[96] World Health Organization. The global burden of disease. 2004 Update: 43.

[97] WHO, Mental Health; New understanding, new hope. Geneva: The World Health Report, 2001.

[98] Murray C, Lopez A. Alternative projections of mortality and disability by cause 1990-2020: Global Burden of Disease. Study. The Lancet. 1997; 349:1498-1504.

[99] Bleher MD, Oren DA "Gender differences in depression." Medscape women's health, 1997; 2-3. Revised from "Women's Increased Vulnerability to Mood Disorders: Integrating psychobiology and epidemiology." Depression, 1995; 3:3-12

5. Loss of energy; feelings of fatigue
6. Feelings of worthlessness, self-reproach, or inappropriate guilt
7. Diminished ability to think or concentrate
8. Recurrent thoughts of death or suicide

The presence of five of the eight symptoms definitively indicates clinical depression; an individual with four is likely depressed. According to the DSM-IV, the symptoms must be present for at least one month to be called depression.

Symptoms of Depression

Depression is manifested both physically and emotionally. The classic physical signs of depression are as follows:

- Headaches
- Fatigue, decreased energy, or a feeling of being "slowed down"
- Digestive problems
- Chronic pain
- Hyperactivity, restlessness, or irritability
- Sleeping disorders
- Loss of concentration; difficulty remembering or making decisions
- Distorted eating patterns—either the urge to consistently overeat or loss of appetite (a significant change in weight is often evident)

The emotional side of depression can include the following:

- Excessive crying
- Persistent sad, anxious, or "empty" mood
- Pessimism; hopelessness
- A sense of worthlessness
- Guilt or self-pity
- Loss of self-esteem
- Loss of enjoyment from normally pleasurable activities
- Decrease in sex drive
- Suicidal tendencies

Types of Depression

Clinical depression is categorized into three types:

1. Major depression manifests a combination of symptoms that interfere with the ability to work, study, sleep, eat, and enjoy once-pleasurable activities. Such a disabling episode of depression may occur only once but more commonly occurs several times in a lifetime.
2. Dysthymia is a less severe type of depression and involves long-term, chronic symptoms that are not disabling but keep someone from functioning well or feeling good. Many people with dysthymia also experience some episodes of major depression.
3. Bipolar disorder is also called manic-depressive disorder. Not nearly as prevalent as other forms of depressive disorders, bipolar disorder is characterized by cyclic mood changes manifesting in severe highs (mania) and

lows (depression). Sometimes the mood switches are dramatic and rapid but more often they are gradual. When in the depressed cycle, an individual can have any or all of the symptoms of depression. When in the manic cycle, the individual may be overactive, over-talkative, and wildly energetic.

Causes of Depression

Depression can often be due to an underlying organic (chemical) or physiological cause. Identification and elimination of the underlying cause should be the primary therapy. The following lists the organic and physiological causes of depression:

- Food allergies
- Heavy metals
- Hypoglycemia
- Hypothyroidism
- Nutritional deficiencies
- Pre-existing physical conditions (cancer, chronic inflammation, chronic pain, diabetes, heart disease, liver disease, lung disease, multiple sclerosis, rheumatoid arthritis)
- Premenstrual syndrome
- Prescription medications (antihistamines, antihypertensive, anti-inflammatory agents, birth control pills, corticosteroids, tranquilizers, and sedatives)
- Sleep disturbances
- Stress/low adrenal function

Uncovering the causes of depression can be attained by precise laboratory testing. The following chart outlines specific lab tests that can be useful diagnostic tools.

Specific Lab Test	Description
ELISA/EIA Food Allergy Testing	This is based on the findings that certain subclasses of IgG have been associated with the *in vitro* degranulation of basophils and mast cells, the activation of the complement cascade, (both of which are important mechanisms in allergy and anaphylaxis) and the observation that high circulating serum concentrations of some IgG subtypes have been measured in certain atopic individuals. The premise behind this testing is that high circulating levels of IgG antibodies are correlated with clinical food allergy signs and symptoms. The ELISA/EIA test itself involves coating a ninety-six-well plate with food antigens, adding a patient's sera and looking for a classic antigen/antibody interaction.
Micro Nutrient Testing for Nutritional Deficiencies	The micronutrient tests measures how micronutrients are actually functioning within the white blood cells. Micro Nutrient's patented testing chemically-defined control media contains the minimal amount of each essential micronutrient that is needed to support optimal lymphocyte growth or mitogenic response.

Neurotransmitter Testing	Medical science has discovered that neurotransmitters are at the foundation of many psychiatric and neurological disorders. Imbalances in neurotransmission, due to excessive or deficient neurotransmitter levels at the synaptic cleft, are associated with depression, insomnia, anxiety, behavioural disorders, memory disorders, and a spectrum of other brain-related functions. Because neurotransmitters play an integral role in these disease states, they are prime targets for treating disorders of the nervous system and mental health concerns. Neurotransmitters are recognized as the primary biochemical messengers of the central and peripheral nervous systems. Studies have demonstrated that urinary neurotransmitter measures are reflective of circulating levels as evidenced by renal neurotransmitter clearance mechanisms. Laboratory methodology for the accurate assessment of urinary neurotransmitter levels has been established. Urinary measures are not recognized as a direct reflection of central activity, however definite associations exist. The ability to measure neurotransmitters has led to the generation of scientific literature that demonstrates urinary neurotransmitter measurements have clinical value as representative biomarkers of various neurological, immunological, and endocrinological conditions.
Adrenal Stress Index	The panel utilizes four saliva samples. Salivary cortisol measurement reflects the free (bioactive) fraction of serum cortisol. The test report shows the awake diurnal cortisol rhythm generated in response to real-life stress. The cortisol-to-DHEA (cortisol/DHEA) relationship highlights the many facets of stress maladaptation. The cortisol/DHEA ratio helps determine the projected time for recovery, and the substances (hormones, supplements, botanicals) that promote this recovery. The cortisol/DHEA ratio regulates a multitude of functions. The panel measures P17-OH levels in order to evaluate the efficiency of the conversion of adrenal precursors into cortisol. Certain adrenal fatigue patients who are genetically predisposed to low production of cortisol will not benefit from exogenous supplementation of pregnenolone or progesterone. The panel includes fasting and non-fasting insulin measurements. The insulin values are used to diagnose insulin resistance-functional insulin deficit (pre-diabetes), as well as to correlate elevated cortisol with insulin to help explain glycemic dysregulation problems.

Complete Female Hormone Panel	Estradiol and progesterone levels and their ratio are an index of estrogen/progesterone balance. An excess of estradiol, relative to progesterone, can explain many symptoms in reproductive age-women. Testosterone levels can also be either too high or too low. Testosterone in excess, often caused by ovarian cysts, leads to conditions such as excessive facial and body hair, acne, and oily skin and hair. Polycystic ovarian syndrome (PCOS) is thought to be caused, in part, by insulin resistance. On the other hand, too little testosterone is often caused by excessive stress, medications, contraceptives, and surgical removal of the ovaries. This leads to symptoms of androgen deficiency including loss of libido, thinning skin, vaginal dryness, loss of bone and muscle mass, depression, and memory lapses. SHBG binds tightly to circulating estradiol and testosterone, preventing their rapid metabolism and clearance and limiting their bioavailability to tissues. SHBG gives a good index of the extent of the body's overall exposure to estrogens.
Thyroid Hormone Testing	A complete thyroid profile includes free T4, free T3, TSH, and TPO and can indicate the presence of an imbalance in thyroid function. Hypothyroidism includes feeling cold all the time, low stamina, fatigue (particularly in the evening), anxiety, depression, low sex drive, weight gain, and high cholesterol. Hyperthyroidism includes heat intolerance, anxiety, palpitations, weight loss tired but wired visual disturbances and insomnia.
Anemia	Low serum iron, hematocrit, and low blood hemoglobin levels can predispose a person to extreme fatigue, contributing to depression.
Celiac Testing	Celiac disease and gluten sensitivity have been linked to mood disorders. The following tests can detect a gluten allergy: Anti-gliadin IgA/IgG antibody Anti-endomysial antibody Anti-tissue transglutiminase (tTG)

Pharmaceutical Medications to Treat Depression

There are three classes of drugs commonly used to treat depression: selective serotonin reuptake inhibitors (SSRIs); tricyclic antidepressants (TCAs), and monoamine oxidase inhibitors (MAOI's).

SSRIs are believed to increase the extracellular level of the neurotransmitter serotonin by inhibiting its reuptake into the presynaptic cell. SSRIs also increase the level of serotonin in the synaptic cleft available to bind to the postsynaptic receptor. They have varying degrees of selectivity for the other monoamine transporters, with pure SSRIs having only weak affinity for the noradrenaline and dopamine transporter.[100]

The majority of the TCAs act primarily as serotonin-norepinephrine reuptake inhibitors (SNRIs) by blocking the serotonin transporter (SERT) and the norepinephrine transporter (NET), respectively, which results in an elevation of the extracellular concentrations of these neurotransmitters, and therefore an enhancement of neurotransmission. Notably, the TCAs have negligible affinity for the dopamine transporter (DAT), and therefore have no efficacy as dopamine reuptake inhibitors (DRIs).[101]

Monoamine oxidase inhibitors (MAOIs) are one of the oldest classes of antidepressants and are typically used when other antidepressants have not been effective. They are used less frequently because they often interact with certain foods and require strict dietary restrictions. MAOIs prevent monoamine oxidase from breaking down the monoamines. This results in an increased amount of active monoamines in the brain. By increasing the amount of monoamines in the brain, the imbalance of chemicals, thought to be important in causing depression, is altered. This helps relieve the symptoms of depression.[102]

Pharmaceuticals Used for Depression

SSRIs	**Dose Range**	**Side Effects**
Citalopram HBr (Celexa)	20-50mg mg 1 time per day (q.d.)	Sexual problems Stomach upset Agitation Weight gain
Escitalopram oxalate (Lexapro)	10-40mg q.d.	(As above)
Paroxetine HCl (Paxil)	20-50mg q.d.	(As above)
Fluouxetine (Prozac)	20-80mg q.d.	(As above)
Sertralane (Zoloft)	25-200mg q.d.	(As above)
Fluvoxamine (Luvox)	50-300mg q.d.	(As above)
Serotonin and Norepinephrine Reuptake Inhibitors (SNRI's)	**Dose Range**	**Side Effects**
Duloxetine (Cymabalta)	20-60mg q.d.	Hypertension, nausea, dizziness, drowsiness
Venlafaxine (Effexor)	37.5mg-300mg q.d.	Can increase diastolic BP and nausea
Desvenlafaxine succinate (Pristiq)	50mg q.d.	Sexual side effects

[100] http://en.wikipedia.org/wiki/Selective_serotonin_reuptake_inhibitor

[101] Tatsumi M, Groshan K, Blakely RD, Richelson E. (1997). "Pharmacological profile of antidepressants and related compounds at human monoamine transporters." Eur J Pharmacol. 340 (2-3): 249–258. doi: 10.1016/S0014-2999(97)01393-9. PMID 9537821.

[102] http://www.netdoctor.co.uk/diseases/depression/monoamineoxidaseinhibitors_000101.htm

TCA	Dose Range	Side Effects
Amitriptyline (Elavil)	25-300mg Before bed (h.s.)	Dry mouth or eyes, bad taste in mouth, photophobia, blurry vision, constipation, urinary hesitancy, cardiovascular risk, orthostatic hypotension, sedation, risk of mortality in overdose
Imipramine (Tofranil)	25-300mg h.s.	(As above)
Nortriptyline (Aventyl)	25-150mg h.s.	(As above)
Clomipramine (Anafranil)	25-75mg 3 times per day with food (t.i.d. cc)	(As above)

MAOI	Dose Range	Side Effect
Phenelzine (Nardil)	15-105mg q.d.	Orthostatic hypotension, sedation interaction with tyramine foods
Parnate (Tranylcypromine)	10-90mg q.d.	(As above)

Nutritional Factors Affecting Depression

Modification of lifestyle, including nutrition, is fundamental to overcoming depression. Nutritional deficiencies are extremely common in depressed patients. Many different nutrients play a critical role in mood regulation. A diet based on whole foods, including a substantial amount of various fresh fruits and vegetables, is fundamental to any health concern, especially depression.

Nutritional deficiencies affecting or even causing depression are numerous. Specifically magnesium, when deficient, can lead to depression, likely by a mechanism that increases inflammation. Other individual deficiencies are listed below:

Behavioural Effects of Some Vitamin Deficiencies[103]

Deficient Vitamin	Behavioural Effects
Thiamine	Korsakoff's psychosis, mental depression, apathy, anxiety, irritability
Riboflavin	Depression, irritability
Niacin	Apathy, anxiety, depression, hyperirritability, mania, memory deficits, delirium, organic dementia, emotional lability
Biotin	Depression, extreme lassitude, somnolence
Pantothenic acid	Restlessness, irritability, depression, fatigue

[103] Encyclopedia of Natural Medicine Revised 2nd Edition Michael Murray ND Joseph Pizzorno ND pg. 387

B6	Depression, irritability, sensitivity to sound
Folic acid	Forgetfulness, insomnia, apathy, irritability, depression, psychosis, delirium, dementia
B12	Psychotic states, depression, irritability, confusion, memory loss, hallucinations, delusions, paranoia
Vitamin C	Lassitude, hypochondriasis, depression, hysteria

Reactive Hypoglycemia

Depression is one of the most common symptoms of reactive hypoglycemia and has been reported to improve after commencement of a dietary program designed to stabilize blood glucose levels.[104] There are four main mechanisms responsible for reactive hypoglycemic depression:

1. As blood sugar levels are increased, so is cortisol secretion. Elevated cortisol levels are directly connected to the development of depression.
2. Low blood sugar levels are implicated in depression, fatigue, and the inability to concentrate.
3. Insulin resistance has been directly connected to reactive hypoglycemia. Neurotransmitter deficiencies are correlated with insulin resistance as insulin is required for the uptake of tryptophan and other amino acid neurotransmitter precursors in the brain.
4. Norepinephrine depletion is caused by the repetitive release of norepinephrine when hypoglycemia is occurring.

In order to stabilize blood sugar levels, specific dietary measures need to be adopted. A nutritional regime that involves consuming six smaller meals per day rather than the standard three meals per day has been shown to dramatically decrease hypoglycemic tendencies. The hypoglycemic patient's diet should consist of one that is high in protein and fats and low in carbohydrates. Protein in moderately high amounts will decrease the release of insulin from the pancreas. If the protein-to-carbohydrate ratio is 0.75 or greater, the insulin release from the pancreas will be slowed down and the subsequent decline in blood glucose following meals will not be as rapid.[105] Macronutrient percentages kept at levels of 40% carbohydrates, 30% protein and 30% fat have been found to balance blood sugar levels substantially.

Food Allergies and Depression

Molecules called exorphins, which are derived from incomplete breakdown during the digestive process, are small proteins that have morphine-like effects. Five exorphins have been discovered in the breakdown products of gluten and eight others in milk.[106] The study of exorphins has been able to identify a possible explanation for some of the reported psychoactive reactions to these proteins, including the sense of "brain fog." Exorphins have also been shown to decrease levels of serotonin, dopamine, and norepinephrine in the central nervous system, contributing to the process of depression. Detection of food allergies can be achieved by the ELISA/EIA Food Allergy Testing or by completing an elimination diet. An elimination diet involves eliminating the most common allergenic foods (gluten,

---

[104] Salzer HM Relative hypoglycemia as a cause of neuro-psychiatric illness J Natl Med Association 1966; 58:12-17

[105] Westphal SA, Gannon MC, Nuttall FQ. Metabolic response to glucose ingested with various amounts of protein. Am J Clin Nutr 1991;52:267-72

[106] Fukudome S, Shimatsu A, Suganuma H, et al. Effect of gluten exorphins A5 and B5 on the postprandial plasma insulin level in conscious rats. Life Sci. 1995;57 (7):729-34

dairy, corn, soy, eggs, peanuts, citrus fruits, sugar, processed foods, alcohol, and shellfish) for a period of twenty-one days and then re-introducing the potential allergens one at a time, three days apart.

Herbal Medicine Indicated for Depression

St. John's wort *(Hypericum perforatum)*

St. John's wort acts pharmacologically to alter brain chemistry in ways similar to antidepressant drugs. Hypericin, hyperforin, and other components (flavonoids) of the plant have been shown to inhibit the breakdown of several neurotransmitters within the brain that maintain normal mood and emotional stability. It appears to improve the signal produced by serotonin after it binds to its receptor sites on the brain cell. Dosage: 300mg-900mg per day

Kava kava *(Piper methysticum)*

Kava kava helps in the treatment of anxiety and depression. Kavalactones are the primary active components. They exhibit sedative, analgesic, anticonvulsant, and muscle relaxant effects. Most sedative drugs work by binding to GABA receptor sites in the brain to promote sedation. Kava lactones do not appear to bind to these receptors but somehow magnify the area near the receptor site in a way that enhances GABA binding and is therefore not addictive.

Maidenhair tree *(Ginkgo biloba)*

Ginkgo increases the blood flow and oxygen supply to the brain. Ginkgo is therefore useful in the prevention and treatment of strokes. It can be used with standard antidepressants and it may enhance their effectiveness. Ginkgo biloba standardized extract contains 24% Ginkgo flavone glycoside at a dose of 40mg three times per day. It should be taken consistently for at least twelve weeks in order to determine the effectiveness.

Specific Nutrients in the Treatment of Depression

5-HTP (5-hydroxytryptophan)

5-HTP, extracted from the seeds of the African plant *Griffonia simplicifolia,* is the intermediate metabolite of the amino acid L-tryptophan in the serotonin pathway. After tryptophan is converted into 5-HTP, the chemical is then converted into another chemical called serotonin (a neurotransmitter which relays signals between brain cells). 5-HTP acts primarily by increasing levels of serotonin within the central nervous system. 5-HTP dietary supplements help raise serotonin levels in the brain. Since serotonin helps regulate mood and behaviour, 5-HTP may have a positive effect on sleep, mood, anxiety, appetite, and pain sensation. Other neurotransmitters and CNS chemicals such as melatonin, dopamine, norepinephrine, and beta endorphin have also been shown to increase following oral administration of 5-HTP. Dosage: 100-600mg per day

Tryptophan

A sufficient supply of the natural amino acid, tryptophan is needed in order for the body to produce serotonin.[107] Studies on tryptophan depletion and the role of serotonin in psychiatric and behavioral disturbances indicate that low tryptophan levels can trigger a corresponding drop in brain serotonin production and can therefore impact mood, impair memory, and increase aggression.[108]

---

[107] 1.Sandyk R. L-tryptophan in neuropsychiatric disorders: a review. Int J Neurosci. 1992 Nov-Dec;67(1-4):127-44.

[108] Bell C, Abrams J, Nutt D. Tryptophan depletion and its implications for psychiatry. Br J Psychiatry. 2001 May;178:399-405.

Tryptophan is available as a safe, well-proven supplement.[109] Supplementing with tryptophan helps normalize levels of serotonin and other neurotransmitters. As a result, it can reverse many of the mood related symptoms of depression including irritability, anxiety, and stress. Dosage: 500mg-1g per day

Essential Fatty Acids

An insufficiency of omega-3 fatty acids in the diet has been linked to depression. This may be related to the impact of dietary fatty acids on the composition of nerve cell membranes. Dietary supplementation with DHA and EPA has proven beneficial for many of the known higher mental functions. Meta-analyses confirm the benefits of Omega-3 fatty acid supplementation in major depressive disorder and bipolar disorder. There are also promising results in schizophrenia with initial benefit for borderline personality disorder. Accelerated cognitive decline and mild cognitive impairment correlate with lowered tissue levels of DHA/EPA and supplementation has improved cognitive function. The brain is the richest source of fatty acids in the human body. Proper nerve cell function is dependent upon membrane fluidity to prevent behavioral, mood, and mental function fluctuations. Dosage: 2000mg-6000mg per day

Folic Acid (Vitamin B9)

Folic acid deficiency alone can cause depression. Several studies have demonstrated that folic acid is effective in the treatment of depression. One of these studies showed benefit from the use of folic acid supplementation in a group of patients suffering from depression. Results showed that 92% of the folic acid group made a full recovery, compared with only 70% of the control group who took the standard prescription drug therapy.[110] Dosage: 500mcg-1mg per day

Vitamin B12 (Methylcobalamin)

A deficiency of vitamin B12 can result in pernicious anemia, depression, anxiety, fatigue, and poor mental function. Vitamin B12 inhibits monoamine oxidase (MAO), an enzyme that metabolizes some of the neurotransmitters that help to elevate mood. Due to these effects, it acts similarly to MAOI medications prescribed for depression but without the negative side effects. B12 is found mostly in animal products such as beef, liver, chicken liver, clams, oysters, and sardines and in smaller amounts in eggs, many fish, and cheeses. Therefore, vegetarians have a higher risk of vitamin B12 deficiency. Dosage: 1g-5g per day taken sublingually

Vitamin D3

Vitamin D is a fat-soluble vitamin that plays a role in many important body functions. It is best known for working with calcium in the body to help build and maintain strong bones. Vitamin D is also involved in regulating the immune system and preventing cancer. Due to the fact that our bodies can produce vitamin D when exposed to sunlight, vitamin D is considered both a vitamin and a hormone. Lack of sunshine during winter months can cause a vitamin D deficiency. Seasonal Affective Disorder (SAD) can surface when there is a deficiency of vitamin D. Dosage: 1000iu-5000iu per day

SAMe (S-Adenosylmethionine)

SAMe is effective and generally well-tolerated in the treatment of depression with results occurring quicker and providing greater benefit than conventional treatments. SAMe is a methyl donor and plays a role in monoamine metabolism, membrane function, and neurotransmission. SAMe is a naturally occurring physiological agent in the human body that forms an integral part of the methylation cycle. It is formed in the body through the combination of the amino acid methionine and adenosine triphosphate (ATP). This compound was first isolated in Italy in 1952 and is now a prescription drug in much of Europe, most commonly prescribed as an antidepressant. Dosage: 400mg-1200mg per day

---

[109] Fernstrom JD. Effects and side effects associated with the non-nutritional use of tryptophan by humans. J Nutr. 2012 Dec;142(12):2236S-44S.

[110] Kelly, GS "Folates: "Supplemental forms and therapeutic applications." Altern. Med. Rev. 1998 Jun; 3(3): 208-20

L-Tyrosine

Tyrosine is a precursor to norepinephrine, the level of which has been found to be deficient in depressed patients. It is possible to increase norepinephrine synthesis through supplementation with L-tyrosine. This is due to one of the enzymes involved in the conversion of tyrosine to norepinephrine being only 75% saturated under normal conditions. Patients who recovered from depression after supplementing with L-tyrosine were found to have increased plasma tyrosine levels than those patients who did not supplement with L-tyrosine. Dosage: 500mg-1000mg per day

Adjunct Therapies for Depression

Sleep

Depression is often characterized by sleep disturbances that precede the onset or recurrence of depression. The following strategies will improve the quality and consistency of sleep in depressed individuals:

- Create a sleep environment that involves eliminating bright lights beginning one hour before bed. This includes any bright lights, computers, televisions, and street lights. Keep the lights very dim in the bedroom. Blackout blinds may need to be utilized.
- Create a nighttime ritual. Each evening at a specific set time the lights should be dimmed and a cup of relaxation tea (chamomile, lavender, lemon balm, passionflower, catnip, or spearmint) can be steeped and sipped along with a relaxation aromatherapy bath (lavender, geranium, chamomile, orange, frankincense, or ylang ylang).
- Go to bed before midnight. Research has shown that going to bed at the same time every night establishes a better quality sleep routine. Additionally, melatonin release begins around 10pm for adults. Therefore, being in bed around that time will allow for adequate secretion of this sleep-inducing hormone.
- Ensure that blood sugar levels are balanced. Some patients require a small amount of protein and carbohydrates in order to maintain balanced blood sugar levels throughout the night.
- Avoid alcohol before bed. Studies have shown that consuming alcohol before bed will actually interrupt the sleep cycle. Alcohol consumed at bedtime, after an initial stimulating effect, may decrease the time required to fall asleep. Because of alcohol's sedating effect, many people with insomnia consume alcohol to promote sleep. However, alcohol consumed within an hour of bedtime appears to disrupt the second half of the sleep period.[111] The subject may sleep fitfully during the second half of sleep, awakening from dreams and returning to sleep with difficulty. With continued consumption just before bedtime, alcohol's sleep-inducing effect may decrease, while its disruptive effects continue or increase.[112] This sleep disruption may lead to daytime fatigue and sleepiness.

Exercise for Depression

There is a great deal of recent scientific evidence demonstrating that regular physical activity leads to significant symptom reduction. Consistent findings show that aerobic exercise, such as brisk walking, for at least thirty minutes three to five times a week at 60% to 80% of one's maximum heart rate results in improved mood in people with depression or anxiety disorder.

Exercise can help to relieve stress, tension, and anxiety. By expelling your excess negative emotions and adrenaline through physical activity, you can enter a more relaxed, calm state of being from which to deal with the issues and conflicts that are causing your anxiety. Exercise is one of the most important coping mechanisms to combat anxiety and stress.

---

[111] Landolt, H.-P., et al. Late-afternoon ethanol intake affects nocturnal sleep and the sleep EEG in middle-aged men. J Clin Psychopharmacol 16(6):428-436, 1996

[112] Vitiello, M.V. Sleep, alcohol and alcohol abuse. Addict Biol (2):151-158, 1997

Exactly how exercise helps in relaxation and stress management is not clear. The benefits of exercise can come from many factors: the decision to take up exercise, the symbolic meaning of the activity, the distraction from worries, the acquisition of mastery over a sport, the effects on self-image and the biochemical and physiological changes that accompany the activity.

Exercise increases blood flow to the brain, releases hormones, stimulates the nervous system, and increases levels of morphine-like substances found in the body (such as beta-endorphin) that can have a positive effect on mood. Exercise may trigger a neurophysiological high that produces an antidepressant effect in some, an anti-anxiety effect in others, and a general sense of "feeling better" in most.

Exercise is only a short-term fix for anxiety. The relaxation induced by the exercise lasts for only four hours or so. The anxiety returns to its previous level within twenty-four hours after a workout. So if you are suffering from chronic anxiety, you will have to exercise every day to see an effect. If you become anxious during the day such as the case if you experience job stress, you may want to exercise first thing in the morning. On the other hand, if you suffer from insomnia, you may want to exercise in the late afternoon. (Note: Exercising too late in the day may make it difficult for you to fall asleep.)

Studies are inconclusive when looking at whether you need to exercise vigorously in order to reduce anxiety. Some studies suggest that exercise should be fairly intense, but not exhausting, to best elicit the tranquilizer effect of exercise. Other researchers have found that light exercise such as walking or swimming decreases anxiety just as effectively as vigorous jogging. Exercises such as golf, tennis, handball, biking, and other sports have shown to help people relax. Choose an exercise (the type and the level of exercise) that work best for you.

Top 5 Strategies for Depression

1. Food Allergy testing
2. Neurotransmitter/Hormone testing
3. Implement exercise program
4. Balance blood sugar levels and consume a healthy whole foods diet
5. Supplement with 5-HTP, B-complex vitamins, Omega 3's, St. John's wort and Vitamin D3

Sandy's Story - Depression

Sandy is a forty-six-year-old female who presented with severe perimenopausal night sweats which were interrupting her sleep. Sandy had been experiencing night sweats for many years but they had gotten progressively worse in the past four months. Sandy also expressed a deep desire to stop taking the antidepressants that she had been on for twelve years. Her depression had been increasing over the past four months and she was also experiencing fatigue and irritability.

Sandy's menstrual cycle was becoming erratic in timing and in flow. She was experiencing heavier flow, shorter cycles of twenty-one days instead of twenty-eight days, and increasing PMS symptoms.

Sandy's typical dietary habits included coffee, very few fresh fruits and vegetables, and high amounts of animal protein as well as a nightly glass of wine.

Sandy's medical doctor had tested Sandy's thyroid as well as FSH and LH levels the previous week, all of which were normal.

Medications:

- Wellbutrin 300mg per day for twelve years

Lab testing:

- Elisa Multi food IgG allergy testing which revealed the following allergies: egg (white and yolk), dairy, walnuts, sesame, and scallops

Management Plan

Sandy was administered the following natural medicine therapies:

- Perimenopausal support: Black cohosh and Vitex- three capsules per day
- Estrogen detoxification: DIM, Calcium D-Glucarate, SGS (standardized to contain 30mg glucoraphanin glucosinolate), Hops extract (0.12% 8-prenylnaringenin) two capsules with breakfast
- Liver cleansing: a low allergy-potential, powdered medical food that provides a combination of protein, natural phytoestrogens, antioxidants, and fiber- two scoops two times per day for four weeks
- Modified Mediterranean Lifestyle Nutrition Plan to balance hormones (See "Specific Guidelines for Nutritional Lifestyle Management in Weight Gain" section)
- Decrease or avoid alcohol and caffeine

Sandy returned for a follow-up four weeks later and reported that she had experienced much improvement in her symptoms. She had a few night sweats but only one or two per night compared to hourly, and this meant she was sleeping much better. Sandy also reported that she had increased energy and fewer PMS symptoms, with only one reported "challenging" day. Sandy also revealed that she had decided to go off the Welbutrin "cold turkey" shortly after her first visit. She was not experiencing any withdrawal effects but was concerned about her ability to remain happy on a long-term basis.

The following changes were made to Sandy's protocol:

- Continue with Perimenopausal support and Estrogen detoxification
- Mood stabilizing agent: 5-HTP, St John's wort, B3,B5, B6 one capsulethree times per day
- Methylcobalamin to increase energy levels 1g per day sublingually

Sandy reported back four weeks later and stated that she was feeling "stable" with her moods although she was still nervous about the depression returning. She was having little or no night sweats and her energy was mostly improved although she did note the odd day of lower energy. She was struggling with nutrition because she has no interest in cooking and has no knowledge of what to cook. Sandy also stated that she had resumed her gym membership and was working out four to five times per week and was feeling very proud of herself.

The following changes were made to Sandy's protocol:

- Finish estrogen detoxification
- Continue with Perimenopausal support
- Increase the mood stabilizing support up to two capsules two times per day
- Liquid vitamin D3 5000iu per day
- Premenstrual formula to be taken ten days prior to the onset of menstruation: vitamin C, B5, B6, magnesium, choline, taurine, bupleurum, peony root, don quai, ginger, licorice root and mint leaf three tablets ten days before the onset of menstruation

- Recommended to purchase a membership to www.eatcleanmenus.com, which is a clean eating menu planning website

Sandy reported back eight weeks later and stated that her mood was completely stable, her energy was restored, sleep was no longer an issue, and there were no night sweats to report. Sandy also stated that she was enjoying cooking with the help of the menu planning membership and found that her whole family was thrilled that she had taken an interest in cooking.

Adrenal Fatigue

The first documented account of adrenal fatigue was in the 1800s in the medical textbooks, listing it as a clinical condition. Throughout early history, it was one of the most prevalent conditions commonly affecting the majority of adults. Conventional physicians were not kept abreast of the seriousness of adrenal fatigue despite the fact that there were very effective diagnostic tools and treatment protocols available. Over the past fifty years, adrenal fatigue has very seldom been diagnosed by conventional practitioners and has often been dismissed and treated with antidepressants along with the recommendation to "relax." Treatments such as these can cause the condition to progress into a complete demise of health for the patient as the natural progression of this pathology takes its course. Even today, adrenal fatigue is not an acknowledged medical condition by mainstream physicians, although some forward-thinking doctors are now recognizing not only the prevalence but also the significance of this condition.

The adrenal glands are comprised of two small glands which are each the size of a large grape, located on top of the kidneys. The main function of the adrenal glands is to provide stress coping and survival responses. Each adrenal gland is made up of two parts or cortices. The inner medulla modulates the sympathetic nervous system through secretion and regulation of two hormones, called epinephrine (adrenalin) and norepinephrine (noradrenalin), which are responsible for the "fight or flight" response. The outer adrenal cortex comprises 80% of the adrenal gland and is responsible for producing over fifty different types of hormones in three major classes – mineralocorticoids, androgens, and glucocorticoids. The main glucocorticoid hormone is cortisol, which is produced in response to stress and is considered to be the primary "stress hormone" in the body. Cortisol is a life-sustaining adrenal hormone essential to the maintenance of homeostasis. It influences, regulates, or modulates many of the changes that occur in the body in response to stress, including, but not limited to:

- Blood sugar (glucose) levels
- Fat, protein, and carbohydrate metabolism to maintain blood glucose (gluconeogenesis)
- Immune responses
- Anti-inflammatory actions
- Blood pressure
- Heart and blood vessel tone and contraction
- Central nervous system activation

Higher and more prolonged levels of circulating cortisol (like those associated with chronic stress) have been shown to have negative effects, such as:[113]

- Impaired cognitive performance
- Dampened thyroid function
- Blood sugar imbalances, such as hyperglycemia

[113] http://www.adrenalfatigue.org/cortisol-and-adrenal-function.html

- Decreased bone density
- Sleep disruption
- Decreased muscle mass
- Elevated blood pressure
- Lowered immune function
- Slow wound healing
- Increased abdominal fat, which has a stronger correlation to certain health problems than fat deposited in other areas of the body. Some of the health problems associated with increased stomach fat are heart attacks, strokes, higher levels of "bad" cholesterol (LDL), and lower levels of "good" cholesterol (HDL), which can lead to other health problems.

Chronically lower levels of circulating cortisol (as in adrenal fatigue) have been associated with negative effects such as:

- Brain fog, cloudy-headedness and mild depression
- Low thyroid function
- Blood sugar imbalances, such as hypoglycemia
- Fatigue–especially in the morning and mid-afternoon
- Sleep disruption
- Low blood pressure
- Lowered immune function
- Inflammation

Aldosterone is the primary mineralcorticoid hormone that is responsible for modulating the cellular mineral balance, especially sodium and potassium. Consequently, aldosterone plays a pivotal role in regulating blood pressure and bodily fluids. Stress causes an increase in the secretion of aldosterone which can lead to sodium retention (contributing to water retention and high blood pressure) and the loss of potassium and magnesium in the early stages of adrenal fatigue.

The adrenal cortex is also responsible for producing small amounts of the androgens, or sex hormones. DHEA (dehydroepiandrosterone), however, is produced in large amounts from the adrenal cortex and is the precursor to many of the adrenal hormones.

Pregnenolone is one of the most important intermediate hormones produced in the hormonal cascade. Pregnenolone leads to the production of progesterone and is one of the intermediary steps in the making of cortisol and aldosterone. Prolonged deficiencies in pregnenolone, which are found in adrenal fatigue, will lead to the reduction of both glucocorticosteroids and mineralocorticoids such as cortisol and aldosterone, respectively.

The adrenal glands are controlled via the hypothalamus-pituitary-adrenal (HPA) axis and are closely linked to the nervous system. The brain perceives stress and then responds by secreting corticotropin-releasing hormone (CRH) from the hypothalamus in the brain. The release of CRH causes stimulation of the pituitary gland to secrete adrenocorticotropic hormone (ACTH), which travels to the adrenal glands to stimulate cortisol production. Cortisol levels follow a rhythmic fashion throughout the day, with healthy levels being highest in the morning and increasingly lower levels as the day progresses. The following chart represents a normal diurnal cortisol rhythm:

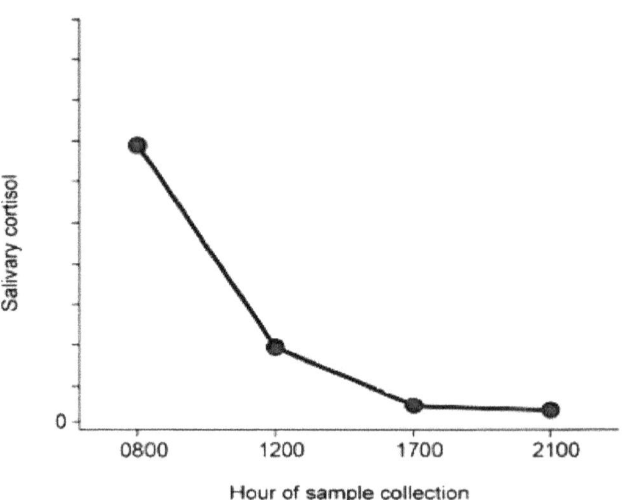

Symptoms Associated with Adrenal Fatigue:

- Always feeling cold
- Anxiety; fearfulness
- Chronic low-grade infections
- Frequent influenza
- Decreased sex drive
- Night sweats
- Needing to go to the bathroom at night
- Depression
- Environmental sensitivities
- Fibromyalgia
- Arthritis
- Headaches
- Hypoglycemia
- Inability to focus or concentrate
- Increased allergies
- Insomnia
- Light-headedness
- Lower back pain in kidney area and sacrum
- Low blood pressure
- Muscular weakness
- Poor memory
- Scanty perspiration
- Sensitivity to light, noise, touch, and movement
- Feeling of exhaustion
- Weight gain or loss
- Feeling overwhelmed by little things
- Nausea
- Lightheaded when rising Lack of energy in the mornings and in the afternoons between 3:00 p.m. and 5:00 p.m.

- Feeling better suddenly for a brief period after a meal
- Often feeling tired from 9:00 p.m. to 10:00 p.m., but resisting going to bed
- Needing coffee or stimulants to get going in the morning
- Cravings for salty, fatty, and high protein food such as meat and cheese
- For women: increased symptoms of PMS; periods are heavy and then stop, or are almost stopped on the fourth day, only to start flowing again on the fifth or sixth day
- Pain in the upper back or neck for no apparent reason
- Feeling better when stress is relieved, such as on a vacation
- Difficulty getting up in the morning

The "father" of stress research, Hans Selye, developed the classic model for adaptation to stress in 1949. His research on rats revealed that in any source of external biological stress, an organism will respond with a predictable biological pattern in an attempt to restore its internal homeostasis. He termed this predictable pattern the General Adaptation Syndrome.

The tree stages of the General Adaptation Syndrome include:

1. **Alarm Stage**: In the Alarm stage, bursts of the hormones cortisol and adrenaline are released in response to a stressor, resulting in the traditional "fight or flight" responses.
2. **Resistance Stage:** In the resistance stage, the body uses high cortisol levels to free up stored energy that helps the body physically resist the stressor. It is now known that a prolonged resistance stage may increase the risk of developing stress-related diseases. If cortisol levels remain elevated, symptoms may include feeling tired but wired, having difficulty sleeping, weight gain around the waist, high blood pressure, hair loss, muscle mass loss and anxiety. Excess cortisol also interferes with the action of other hormones like progesterone, testosterone and thyroid which further creates more imbalances and increasing symptoms.
3. **Exhaustion Stage:** At this stage, the adrenals are either depleted from producing too much cortisol or are reacting to the detrimental effects of high cortisol. This reduces the cortisol production significantly. Symptoms of low cortisol include fatigue (especially morning fatigue), increased susceptibility to infections, decreased recovery from exercise, allergies, and low blood sugar, a burned out feeling, depression and low sex drive.

Causes of Adrenal Fatigue

In western society, chronic stress is very common and seemingly accepted as "normal." The most common causes of chronic stress are work pressure, career change, death of a loved one, moving homes, illness, and marital disruption. Adrenal fatigue occurs when the amount of stress overextends the capacity of the body to compensate and recover.

Stressors that can lead to Adrenal Fatigue include:[114]

- Anger
- Chronic fatigue
- Chronic illness
- Chronic infection—A commonly overlooked cause of adrenal fatigue is chronic or severe infection that gives rise to an inflammatory response. Such infection can occur sub-clinically with no obvious signs at all. Parasitic and bacterial infections including Giardia and H. pylori are often the main causes.
- Chronic pain

[114] Adrenal Fatigue By: Michael Lam, MD, MPH www.DrLam.com

- Depression
- Excessive exercise
- Fear and guilt
- intolerance
- blood sugar
- Mal-absorption
- Mal-digestion
- Toxic exposure
- Severe or chronic stress
- Surgery
- Working late hours
- Sleep deprivation
- Excessive exercise
- Excessive sugar in diet
- Excessive caffeine intake from coffee and tea
- Chronically infected root canal

The following questionnaire is a key diagnostic tool used to evaluate the involvement of adrenal gland function in any disease state and is also used to aid in the diagnosis of adrenal fatigue. The questionnaire should be used in conjunction with specific laboratory testing to determine a definitive diagnosis of adrenal fatigue.

Adrenal Health Questionnaire[115]

Read each statement and decide its degree of severity based on the severity ranking system below.

0= Never

1= Occasionally (1-4 times per month)

2= Moderate in severity and occurs moderately frequently (1-4 times per week)

3= Intense in severity and occurs frequently (more than 4 times per week)

1. I get dizzy or see spots when standing up rapidly from a sitting or lying position.
2. I urinate more frequently than others and may need to get up at night.
3. I feel as though I might faint or black out.
4. I have chronic fatigue.
5. I have mitral valve prolapse or get heart palpitations.
6. I often have to force myself in order to keep going.
7. I have difficulty getting up in the morning.
8. I have low energy before the noon meal (approximately 11:00 a.m.).
9. I have low energy in the late afternoon between 3:00 p.m. and 5:00 p.m.
10. I usually feel better after 6:00 p.m.
11. I often feel best late at night because I get a"second wind."
12. I have trouble getting to sleep.
13. I tend to wake early (approximately 3:00 a.m. to 5:00 a.m.) and have trouble getting back to sleep.

[115] Fundamentals of Naturopathic Endocrinology Michael Friedman, MD pg. 218-220

14. I have vague feelings of being generally unwell for no apparent reason.
15. I get swelling in the extremities, such as the ankles.
16. I need to rest after times of mental, physical, or emotional stress.
17. I feel more tired after exercise or being physical, either soon after or the next day.
18. My muscles feel weak and heavy more that I think they should.
19. I have chronic tenderness in my back area near the bottom of my rib cage.
20. I have a weak back and/or weak knees.
21. I have restless extremities.
22. I am allergic to many things, such as foods, animals, and pollens.
23. My allergies are getting worse.
24. I get bags or dark circles under my eyes which may be worse in the morning.
25. I have multiple chemical sensitivities.
26. I have asthma or get regular bouts of bronchitis, pneumonia, or other respiratory infections.
27. I have dermatographism (a white line appears on my skin if I run my fingernail over it and the line persists for one minute).
28. I have an area of pale skin around my lips.
29. The skin on the palms of my hands and soles of my feet tend to be red/orange in color.
30. I tend to have dry skin.
31. I tend to get headaches and a sore neck and shoulders.
32. I am sensitive to bright light.
33. I frequently feel colder than others around me.
34. I have decreased tolerance to cold.
35. I have Raynaud's syndrome (extremely cold hands/feet).
36. My temperature tends to be below normal when measured with a thermometer.
37. My temperature tends to fluctuate during the day.
38. I have low blood pressure.
39. I become hungry, confused, or shaky if I miss a meal.
40. I crave sugar, sweets, or desserts.
41. I use stimulants, such as tea or coffee, to get started in the morning.
42. I crave food high in fat and feel better with high-fat foods.
43. I need caffeine (chocolate, tea, coffee, colas) to get me through the day.
44. I often crave salt and/or foods high in salt, such as potato chips.
45. I feel worse if I eat sweets and no protein for breakfast.
46. I do not eat regular meals.
47. I eat fast food often.
48. I am sensitive to pharmaceutical or nutritional supplements.
49. I have taken steroid medications for a long term or at a high dose.
50. I have symptoms that improve after I eat.
51. I tend to be thin and find it difficult to put weight on.
52. I have feelings of hopelessness and despair or have been diagnosed with depression.
53. I lack motivation because I do not feel I have the energy to get things done.
54. I have decreased tolerance toward other people and tend to get irritated by them.
55. I get more than two colds per year.
56. It takes me a long time to recover from illness.
57. I get rashes, dermatitis, eczema, psoriasis, or other skin conditions.
58. I have an autoimmune disease.
59. I have fibromyalgia.
60. I have had mononucleosis or been diagnosed with Epstein Barr virus.

61. I do not exercise regularly.
62. I have a history of large amounts of stress in my life.
63. I tend to be perfectionist.
64. My health is negatively affected by stress.
65. I tend to avoid stressful situations for the sake of my health.
66. I am less productive at work that I used to be.
67. My ability to focus mentally is generally impaired.
68. Stressful situations hinder my ability to focus.
69. Stress causes me to become overly anxious.
70. I startle easily.
71. It can take me days or weeks to recover from a stressful event.
72. I tend to get digestive disturbances when tense.
73. I tend to get unexplained fears and phobias.
74. My sex drive is very low or non-existent.
75. My relationships at work and or home tend to be strained.
76. My life contains insufficient time for fun and enjoyable activities.
77. I have little control over my life and I feel "stuck."
78. I tend to get addicted easily to drugs, alcohol, or foods.
79. I suffer from post-traumatic distress disorder.
80. I have or have had an eating disorder.
81. I have gum disease and/or tooth infections or abscesses.
82. I have symptoms of premenstrual syndrome (PMS)- *for women only*
83. My periods are irregular and/or affected by stress- *for women only*

Interpretation:

Total score:

Under 40: very slight or no adrenal fatigue

41-80: mild adrenal fatigue

81-120: moderate adrenal fatigue

Above 120: severe adrenal fatigue

The following are three additional tests that can be performed in order to further determine the function or lack of function of the adrenal glands:

ADRENAL FUNCTION TEST #1-Postural Hypotension:

Postural hypotension (also known as orthostatic hypotension) is a drop in blood pressure that occurs upon rising from a horizontal position. It is commonly expressed as a feeling of dizziness or lightheadedness, a "head rush," or "standing up too fast."

To do this test, a blood pressure cuff is required. Lie down and rest for five minutes. Take a blood pressure reading while still horizontal. Then, stand up and take another reading.

Normally, a healthy blood pressure reading should rise ten to twenty points. If it drops, particularly by ten points or more, hypoadrenia is indicated. Generally, the bigger the drop, the greater the adrenal insufficiency.

ADRENAL FUNCTION TEST #2-Iris Contraction Test

For this test, a weak flashlight or penlight and a mirror are both needed. In a dark bathroom or closet, wait a minute for the eyes to adjust to the dark. This will allow the pupils to dilate (open) fully. Then, shine the flashlight into the eyes and watch the reaction of the pupils for at least thirty seconds.

The light should cause the iris to contract, making the pupils (the dark spot in the center of your eye) smaller. Normally, they should stay that way, but if adrenal gland fatigue is occurring, the iris will be weak and will not be able to hold the contraction. It will either waver between being contracted and relaxed, or will contract initially, but then open up after ten to thirty seconds.

As with the postural hypotension test, the degree to which you "fail" this test is an indicator of the degree of adrenal insufficiency you are experiencing.

ADRENAL FUNCTION TEST #3-Sergent's Adrenal White Line

With the fingernail or the dull end of a spoon, draw a line across the belly. In moderate to severe cases of adrenal fatigue, the line will stay white, and even get wider over the course of time. The "normal" reaction would be for the line to almost immediately turn red.

This test has historically been used to indicate severe adrenal fatigue and Addison's disease. Milder cases of adrenal fatigue may not exhibit this sign.

The following lab tests will confirm a definitive diagnosis of adrenal fatigue. The ELISA test is included to determine if any food allergies are present. Eliminating positive allergens will improve adrenal function and remove a major body burden.

Specific Lab Test	Description
ELISA/EIA Food Allergy Testing	This is based on the findings that certain subclasses of IgG have been associated with the *in vitro* degranulation of basophils and mast cells, the activation of the complement cascade, (both of which are important mechanisms in allergy and anaphylaxis) and the observation that high circulating serum concentrations of some IgG subtypes have been measured in certain atopic individuals. The premise behind this testing is that high circulating levels of IgG antibodies are correlated with clinical food allergy signs and symptoms. The ELISA/EIA test itself involves coating a ninety-six-well plate with food antigens, adding a patient's sera and looking for a classic antigen/antibody interaction.
Adrenal Stress Index	The panel utilizes four saliva samples. Salivary cortisol measurement reflects the free (bioactive) fraction of serum cortisol. The test report shows the awake diurnal cortisol rhythm generated in response to real-life stress. The cortisol/DHEA relationship highlights the many facets of stress maladaptation. The cortisol/DHEA ratio helps determine the projected time for recovery, and the substances (hormones, supplements, botanicals) that promote this recovery. The cortisol/DHEA ratio regulates a multitude of functions. The panel measures P17-OH levels in order to evaluate the efficiency of the conversion of adrenal precursors into cortisol. Certain adrenal fatigue patients who are genetically predisposed to low production of cortisol will not benefit from exogenous supplementation of pregnenolone or progesterone. The panel includes fasting and non-fasting insulin measurements. The insulin values are used to diagnose insulin resistance-functional insulin deficit (pre-diabetes), as well as to correlate elevated cortisol with insulin to help explain glycemic dysregulation problems.

Interpretation of The Adrenal Stress Index Test for DHEA and Cortisol Levels[116]

Levels of DHEA and cortisol vary according to the level of stress and for how long that stress has been applied. Increasing cortisol production is the normal response to stress and is highly desirable, so long as the stress is removed and the adrenal glands can recover.

Ongoing, unremitting stress means the adrenal gland and the whole body is in a constant state of alert and does not get time to recover, and eventually functionally fails. Therefore, there are several stages of adrenal function gradually leading to failure:

1. **Normal levels of cortisol and normal levels of DHEA**. Normal result, indicating a normal adrenal gland.
2. **High levels of cortisol and normal levels of DHEA.** This indicates a normal short-term response to stress.
3. **High levels of cortisol and high levels of DHEA.** The adrenal gland is functioning normally but the patient is chronically stressed. If the stress is removed, the adrenal gland will recover completely.
4. **High levels of cortisol and low levels of DHEA.** The body cannot make enough DHEA to balance the cortisol. This is the first sign of adrenal exhaustion and the first abnormal response to chronic stress. The patient needs a long break from whatever that chronic stress may be. The most common chronic stress is hypoglycemia, but the stress could also be caused by insomnia or mental, physical, or emotional overload. DHEA can be supplemented to make the patient feel better but it must be part of a package of recovery, without which worsening can be expected.
5. **Low levels of cortisol and low levels of DHEA.** The gland is so exhausted that it can't make cortisol or DHEA. By this time, patients are usually severely fatigued.
6. **Low levels of cortisol and borderline or normal levels of DHEA.** This probably represents the gland beginning to recover after a long rest. DHEA may be used to help patients feel better while they continue their program of rest and rehabilitation.

Note:

In Addison's disease, there is complete failure of the adrenal gland not because of chronic stress but because of autoimmunity. This is a life-threatening disorder and it indicates that the patient is severely ill. The main clinical symptom is severe postural hypotension (dizziness when rising to an upright position) and chronic hypoglycemia.

Addison's disease is tested for by a short synacthen test in which cortisol levels are measured before and after an adrenal gland stimulant ACTH. Many patients with chronic fatigue syndrome are given this test, which is found to be normal, resulting in the patient being told their adrenal gland is fine and no action is required. The problem with this test is that it only shows whether the adrenal gland is completely non-functioning. It does not diagnose *partial* adrenal failure or adrenal stress and no measurements of DHEA are made. This makes it potentially misleading.

Nutritional Factors Affecting Adrenal Fatigue

During adrenal fatigue, the cells of the body respond to stress by speeding up cellular metabolism and subsequently burning precious nutrients at a much higher pace. Very quickly the cells use up much of the body's supply of stored nutrients and deficiencies may ensue, further exacerbating the issues. Nutrition becomes a critical part of the healing and a diet abundant in good quality food is crucial. In addition, not only is the quality of the food important, but also the timing in which it is consumed. The adrenal hormone cortisol aids in maintaining balanced blood sugar levels to meet the body's constant demand for energy. During adrenal fatigue, cortisol levels drop lower than normal, making it very difficult to maintain balanced blood sugar levels. As a result, hypoglycemia (low blood sugar) often accompanies adrenal fatigue.

[116] http://www.prohealth.com/ME-CFS/library/showArticle.cfm?libid=14383&B1=EM031109C

Eating Patterns

- It is crucial to eat before 10:00 a.m. to replenish glycogen (stored blood sugar) levels.
- Eat lunch early, between 11:00 a.m. and 11:30 a.m., as the body quickly uses up the nutrients from the morning meal.
- Have a nutritious snack between 2:00 p.m. and 3:00 p.m. in order to prevent the typical hypoglycemic tendencies that occur between 3:00 p.m. and4:00 p.m.
- Dinner should be eaten between 5:00 p.m. and 6:00 p.m.
- Just before bed, a small snack may be required to prevent panic attacks, sleep disturbances, and anxiety reactions throughout the night.

Foods to Consume

- Combine a fat, protein, and carbohydrate at every meal and snack.
- The diet should consist of 30% to 40% vegetables (50% should be raw or lightly cooked), 30% to 40% whole grains (brown rice, millet, barley, oats, quinoa, amaranth, and buckwheat), 10% to 20% animal proteins (wild fish, organic poultry, and wild game), 10% to 15% beans, seeds (raw only), and nuts (raw only), and 5% to 10% fruits.
- Celtic sea salt can be added to foods in moderation to improve adrenal function.
- Add one to two tablespoons of essential oils into grains, vegetables, and proteins daily.

Foods to Avoid

- Refined sugar including cakes, pies, doughnuts, cookies, and other foods containing white flour, sugar, and chocolate.
- Stimulating beverages such as coffee, colas, black tea, hot chocolate.
- Avoid alcohol
- Eating fruit in the morning (the naturally-occurring fructose in the fruit will cause a spike in blood sugar and an eventual drop, which is exacerbated in the morning).
- Processed foods that rob the cells of the body of the critical energy needed to heal. In addition, processed foods put extra stress on the liver, which is often already sluggish in adrenal fatigue.

Herbal Medicine Indicated for Adrenal Fatigue

There is a class of herbs known as "adaptogens." An herb classified as an adaptogen has the unique ability to aid in the body's response system to stress. These herbs allow the body to better adapt to stress and provide a buffering or balancing action that counteracts an exaggerated adrenal response to stress. Adaptogens affect both the adrenal gland function directly as well as the HPA axis (Hypothalamus-pituitary-adrenal axis). There are six main herbs that fall into this category:

Licorice Root *(Glycyrrhiza glabra)*

Licorice is one of the most well-known adaptogenic herbs, with use dating back thousands of years.[117] The action of licorice comes from the triterpenes, glycyrrhizin, and its aglycone component, glycyrrhetinic acid. The triterpenes are metabolized to a similar structure as the adrenal cortical hormones, which may be responsible for licorice root's anti-inflammatory action. Glycerrhizin inhibits liver damage and increases antibody production through a stimulation

[117] Fundamentals of Naturopathic Endocrinology Michael Friedman, MD pg. 127

of interleukin.[118] Glycyrrhetinic acid has been shown to be similar in structure to corticosteroids and therefore have adrenocortico mimetic actions. Research has shown that licorice can increase cortisol levels and help to resolve issues with low blood pressure. Through its effects on the kidneys, it also improves the body's ability to retain sodium and magnesium and subsequently reduces issues with frequent urination.

There has been much research on the concern that licorice can increase blood pressure. This is due to the fact that licorice blocks the conversion of cortisol into cortisone, which can produce higher amounts of circulating cortisol. Most patients with adrenal fatigue typically have low blood pressure but simple monitoring of blood pressures levels will allow for the successful and safe administration of licorice root.

Ashwagandha Root *(Withania somnifera)*

Ashwagandha is an ancient Indian herb with therapeutic actions dating back to at least 1000 BC. Ashwagandha is commonly called Indian ginseng, although it is not related to any species of ginseng, it does, however, have similar therapeutic effects. Traditionally, ashwagandha has been prescribed in the healing of a wide variety of illnesses and has been touted as a tonic for restoring strength and vigor. Research has shown that ashwagandha can influence hormone activity by providing support to the HPA axis function. As an adaptogen, it also aids in the adaptability to both physical and chemical stress by increasing catecholamine production.[119] More than thirty-five active constituents have been identified in ashwagandha but it is the alkaloids and steroidal lactones that are responsible for many of its effects.

Ashwagandha studies have shown that the plant protects against the physical ravages of stress, preventing adrenal mass increase and vitamin C depletion. In addition, stress-induced increases of both blood urea nitrogen and lactic acid are avoided.[120]

Rhodiola *(Rhodiola rosea/Rhodiola crenulata)*

Rhodiola comes from the mountainous regions of Siberia. It is thought to strengthen the nervous system, fight depression, enhance immunity, elevate the capacity for exercise, enhance memory, aid weight reduction, increase sexual function, and improve energy levels. It has long been known as a potent adaptogen. Since rhodiola administration appears to impact central monoamine levels, it might also provide benefits and be the adaptogen of choice in clinical conditions characterized by an imbalance of central nervous system monoamines.

There have also been claims that this plant has great utility as a therapy in asthenic conditions (decline in work performance, sleep disturbances, poor appetite, irritability, hypertension, headaches, and fatigue), developing subsequent to intense physical or intellectual strain, influenza and other viral exposures, and other illness. Two randomized, double-blind, placebo-controlled trials of the standardized extract of rhodiola root provide a degree of support for these claimed adaptogenic properties.[121]

Siberian Ginseng Root *(Eleutherococcus senticosus)*

Siberian ginseng first became medically recognized for its therapeutic benefits in the 1950s and 1960s when Dr. Brekham studied the attributes of this herb. Eleutherosides have been found to be the main active constituent in Siberian ginseng. Beta-sitosterol, which possesses anti-cancer, anti-inflammatory, and anti-hyperglycemic properties, is the other active constituent. In addition, the lignans that are produced in this herb are responsible for its immunostimulating effects. The eleutherosides were found to have specific binding affinity for adrenal receptor sites, including glucorticoid, mineralcorticoid, and progestin receptors. Siberian ginseng is typically useful in states

---

[118] Fundamentals of Naturopathic Endocrinology Michael Friedman, MD pg 127

[119] Archana R Namasivayam A. Antistressor effect of Withania somnifera. J Ethnopharmacol 1998 Oct; 62 (3): 209-14

[120] Archana R Namasivayam A. Antistressor effect of Withania somnifera. J Ethnopharmacol 1998 Oct; 62 (3): 91-93

[121] http://www.herbwisdom.com/herb-rhodiola.html

of exhaustion as it is considered to be one of the more stimulating adaptogens and is also useful in depression and debility.

Siberian ginseng has a wide range of therapeutic benefits including rejuvenating adrenal function, increasing resistance to all forms of stress, normalizing metabolism, regulating neurotransmitters, and counteracting mental fatigue.

Schisandra *(Schisandra chinensis)*

Schisandra has been traditionally used to promote energy and alleviate exhaustion and immune system disturbances caused by stress. Schisandra has also been taken to strengthen the sex organs and promote mental function. The herb counteracts testosterone-induced atrophy of the adrenal glands in animal studies. Ingestion of the fruit of schisandra has been shown to increase adrenal and spleen function in animals.

As many as thirty lignans have been identified in schisandra that are responsible for increasing metabolism of deoxycholic acid, which is a risk factor for hepatocarcinogenesis. For this reason, schisandra is used in cases of poor liver function, hepatitis, and liver cancer. Due to the fact that it increases the secretion of sexual fluids in both males and females, it is useful in cases of low libido. In addition, schisandra balances fluid and relieves urinary frequency as it tones and strengthens kidney function. It is also useful in cases of excessive thirst and night sweats and in cases of insomnia, as it acts to calm the body. Mental illness, memory lapse, and irritability also improve significantly with the use of schisandra. It is considered to be a deep immune activator.

Specific Nutrients in the Treatment of Adrenal Fatigue

Vitamin C

Vitamin C, also known as ascorbic acid, is the primary vitamin for adrenal gland function. With increasing levels of cortisol, the need for vitamin C rises. Vitamin C is critical to the manufacture of adrenal steroid hormones and the homeostasis of the adrenal hormone cascade. Vitamin C is used along the entire adrenal pathway and has antioxidant functions within the adrenal cortex.

Naturally occurring vitamin C always occurs with bioflavonoids. The addition of bioflavonoids to supplemental ascorbic acid more than doubles the effectiveness of the vitamin C. Bioflavonoids are essential if ascorbic acid is to be fully metabolized and utilized by the cells of the body. The best found ratio is one to two bioflavonoids to ascorbic acid.

Vitamin C is a water-soluble vitamin and is utilized and excreted by the body very quickly. Therefore, doses should be administered several times throughout the day. Individual dosing needs can be determined through a bowel tolerance functional test. Start by taking 1000mg of vitamin C (this should include 500mg of bioflavonoids) and continue this dose every hour until bowel movements become watery. Decrease the dose by 1000mg and continue with that level each day in divided doses.

Vitamin B Complex

As coenzymes, the B vitamins are essential components in most major metabolic reactions. They play an important role in energy production, including the metabolism of lipids, carbohydrates, and proteins. B vitamins are also important for blood cells, hormones, adrenal gland, and nervous system function. As water-soluble substances, B vitamins are not generally stored in the body in any appreciable amounts (with the exception of vitamin B-12). Therefore, the body needs an adequate supply of B vitamins on a daily basis. Dosage: 100 mg-200mg per day with food

Vitamin B5 (Pantothenic Acid)

Vitamin B5 is essential for healthy adrenal and immune function. In particular, B5 serves as the starting material for the synthesis of coenzyme A, which acts as the carrier of acyl groups in oxidation, acetylation, and decarboxylation reactions and it is instrumental in the synthesis of fatty acids and adrenal hormones. Thus, B5 is important for energy production as acetyl CoA is converted from B5 and is crucial for the conversion of glucose into energy. Dosage: 500mg-1500mg per day with food

Vitamin B6 (Pyridoxine HCl)

Vitamin B6 and its bioactive form, pyridoxal 5'-phosphate (P5P), are essential for such processes as amino acid metabolism, neurotransmitter synthesis, and glycogen breakdown. Vitamin B6 is a co-factor in several of the enzymatic pathways in the adrenal cascade. It is also involved in heme synthesis, conversion of tryptophan to niacin, and proper metabolism of fatty acids. Due to the fact that the conversion of pyridoxine to P5P occurs in the liver, a compromise in liver function can have deleterious effects on P5P levels in the body, placing one at risk of vitamin B6 deficiency. Recollection of dreams often significantly improves when vitamin B6 deficiency levels are corrected. Dosage: 50-100mg per day with food

Magnesium

Adequate magnesium is critical to adrenal gland fatigue recovery. Magnesium is essential to the production of enzymes and the energy necessary for the adrenal hormonal pathway. Magnesium is a mineral that functions as a coenzyme for nerve and muscle function. It is essential for the formation of bones, regulation of body temperature, energy metabolism, and DNA and RNA synthesis. The need for magnesium increases during periods of heightened stress because it is a cofactor for several regulatory enzymes, especially those involved with energy production and nervous system function. Clinical studies have shown that magnesium supplements decrease anxiety and chronic stress. Dosage: 400-600mg per day

Pregnenolone

Pregnenolone is the first hormone to be made from cholesterol in the adrenal pathway. It can be converted into several other adrenal hormones including DHEA, sex hormones, aldosterone, and cortisol. In advanced cases of adrenal fatigue, it is often required to begin replacing chronically deficient adrenal hormones. Beginning with pregnenolone will allow the body the opportunity to determine which hormones the pregnenolone will be converted into based on specific needs. Often the body naturally converts the pregnenolone into sex hormones which are severely decreased in adrenal fatigue. A specific function of the sex hormones is to act as antioxidants and protect the body from the oxidative damage from high levels of circulating cortisol, which is a key factor in rapid aging. Dosage: 20-30mg of the bioidentical cream per day

DHEA (Dehydroepiandrosterone)

DHEA levels often become depressed during adrenal fatigue. DHEA is one of the main androgen hormones secreted by the adrenal glands and is the precursor to many of the adrenal sex hormones. It is an important hormone base from which testosterone, progesterone, and corticosterone, either directly or indirectly, can be derived. After age forty, the amount produced in the body starts to decline. Very little is left by age seventy. Research indicates that taking DHEA supplements may help to prevent cancer, arterial disease, multiple sclerosis, and Alzheimer's disease. DHEA may even be useful in the treatment of lupus and osteoporosis, may help to improve memory, and may enhance the activity of the immune system. DHEA should only be used in extreme cases, the patient should be closely monitored, and levels should be tested regularly. Dosage: DHEA for chronic fatigue, 5-25 mg (only if testing shows that levels are low) helps with energy production and the effects of stress

Adrenal Cell Extracts

The adrenal cell extracts restore, support, and transform adrenal fatigue. They enhance adrenal activity and speed recovery. Adrenal cell extracts are not replacement hormones but rather contain the essential constituents for adrenal repair, including cellular contents such as the nucleic acids RNA and DNA. In addition, cell extracts contain concentrated nutrients in the form and proportion used by the adrenals to properly function and recover. They contain only minute amounts of the actual hormones in the adrenal gland. Dosage: varies depending on individual preparations

Phosphorylated Serine (PS)

PS is of extremely beneficial use in stage two adrenal dysfunction when cortisol levels are high. PS has the unique ability to decrease circulating cortisol and allow for a dramatic decrease in symptoms such as anxiety and insomnia. It is important to obtain lab testing to determine when to administer PS, as it should be taken one hour before cortisol levels are elevated. Dosage: 500mg-1000mg one hour before elevated cortisol levels

Adjunctive Therapy for Adrenal Fatigue: Sleep

Sleep is crucial to full adrenal fatigue recovery. The timing and quality of sleep patterns are inherently involved in the healing process. Although insomnia can be a common symptom of adrenal fatigue, establishing regular sleep patterns will alleviate adrenal fatigue.

- It is important to be in bed by 10:30 p.m. and asleep by 11 p.m. to avoid the pitfall of the second wind commonly experienced by adrenal fatigue patients. Staying up past this time will only further exacerbate the adrenal fatigue.
- Take advantage of the restorative power of sleep between 7:00 a.m. and 9:00 a.m. as time permits, to aid in the healing of adrenal fatigue.
- Get enough varied physical exercise during the day.
- Avoid the use of any stimulants, such as coffee and other caffeine-containing stimulants, which can interrupt sleep patterns for several hours.
- Avoid photo stimulation after 8:00 p.m. by turning off the TV, computer, or any other electronic devices.

Top 5 Strategies for Adrenal Fatigue

1. Adrenal Stress Index testing
2. Food Allergy testing
3. Maintaining blood sugar balance is crucial as well as optimizing nutrition through a whole food diet
4. Take a stress inventory and reduce/eliminate changeable stressors
5. Supplement with B-complex vitamins, Vitamin C, Adrenal extracts and a combination of Rhodiola, Ashwagandha, Licorice root, Schisandra and Siberian ginseng

Cheryl's Story - Adrenal Fatigue

Cheryl is a fifty-year-old woman who presented with relentless fatigue. Cheryl stated that the fatigue began as a decrease in motivation three years prior. Cheryl also noticed that her sleep had become quite challenging and she was waking frequently throughout the night. Cheryl was still having regular menstrual cycles but she noted that the flow had become heavier in the past year and she was beginning to experience some night sweats. Cheryl had gained ten pounds in the previous four months with no change to her diet or exercise regime.

Cheryl consumed one to two diet sodas and two to three cups of coffee per day as well as five to six alcoholic beverages each weekend. She often chose salty foods over fresh foods. She mentioned that she craved salt. She did not consume any fast food and ate at regular intervals throughout the day. Cheryl's diet diary revealed that she consumed a very large amount of whole grain carbohydrates. Cheryl exercised regularly although she found it very challenging to remain motivated.

Lab testing:

- Low morning cortisol levels
- Elevated cortisol levels throughout the day
- Low testosterone levels
- Erratic fluctuations in estrogen levels throughout the month
- Low to normal DHEA

Management Plan

Cheryl was administered the following natural medicine therapies:

- Estrogen detoxification: Isoflavones, turmeric, rosemary, resveratrol, B6, B12, folic acid three times per day
- Adrenal support: L-histidine, N-acetyl-tyrosine, rhodiola rosea two capsules two times per day
- Cortisol management: ashwagandha, L-theanine, phosphatidylserine one capsule before bed
- Modified Mediterranean Lifestyle Nutrition Plan to balance hormones (See "Specific Guidelines for Nutritional Lifestyle Management in Weight Gain" section)

Cheryl reported back four weeks later and stated that she had much less daytime fatigue. She also noted that she was going to bed earlier because she was more tired in the evenings. Cheryl had just started noticing an improvement in her sleep about one week previously. She was now sleeping five hours per night instead of two hours. She had improved her nutrition, was no longer consuming aspartame, and had dramatically lessened her consumption of both caffeine and alcohol. Cheryl said her biggest improvement was her return of motivation, which was thrilling to her. She also took note of some hormonal acne that she was experiencing along her jaw line and had been suffering with for many years.

The following changes were made to Cheryl's protocol:

- Continue with the previously-mentioned remedies
- Vitex agnus castus fluid extract- 5mL each morning for acne treatment

Cheryl returned four weeks later to report that she was feeling much better overall. Her sleep was good most of the time and she had no night sweats to report. Cheryl stated that her motivation was completely back to normal and that she was no longer experiencing fatigue.

Cheryl was recommended to continue with the current protocol.

Cheryl returned eight weeks later to report that her sleep had become an issue once again. Other than the relentless insomnia, she felt great and had no issues. Cheryl had lost a total of fifteen pounds and she was very happy about this.

The following protocol was administered:

- Discontinue the use of all previous remedies except dietary recommendations
- Neurotransmitter support required for sleep: vitamin B6, Thera Mix 4 Proprietary Blend (475mg) of: Taurine and 4-amino-3-phenylbutyric acid two capsules before bed
- Estrogen support: Isoflavone Complex Herbal Proprietary Blend-Pueraria lobata (Kudzu, root), red clover (flowering tops, standardized to 8% isoflavones) and Novasoy™ Isoflavone, black cohosh concentrate, bacopa monnieri (standardized to 20% bacosides, leaf), cranberry (fruit), dong quai (root), schisandra (standardized to 0.9% schisandrins, fruit and seeds), sage (salvia officinalis leaf), and hops (aerial parts) one capsule three times per day

- Progesterone support: rehmannia (root), bupleurum (root), passion flower (aerial parts), peony (root), coleus forskohlii (root, standardized to 10% forskohlin), dioscorea villosa (root), and chasteberry extract (fruit) one capsule three times per day

Cheryl returned eight weeks later and reported that she was feeling fantastic. She was finally able to sleep consistently and she had remained symptom-free for the previous six weeks. She was recommended to stay on her protocol to support her through menopause.

Thyroid Disorders

Imbalances of the thyroid are connected to many female hormone issues. These can include breast cancer, uterine fibroids, ovarian cysts, endometriosis, infertility, postpartum depression, miscarriage, PMS, amenorrhea, and menorrhagia. Hypothyroidism, or underactive thyroid, is often linked with adrenal fatigue, estrogen dominance, and progesterone deficiency. A dysfunctional thyroid can affect almost every aspect of health. It is one of the most under-diagnosed hormonal imbalances of aging, together with estrogen dominance and metabolic syndrome.

More than ten million Americans have been diagnosed with thyroid disease, and another thirteen million people are estimated to have undiagnosed thyroid problems. About 10% of the adult population is afflicted with this frequently-overlooked disease of epidemic proportions.

The butterfly-shaped thyroid gland is located in the neck and covers the anterior surfaces of the second to fourth tracheal rings. The thyroid gland is made up of loose, grape-like clusters of tissue with many blood vessels. The thyroid depends upon iodine to combine with the amino acid tyrosine to then be converted into the thyroid hormones T3 and T4. T3 is produced in small amounts from the thyroid, but most significantly, it is converted in the liver and kidneys from T4. T4 secretion is controlled by the pituitary secretion of TSH (thyroid stimulating hormone).[122]

The thyroid hormone, like other hormones, is regulated by an extensive negative feedback system. The system starts in the hypothalamus of the brain that releases thyrotropin-releasing hormone (TRH). TRH signals the pituitary gland to release thyroid stimulating hormone (TSH). TSH in turn instructs the thyroid gland to make thyroid hormones and release them into the bloodstream. When the level of thyroid hormone in your body is high, a negative feedback system exists to reduce the production of TSH, and vice-versa. Therefore, a high TSH is indicative of hypothyroidism, while a low TSH can be indicative of hyperthyroidism.[123]

The following illustration depicts the location of the thyroid gland:[124]

[122] Fundamentals of Naturopathic Endocrinology Michael Friedman, MD pg. 93

[123] Adrenal Fatigue: Michael Lam, MD, MPH www.DrLam.com

[124] http://www.google.ca/images/thyroid gland

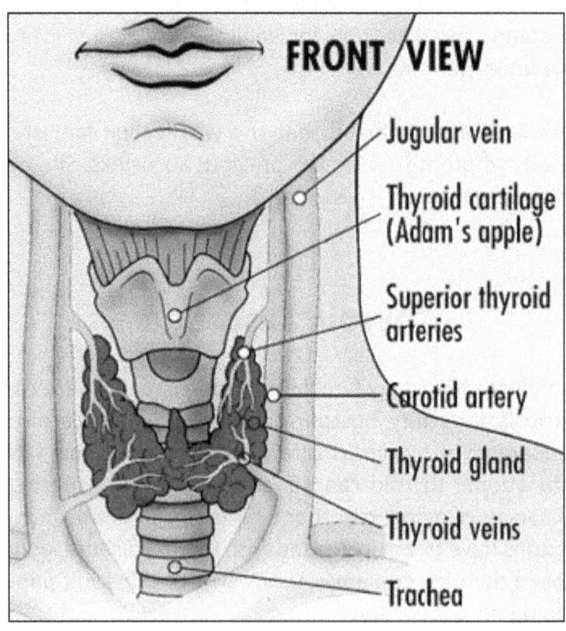

Hypothyroidism can be classified into four grades:

1. Grade 1 has low T3 and low T4
2. Grade 2 has normal T3 and T4 but elevated TSH (above 3.0)
3. Grade 3 has normal T3, T4, and TSH but an aggravated TSH response to TRH challenge
4. Grade 4 has elevated antimicrosomal antibodies and antithyroglobulin antibodies

Hyperthyroidism is a condition in which the thyroid gland makes too much thyroid hormone. The condition is often referred to as an "overactive thyroid." Levels of TSH below 0.3 can indicate hyperthyroidism.

Symptoms of Thyroid Imbalance[125]

Hypothyroid State	Hyperthyroid State
General Symptoms	General Symptoms
a.m. underarm temperature lower than 97.8° F	a.m. underarm temperature higher than 98.2° F
Carpal tunnel syndrome, tendonitis, joint stiffness and swelling, muscle weakness, fibromyalgia, muscle and joint pain, increased rheumatoid arthritis	Fatigue and weakness
Puffy face, especially around the eyes, swelling of hands and feet, weight gain, difficulty losing weight	Weight loss, increased appetite
Slower speech, thick tongue, deep, hoarse voice	Hyperactive state, racing thoughts, nervousness

[125] Complete Natural Medicine Guide to Women's Health Sat Dharam Kaur, ND pg. 417-18

Feels cold all the time, hard to stay warm	Feels warm most of the time, intolerant to heat
Frequent or chronic infections, particularly fungal or viral	Osteoporosis, increased calcium loss in urine
Low DHEA, DHEA-S and pregnenolone	High DHEA-S and pregnenolone sulfate

Hypothyroid State	Hyperthyroid State
Reproductive System	Reproductive System
Low libido	Low or very high libido
PMS, prolonged heavy period, longer menstrual cycle	Irregular periods, usually more frequent, light menstrual flow
Failure to ovulate, infertility, easy miscarriage	Infertility
Premature delivery, stillbirth	
Production of breast milk when not nursing, elevated prolactin	
Decreased sex hormone binding globulin-means more available estrogen, estrogen dominance	Increased sex hormone binding globulin-means less available estrogen
Severe menopausal symptoms	Increased menopausal symptoms
Can have increased susceptibility to breast cancer and other cancers	Increased susceptibility to fibrocystic breast disease, breast cancer, and other cancers

Hypothyroid State	Hyperthyroid State
Cardiovascular System	Cardiovascular System
Slow pulse (less than sixty beats per minute)	Fast pulse (more than one hundred beats per minute), heart palpitations
Low blood pressure	High blood pressure (systolic, shortness of breath)
Sleep apnea	Swollen, red, bulging eyes
High cholesterol, high LDL, and triglycerides, low HDL, macrocytic anemia	Reduced platelets causing easy bleeding
High homocysteine and lipoprotein (a)	Enlarged heart, angina, increased risk of heart disease, increased risk of mitral valve prolapse
	Palpable goiter (swelling) of thyroid gland in throat, atrial fibrillation (fluttering beats), arrhythmia

Hypothyroid State	Hyperthyroid State
Hair, Skin, and Nails	Hair, Skin, and Nails
Hair is dry, brittle, falling out, loss of lateral 1/3 of eyebrow	Hair loss, thinning, greasiness
Dry scaly skin, tendency to eczema, psoriasis, no perspiration	Increased perspiration, vitiligo (white patches)
Yellowing of the skin, especially on the palms	Raised thickened skin over shins
Thin brittle nails with transverse grooves	Soft nails, easily torn, clubbing of fingertips

Hypothyroid State	Hyperthyroid State
Nervous System	Nervous System
Mental-emotional symptoms	Mental-emotional symptoms
Fatigue and muscle weakness, anemia	Over activity, insomnia, eyes sensitive to light
Depression, memory loss, poor concentration	Confusion, disorganized thinking, depression
Slow thinking, emotional instability, agoraphobia, anxiety, irritability, apathy, dementia	Nervousness, anxiety, panic attacks, irritability, mood swings, paranoia, aggression, psychosis
Slow reflexes, particularly Achilles tendon reflex	Shakiness and tremor (especially in hands)

Hypothyroid State	Hyperthyroid State
Gastrointestinal Tract	Gastrointestinal Tract
Constipation, frequent headaches	Frequent bowel movements, diarrhea, increased thirst
Low stomach acid, mineral deficiencies-poor zinc absorption	Increased need for vitamins and minerals; zinc and calcium deficiency

Causes of Hyperthyroidism

Causes of hyperthyroidism:

- About 95% of people diagnosed with hyperthyroidism are found to have a condition called Graves' disease.
- Most of the remaining persons have a condition called nodular thyroid disease.
- A less frequent cause is inflammation of the thyroid gland, which is called thyroiditis.
- Uncommon causes include hormone producing tumors of the pituitary gland or ovary and iodine- induced hyperthyroidism from iodine-containing drugs.

In Graves' disease, the immune system mistakenly directs an immune "attack" against its own healthy cells. Antibodies are manufactured and misdirected against the thyroid gland, mimicking the action of the hormone from the brain (thyroid stimulating hormone) that normally controls the thyroid function. These antibodies act like a switch put into a permanent "on" position. Thyroid cells are continually stimulated to produce and release thyroid hormone, even after blood levels are already high.

Causes of Hypothyroidism

- High or low cortisol, low DHEA
- Estrogen dominance, HRT, BCP
- Progesterone deficiency
- Extreme hormonal fluctuations such as pregnancy, childbirth, and menopause
- Increased or prolonged stress
- Sluggish liver
- Iron deficiency anemia
- Nutritional deficiencies (zinc, selenium copper, manganese, magnesium, vitamins A, B2, B3, B6, B12, C, and E)
- Iodine deficiency
- Heavy metal toxicity (lead, cadmium, and mercury interfere with the conversion of T4 into T3 in the liver)
- Injury to the cervical vertebrae
- Accumulating fluoride levels
- Radiation from x-rays
- Food allergies (gluten, animal protein, and dairy)
- Candida overgrowth and bowel toxicity

Lab Testing

Standard laboratory tests have been established for thyroid disease although there are additional hormones that need to be evaluated when examining the many aspects of thyroid imbalances.

The basal body temperature test can be used as an indication to the presence of a thyroid disorder. Hormones secreted by the thyroid gland reflect the metabolic rate as the body temperature is examined. This is deemed as the most sensitive thyroid test.

Basal Body Temperature Test

1. Shake down the thermometer to below 95°F and place it by your bed before going to bed at night.
2. On waking, place the thermometer in the armpit for a full ten minutes. It is important to move as little as possible; lying and resting with closed eyes is best. Do not get up until the ten minutes have passed.
3. After ten minutes, read and record the temperature and date.
4. Record the temperature for at least three mornings at the same time of day.

A normal temperature is 97.8°F to 98.2°F or 36.6°C to 36.8°C with fluctuations that occur with the menstrual cycle. Menstruating women must perform the test on the second, third, and fourth days of the menstrual cycle. Post-menopausal women can perform the tests on any day. If your temperature is consistently lower than this, there may be an indication of hypothyroidism. If the temperature is consistently higher, this may be an indication of hyperthyroidism.

The following laboratory testing is recommended for thyroid conditions:

Thyroid Hormone Testing	A complete thyroid profile includes free T4, free T3, TSH, and TPO and can indicate the presence of an imbalance in thyroid function. Hypothyroidism includes feeling cold all the time, low stamina, fatigue (particularly in the evening), anxiety, depression, low sex drive, weight gain, and high cholesterol. Hyperthyroidism includes heat intolerance, anxiety, palpitations, weight loss, tired but wired visual disturbances, and insomnia.
Anemia	Low serum iron, hematocrit, and low blood hemoglobin levels can predispose a person to extreme fatigue, contributing to depression.
Adrenal Stress Index	The panel utilizes four saliva samples. Salivary cortisol measurement reflects the free (bioactive) fraction of serum cortisol. The test report shows the awake diurnal cortisol rhythm generated in response to real-life stress. The cortisol/DHEA relationship highlights the many facets of stress maladaptation. The cortisol/DHEA ratio helps determine the projected time for recovery, and the substances (hormones, supplements, botanicals) that promote this recovery. The cortisol/DHEA ratio regulates a multitude of functions. The panel measures P17-OH levels in order to evaluate the efficiency of the conversion of adrenal precursors into cortisol. Certain adrenal fatigue patients who are genetically predisposed to low production of cortisol will not benefit from exogenous supplementation of pregnenolone or progesterone. The panel includes fasting and non-fasting insulin measurements. The insulin values are used to diagnose insulin resistance-functional insulin deficit (pre-diabetes), as well as to correlate elevated cortisol with insulin to help explain glycemic dysregulation problems.
Complete Female Hormone Panel	Estradiol and progesterone levels and their ratio are an index of estrogen/progesterone balance. An excess of estradiol, relative to progesterone, can explain many symptoms in reproductive age-women. Testosterone levels can also be either too high or too low. Testosterone in excess, often caused by ovarian cysts, leads to conditions such as excessive facial and body hair, acne, and oily skin and hair. Polycystic ovarian syndrome (PCOS) is thought to be caused, in part, by insulin resistance. On the other hand, too little testosterone is often caused by excessive stress, medications, contraceptives, and surgical removal of the ovaries. This leads to symptoms of androgen deficiency including loss of libido, thinning skin, vaginal dryness, loss of bone and muscle mass, depression, and memory lapses. SHBG binds tightly to circulating estradiol and testosterone, preventing their rapid metabolism and clearance and limiting their bioavailability to tissues. SHBG gives a good index of the extent of the body's overall exposure to estrogens.
Dried Urine - Iodine	Iodine is an essential component of the thyroid hormones T4 and T3. About 90% of iodine consumed from any source (e.g., diet, supplements, medication) is eliminated in urine within twenty-four to forty-eight hours; therefore, urine is an excellent source to determine an individual's iodine status. When urine iodine levels are outside optimal ranges (too low or high), thyroid hormone synthesis can be abnormal. Therefore, information about urinary iodine status can provide clues to thyroid dysfunction and the means to correct it.

Conventional Pharmaceuticals for Hyperthyroidism

- PTU (propylthiouracil) blocks the conversion of T4 to T3.
- RAI (radioactive iodine) is the conventional treatment of choice for Graves' disease and results in non-reversible hypothyroidism.
- Surgery is another permanent cure for hyperthyroidism is to surgically remove all or part of the thyroid. Surgery is not used for this disease as frequently as the other treatments.

Conventional Pharmaceuticals for Hypothyroidism

- Armor thyroid is used by both conventional and natural medicine practitioners. It is made from the desiccated thyroid from a pig. It contains both T4 and T3 and therefore initiates a better response from many individuals. Dosing with armour can be arduous due to its small therapeutic window which is why many conventional physicians dismiss its usage.
- Levothyroxine (Synthroid, Levothyroid) is the most commonly prescribed drug treatment for hypothyroidism and is a synthetic form of T4. It supresses the function of the thyroid gland and once administered, it will often need to be taken for life. One third of all women taking Synthroid still experience hypothyroid symptoms. Many women have difficulty converting T4 into T3 and therefore Synthroid will be of no therapeutic benefit.

Nutritional Factors Affecting Thyroid Disorders

1. Avoid gluten in the case of autoimmune hypothyroidism (Graves' disease). Gluten will act as an inflammatory agent in the case of autoimmune hypothyroidism. Testing for celiac disease is this case is also recommended but regardless of the outcome of the testing, strict gluten avoidance is recommended.
2. Eat nutrient dense food, preferably organic (to avoid pesticides and other chemicals that place additional stress on the body), including plenty of fruits, vegetables, and cold water fish.
3. Hypothyroidism: Avoid goitrogens food (especially raw) – turnips, cabbages, mustard greens, radishes, horseradish, kale, cassava root, soybeans, peanuts, pine nuts, millet, peaches, pears, spinach, and turnips. If eaten, make sure they are well-cooked (goitrogens reduce thyroid activity by blocking iodine utilization when raw, and cooking inactivates this action).
4. If iodine deficiency is suspected, include kelp, organic/unprocessed sea salt on diet.
5. Avoid processed and refined foods, especially sugar, white flour, and foods containing a lot of additives (food dyes, flavoring as MSG, food coloring, and especially artificial additives).
6. Include food such as whole grains, green vegetables, lean meat, brown rice, and other foods that are rich in B vitamins. Some B vitamins (B2, B3, and B6) are needed for production/conversion of thyroid hormones; they also help build resistance to stress and participate in productions of energy, cell proliferation, and the metabolism of fats, proteins, and carbohydrates.
7. Lima beans, tomatoes, and salmon are high in potassium and vitamin B5. Potassium can help alleviate symptoms of excess adrenaline (avoiding salt to support the sodium–potassium balance) and vitamin B5 (considered the anti-stress vitamin) helps with the functioning and production of the adrenal glands hormones.
8. If possible, buy organic products to reduce intake of pesticide residues and other chemicals, and hormones in animal-foods.
9. Hypothyroidism: Eat sea vegetables such as kelp, dulse, nori, hiziki, and wakami as a source of iodine.

Herbal Medicine Indicated for Thyroid Disorders

Herbal Medicine Indicated for Hyperthyroidism

Lemon Balm *(Melissa officinalis)*

Lemon balm is useful in the treatment of hyperthyroidism as it inhibits TSH and auto-antibodies binding to thyroid TSH receptors, which is likely due to its flavonoids and polyphenols. The active medicinal ingredients in lemon balm include citronella, citral, tannins, and geraniol. Preparations containing lemon balm should clearly list lemon balm or melissa officinalis as an ingredient rather than lemongrass or lemon oil. Used as essential plant oil, as a tincture, or as a tea composed of dry leaves, lemon balm treats anxiety, depression, palpitations, respiratory congestion, allergic reactions, menstrual pain, and nervousness. Lemon balm is used to mildly reduce thyroid hormone levels and symptoms associated with hyperthyroidism. Lemon balm promotes immune system health by fighting bacteria and viruses, which is demonstrated by its ability to reduce fever, spasms, flatulence, and cramps. Lemon balm also promotes detoxification by stimulating liver and gall bladder function. Lemon balm is widely used in Europe as an injection along with lycopus virginicus or bugleweed for treating Graves' disease. Lemon balm is also used as a tonic or tea to reduce and manage symptoms in Graves' disease. Lemon balm slows pituitary function, lowering TSH levels, which, in turn, reduces thyroid hormone levels. Paradoxically, lemon balm is also used to raise thyroid hormone levels in patients with hypothyroidism. Lemon balm strengthens rather than stimulates thyroid function, restoring normal levels to patients with autoimmune thyroid disease.

Motherwort *(Leonorus cardiaca)*

Motherwort is classically used for the treatment of anxiety, depression, heart palpitations, and tachycardia, making it highly appropriate for symptomatic relief in hyperthyroid disease. Chemical analytical and animal studies confirm the herb's sedative, anxiolytic, anti-arrhythmic, and antispasmodic effects. The German Commission E supports the use of motherwort for the treatment of cardiac disorders associated with anxiety and for the symptomatic relief of hyperthyroidism. The alkaloids in motherwort, specifically leonurine, act as a central nervous depressant and hypotensive.

Bugleweed *(Lycopus virginicus)*

The German Commission E Herbal Regulatory Authority monograph recommends the use of bugleweed for people with hyper-functioning thyroid glands. Bugleweed's activity is thought to be mediated by a reduction in thyroid-stimulating hormone (TSH) and thyroxine (T4), inhibition of the conversion of T4 to T3, and inhibition of the receptor-binding and biological activity of Graves' immunoglobulins. In a clinical trial of 905 patients with hyper-functioning thyroid glands, symptoms such as restlessness, palpitations, and headaches improved in 87% of those treated with bugleweed.[126] Bugleweed works as a vascular sedative and is indicated for a rapid pulse and a weak heart, which are typical with hyperthyroidism.

Herbal Medicine Indicated for Hypothyroidism

Bladderwrack *(Fucus vesiculosos)*

Bladderwrack contains three main constituents: iodine, alginic acid, and fucoidan. The iodine in bladderwrack helps those people deficient in this trace mineral to regulate and improve thyroid function, thus it is beneficial for hypothyroidism and goiter. It works as an anti-inflammatory and possesses anti-rheumatic properties to relieve arthritis and rheumatism. Bladderwrack's anti-bacterial properties help ward off bacteria and viruses. The alginic acid constituent, a type of dietary fiber, is useful in relieving constipation, diarrhea, and heartburn. The fucoidan constituent, another type of fiber, contributes to lowering cholesterol and glucose levels. The symptoms of iodine deficiency can

[126] http://www.restorativemedicine.org/pages/hyperthyroidism.html

be relieved with seaweed therapy (bladderwrack) at five grams per day. It contains weak hormone activity with the compound diiodotyrosine, which is the building block for T3 and T4 production.

Ashwagandha *(Withania somnifera)*

Ashwagandha (Withania somnifera) directly affects production of thyroid hormones. Animal studies during the late 1990s demonstrated its ability to directly act on thyroid tissue to bring about a rise in serum levels of thyroid hormones. Serum levels of the thyroid hormone can also be raised in humans and so excessive dosages should be avoided. Studies have been conducted to investigate the effects of ashwagandha on thyroid and liver function. Mice given high doses (1.4g/kg) of the root extract showed significant increases in serum levels of T3 and T4. Furthermore, the extract was shown to reduce hepatic lipid peroxidation significantly while increasing the activity of superoxide dismutase and catalase. These results indicate that ashwagandha stimulates both thyroid and hepatic antioxidant activity. [127]

Coleus *(Coleus Forskohlii)*

Increased cellular cyclic AMP results in inhibition of platelet activation, decreased likelihood of blood clots, reduced release of histamine, decreased allergy symptoms, increased force of contraction of the heart, relaxation of the arteries and other smooth muscles, increased thyroid function, increased fat metabolism, and increased energy, along with possible weight loss. Cyclic AMP and the chemicals it activates comprise a second messenger system that is responsible for carrying out the complex and powerful effects of hormones in the body. Coleus (Coleus forskohlii) contains forskohlin, which is specifically able to mimic the effect of TSH in thyroglobulin (TG) production and promote secretion of T3 and T4.

Guggul *(Commiphora mukul)*

Guggul (Commiphora mukul) is considered a rejuvenating herb and a stimulant in Ayurvedic medicine. The resin of the Commiphora mukul tree, termed "guggul" or "guggulipid," has been associated with thyroid stimulating activity. Guggul causes the thyroid to increase iodine uptake and increase production of thyroid hormones. Studies in both animals and humans have shown that guggul can also modulate cholesterol levels. [128]

Specific Nutrients in the Treatment of Thyroid Disorders

Iodine and Tyrosine

Iodine deficiency is well accepted as the most commonly preventable cause of mental retardation in the world and the most common cause of endocrinopathy (goiter and primary hypothyroidism). Iodine deficiency is most critical in pregnancy due to the consequences for neurological damage during stages of fetal development and lactation. The safety of therapeutic doses of iodine above the established safe limit of 1.0 mg may be evident in the lack of obvious toxicity in the Japanese population that consumes twenty-five times the median intake of iodine consumption in the United States. The Japanese population suffers no demonstrable increased incidence of autoimmune thyroiditis or hypothyroidism. Studies using 3 to 6mg doses to effectively treat fibrocystic breast disease may reveal an important role for iodine in maintaining normal breast tissue architecture and function. Iodine may also have important antioxidant functions in breast tissue and other tissues that concentrate iodine via the sodium iodide symporter. L-tyrosine is an amino acid necessary for the synthesis of thyroxine (T4) and triiodothyronine (T3). In the process of thyroid hormone synthesis, iodine binds to two positions on the tyrosyl ring of tyrosine. Thus, a deficiency of this important amino acid could contribute to low thyroid hormone levels. Studies have found that tyrosine may be beneficial for

---

[127] Kohrle J, Spanka M, Irmscher K, Heschrd. Flavanoid Effects on Transport Metabolism and Action of Thryoid Hormones. Prog. Clin. Biol. Res. 1988;280:323-40

[128] http://www.restorativemedicine.org/pages/hypothyroidism_moderate.html

treating fatigue, which is a common symptom of low thyroid activity. Iodine is necessary for the formation of T4, but appears to have no effect on peripheral conversion of T4 to T3. Goitrogenic foods can cause a relative iodine deficiency by binding to iodine, making it inaccessible for thyroid hormone synthesis.

Trace Minerals

All the essential minerals bound to citric acid, including copper and iron, are required for proper thyroid hormone balance. Besides providing a well-absorbed chelate, citric acid has potential health benefits of its own. As an important Krebs cycle intermediate, it is essential for metabolism in all living organisms. Citric acid has been shown to inhibit urinary precipitation of calcium oxalate and phosphate crystals, preventing the formation of kidney stones. Specifically, zinc (50mg per day) and selenium (200 mcg per day) are an essential part of the conversion of T4 into T3 occurring in the liver.

Vitamin C and the B vitamins riboflavin (B2), niacin (B3), and pyridoxine (B6) are also necessary for normal thyroid manufacture.

Armour Thyroid

Armour Thyroid is a natural, porcine-derived thyroid hormone replacement containing both T4 and T3. Armour thyroid is used in the treatment of hypothyroidism. Thyroid glands are collected from USDA-approved grain-fed pigs. The thyroids are processed, dried, powdered, and compounded to produce Armour Thyroid tablets. Since the amount of thyroid hormone present in the thyroid gland may vary from animal to animal, the T4 and T3 are measured in both the raw material and in the actual tablets. This ensures that Armour Thyroid tablets are the same from tablet to tablet.

A dosage conversion table for all other similar medications is provided below for guidance[129]

Drug	**Thyroid Tablets, USP (Armour® Thyroid)**	**Liotrix Tablets, USP (Thyrolar®a)**	**Liothronine Tablets, USP (Cytomel®b)**	**Levothyroxine Tablets, USP(Unithroid®c, Levoxyl®d, Levothroid®e, Synthroid®f)**
Approx. Dose Equivalent	1/4 grain (15 mg)	1/4		25 mcg (.025 mg)
Approx. Dose Equivalent	1/2 grain (30 mg)	1/2	12.5 mcg	50 mcg (.05 mg)
Approx. Dose Equivalent	1 grain (60 mg)	1	25 mcg	100 mcg (0.1 mg)
Approx. Dose Equivalent	1 1/2 grains (90 mg)	1 1/2	37.5 mcg	150 mcg (0.15 mg)
Approx. Dose Equivalent	2 grains (120 mg)	2	50 mcg	200 mcg (0.2 mg)
Approx. Dose Equivalent	3 grains (180 mg)	3	75 mcg	300 mcg (0.3 mg)

[129] http://armourthyroidcanada.com/faq.html

Top 5 Strategies for Hypothyroid

1. Complete Hormone testing including adrenal hormones, all thyroid hormones, thyroid antibodies, Progesterone, Estrogen, Testosterone and Vitamin D3
2. Food Allergy testing/Celiac testing
3. Strict gluten elimination (regardless of intolerance)/Optimize nutrition through whole foods diet/ Avoid raw goitrogens in large quantities
4. Restore adrenal health before implementing thyroid remedies
5. Supplement with Selenium, Zinc, Tyrosine, Iodine, Vitamin D3, Guggul and Armour thyroid

Teresa's Story - Thyroid Disorder

Teresa is a forty-two-year-old female who presented with the main complaint that she had the inability to lose weight. She stated that she had been dieting her entire life and it was a constant struggle. Teresa is five feet two inches in height and weighs 254 pounds. She exercises approximately six days per week with a mixture of several different types of exercise regimes. She had been exercising for about five years and although she thoroughly enjoyed it, she did not see any weight loss results.

Teresa's diet is generally good, following a well-balanced diet most of the time with the occasional break in regime. Upon review of her diet diary it was noted that she was consuming an excess of grains, dairy, and nuts. She was relying on granola bars for snacks, which are unknowingly weight-inducing.

Lab testing:

- Fasting insulin levels were slightly elevated
- TSH levels were elevated
- Free T3 and Free T4 were normal
- TPO (thyroid antibodies) were normal

Management Plan

Teresa was administered the following natural medicine therapies:

- Soft heat infrared sauna therapy thirty minutes four times per week for additional calorie burning and detoxification
- Thyroid support: iodine (as potassium iodide), zinc (as zinc picolinate), copper (as copper chelate), L-tyrosine, thyroid glandular- two capsules two times per day
- Chromium citrate two capsules two times per day
- Conjugated Linoleic Acid (CLA) one capsule three times per day
- Modified Mediterranean Lifestyle Nutrition Plan to balance hormones (See "Specific Guidelines for Nutritional Lifestyle Management in Weight Gain" section)

Teresa reported back three weeks later to state that she was doing well with the remedies and had started to lose a small amount of weight. She also reported that her long-standing rosacea was starting to clear up after no improvement for years.

Teresa was recommended to stay on the same protocol.

Teresa reported back eight weeks later. Bio Impedance Analysis (BIA) testing revealed that she had lost eight pounds of fat without affecting her lean body mass. Teresa was thrilled with these results, as she had not lost any weight in years. Teresa had gone to her own medical doctor and had her TSH retested and it was now back into the normal range. Teresa was recommended to stay on the protocol.

Estrogen Dominance

Dr. John Lee, the world's authority on natural hormone therapy, coined the phrase "estrogen dominance." This condition occurs when deficient, normal, or excessive estrogen levels are not equally balanced with progesterone. Estrogen and progesterone work synergistically with each other to achieve and maintain hormonal balance in the body. The main cause of many hormonal issues is not the absolute deficiency of estrogen or progesterone but rather when estrogen dominates the hormonal pathway over progesterone.

Presently, the average female begins puberty at approximately age twelve. She seldom lactates, has few children, and menstruates about 350 to 400 times during her lifetime. This frequent menstruation of the modern-day female has been associated with the increased occurrence of a variety of hormonal conditions, including infertility, cancer, fibroids, anemia, migraines, mood swings, abdominal pain, fluid retention, and endometriosis. In stark contrast, one hundred years ago, the average female started her menses at approximately age sixteen. It was common to not only have more children but to conceive at a younger age. She therefore spent more time lactating and had fewer menstrual cycles. In total, women at that time experienced the menstrual cycle only about 100 to 200 times in their lifetimes.

From age thirty-five to fifty (perimenopause), there is a 75% reduction in production of progesterone in the body. Estrogen, during the same period, only declines about 35%. In North America, the prevalence of estrogen dominance syndrome approaches 50% in women over thirty-five years old. By menopause, the total amount of progesterone made is extremely low, while estrogen is still present in the body at about half its pre-menopausal level.

With the gradual drop in estrogen but severe drop in progesterone, there is insufficient progesterone to counteract the amount of estrogen in the body. According to Dr. John Lee, the key to hormonal health is achieving the balance of progesterone and estrogen. For optimum health, the progesterone to estrogen ratio should be approximately between two hundred and three hundred to one of progesterone to estrogen.

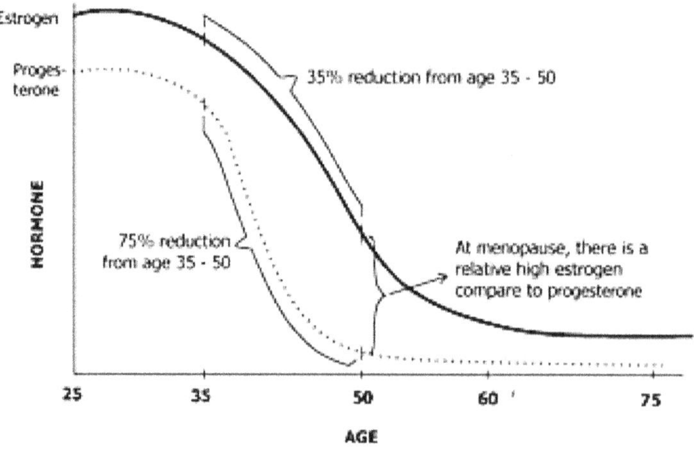

The symptoms and conditions associated with estrogen dominance are: [130]

- Acceleration of the aging process
- Allergies, including asthma, hives, rashes, and sinus congestion
- Autoimmune disorders such as lupus erythematosis and thyroiditis, and possibly Sjoegren's disease
- Breast cancer
- Breast tenderness; fibrocystic breasts
- Cervical dysplasia
- Cold hands and feet as a symptom of thyroid dysfunction
- Copper excess
- Decreased sex drive
- Depression with anxiety or agitation
- Dry eyes
- Early onset of menstruation
- Endometrial (uterine) cancer
- Fat gain, especially around the abdomen, hips, and thighs
- Fatigue
- Foggy thinking
- Gallbladder disease
- Hair Loss
- Headaches
- Hypoglycemia
- Increased blood clotting (increasing risk of stroke)
- Infertility
- Irregular menstrual periods
- Irritability
- Insomnia
- Magnesium deficiency
- Memory loss
- Mood swings
- Osteoporosis
- Polycystic ovaries
- Premenopausal bone loss
- PMS
- Prostate cancer (men only)
- Sluggish metabolism
- Thyroid dysfunction mimicking hypothyroidism
- Uterine cancer
- Uterine fibroids
- Water retention, bloating
- Zinc deficiency

Causes of Estrogen Dominance

During a normal menstrual cycle, estrogen is the naturally dominant hormone for the first two weeks leading up to ovulation. In the last two weeks of the menstrual cycle, estrogen is naturally balanced by progesterone. As a woman

[130] http://www.johnleemd.com/store/estrogen_dom.html

enters perimenopause and begins to experience anovulatory cycles (cycles where no ovulation occurs), estrogen can often go unopposed, causing hormonal imbalance. Anovulatory cycles are, however, only one potential factor in estrogen dominance. In industrialized areas such as North America, there can be many other causes leading to estrogen dominance, including:

1. **Exposure to In Utero Xenoestrogens**: When symptoms of anovulation or progesterone deficiency are noted in puberty, exposure to xenoestrogens in utero can be a factor. Five hundred thousand to eight hundred thousand follicles are created in the embryo, each enclosing an immature ovum when a female embryo develops in the womb. Outward changes to the pregnant mother may not be obvious when exposed to toxic estrogen-like chemicals. However, the fragile ovarian follicles are extremely sensitive to environmental pollutants, which can be toxic. The fetus is therefore increasingly affected by environmental toxins, which may then damage its ovarian follicles.
2. **Exposure to Petrochemical Compounds**: Petrochemical compounds are found in general consumer products such as creams, lotions, soaps, shampoos, perfumes, hair sprays, and room deodorizers. These compounds have estrogen-like chemical structures and may have estrogen-mimicking effects. Other sources of xenoestrogens include car exhausts, petro chemically derived pesticides, herbicides, and fungicides, solvents and adhesives such as those found in nail polish, paint removers, and glues, dry-cleaning chemicals, and practically all plastics and industrial waste such as PCBs and dioxins. Synthetic estrogens from urine of women taking HRT and birth control pills are flushed down the toilet and eventually find their way into the food chain and back into the body. They are fat-soluble and non-biodegradable.[131]
3. **Exposure to Industrial solvents**: Solvents are a family of chemicals that are often overlooked as a common source of xenoestrogens. These chemicals enter the body through the skin and accumulate quickly in the lipid-rich tissues such as myelin (nerve sheath) and adipose (fat). Some common organic solvents include alcohol, such as methanol, aldehydes, such as acetaldehyde, glycol, such as ethylene glycol, and ketones, such as acetone. They are commonly found in cosmetics, fingernail polish and fingernail polish remover, glues, paints, varnishes, and other types of finishes, cleaning products, carpets, fiberboards, and other processed woods. Pesticides and herbicides such as lawn and garden sprays and indoor insect sprays are also sources of minute amounts of xenoestrogens. While the amount may be small in each, the additive effect from years of chronic exposure can lead to estrogen dominance.[132]
4. **Exposure to Hormone Replacement Therapy (HRT):** The hormones used in HRT are different in structure to the hormones naturally found in humans. This differing structure is processed in a lab in order to patent the medication and therefore make an economic profit. One of the most popular HRT drugs is called Premarin and has been the mainstay choice of doctors prescribing HRT. Premarin contains 48% estrone and only a very small amount of progesterone, which is insufficient to have a significant opposing effect. The excessive estrogen from HRT can lead to an increased chance of DNA damage and can result in endometrial and breast cancer.
5. **Exposure to Xenoestrogens in Commercially Raised Cattle and Poultry:** Twenty-five million pounds per year, or half the antibiotics used in the United States each year, are used in livestock. These antibiotics enter our food supply and result in hormone disruption as we consume them as meat. In poultry farms, it now only takes six weeks to grow a chicken to full size, compared to four months in 1940. Feed containing a cocktail of hormone-disrupting toxins including pesticides, antibiotics, and drugs is used to combat disease and is necessary due to the overcrowded conditions of animal warehouses.
6. **Exposure to Commercially Grown Fruits and Vegetables Containing Pesticides**: Over the years, but especially over the past 50 years several billion pounds of pesticides have been released into the environment. These pesticides are similar in structure to estrogen and therefore can disrupt our hormonal system.

[131] http://www.drlam.com/articles/Estrogen_Dominance.asp

[132] http://www.drlam.com/articles/Estrogen_Dominance.asp

Pesticides that were previously banned make their way back to our food supply illegally. Approximately five billion pounds of chemicals have been added to the world each year in the form of pesticides, herbicides, fungicides, and other biocides. It is estimated that the average person eats seventy-five pounds of illegal pesticides per year just by following the guidelines of eating five servings of fruits and vegetables a day, if purchasing them from non-organic sources.[133]

7. **Overproduction of estrogen**. Excessive estrogen can arise from ovarian cysts or tumors.
8. **Stress.** The effects of chronic stress cause a reduction in progesterone levels and leads to adrenal gland exhaustion. This causes the hormonal pathway to favor estrogen over progesterone. The adrenal glands are further depleted as excessive estrogen causes insomnia and anxiety. The cycle continues, as there is a further reduction in progesterone output and even more estrogen dominance results. After a few years in this vicious cycle, the adrenal glands become exhausted. This dysfunction leads to blood sugar imbalance, hormonal imbalances, and chronic fatigue.
9. **Obesity.** Fat has an enzyme that converts adrenal steroids to estrogen. The higher the fat intake, the higher the conversion of fat to estrogen. Studies have shown that estrogen and progesterone levels fell in women who switched from a typical high-fat, refined-carbohydrate diet to a low-fat, high-fiber and plant-based diet even though they did not adjust their total calorie intake.
10. **Liver diseases**. Estrogen breakdown is reduced in individuals suffering from liver diseases, such as cirrhosis from excessive alcohol intake. Estrogen levels increase in the body when the liver is unable to complete the detoxification process due to conditions, drugs or alcohol that can impair liver function.
11. **Deficiency of Vitamin B6 and Magnesium**. These are important constituents of hormonal balance and are necessary for the neutralization of estrogen in the liver. Too much estrogen also tends to create deficiencies of zinc, magnesium, and B vitamins. Increased consumption of sugar, fast food, and processed food leads to a depletion of magnesium.
12. **Increase in caffeine consumption.** Caffeine intake from all sources has been linked to higher estrogen levels. This is true regardless of age, body mass index (BMI), and caloric intake, smoking, and alcohol habits. Studies have shown that women who consumed at least 500 mg of caffeine daily, the equivalent of four or five cups of coffee, had nearly 70% more estrogen during the early follicular phase than women who consume no more than 100 mg of caffeine daily, or less than one cup of coffee. Tea is not much better as it contains about half the amount of caffeine as coffee. The exception is herbal teas, which contain no caffeine.

Diagnosing Estrogen Dominance

The diagnosis of estrogen dominance can be achieved through lab testing.

Complete Female Hormone Panel	Estradiol and progesterone levels and their ratio are an index of estrogen/progesterone balance. An excess of estradiol, relative to progesterone, can explain many symptoms in reproductive age-women. Testosterone levels can also be either too high or too low. Testosterone in excess, often caused by ovarian cysts, leads to conditions such as excessive facial and body hair, acne, and oily skin and hair. Polycystic ovarian syndrome (PCOS) is thought to be caused, in part, by insulin resistance. On the other hand, too little testosterone is often caused by excessive stress, medications, contraceptives, and surgical removal of the ovaries. This leads to symptoms of androgen deficiency including loss of libido, thinning skin, vaginal dryness, loss of bone and muscle mass, depression, and memory lapses.

[133] http://www.drlam.com/articles/Estrogen_Dominance.asp

	SHBG binds tightly to circulating estradiol and testosterone, preventing their rapid metabolism and clearance and limiting their bioavailability to tissues. SHBG gives a good index of the extent of the body's overall exposure to estrogens.

Nutritional Factors Affecting Estrogen Dominance

The following table illustrates the specific dietary recommendations to reduce estrogen dominance:

Food Group	Foods To Include	Foods to Exclude
Legumes	All legumes and legume products, especially soy products	None
Vegetables	All, especially cruciferous (see additional note #1) and sea vegetables (various seaweeds)	None
Fruits	All whole and dry fruits especially lemons and limes	None
Grains	All whole grains and whole-grain products especially rye	Non-whole grains, refined flours, refined flour products
Nuts/Seeds	All nuts and seeds and their butters, especially flax seeds, walnuts, and pumpkin seeds (in their raw form only)(See additional note #2)	None
Fish	All, especially cold water fish: salmon, sardines, tuna, and halibut are an excellent source of omega-3 fatty acids	Salted or cured fish
Eggs	From organically raised hens	Non-organic eggs
Poultry/Meat	Organic meats and poultry (See additional note #3)	Non-organic meats and poultry, salted and cured meats
Dairy	Organic dairy products and soy, nut and grain dairy substitutes	Non-organic dairy products
Oils	Organic cold-pressed, unrefined, seed and nut oils, especially flax seed, walnut, sesame, canola, and olive oil (See additional note #4)	Refined vegetable oils, butter, lard, margarine, shortening, and saturated or hydrogenated fats
Beverages	Mineral or filtered water, herbal tea, fresh fruit juice	Alcohol, coffee
Sweeteners	Brown rice syrup, fruit sweetener, molasses, stevia	Reined or artificial sweeteners, chocolate
Spices and Herbs	Especially nutmeg, anise, thyme, sage, fennel, caraway, turmeric	High sodium foods and salt

Additional Notes:

1. Cruciferous vegetables include: broccoli, cauliflower, all cabbages, Brussels sprouts, kale, bok choy, arugula, mustard greens, and watercress.
2. Omega-3 and some omega-6 fatty acids help to counteract symptoms associated with hormonal imbalance and should be consumed daily.
3. Non-organically raised livestock are often given hormones to improve their growth; unfortunately, these hormones can be passed on to the consumer and negatively influence hormone balance.
4. Important: Do not cook with oils that are not specified for cooking or baking, such as flaxseed or walnut oils. Olive, canola, and sesame oils are good choices for cooking or baking. Use flaxseed, olive, sesame, or walnut oils for homemade salad dressings. These provide valuable omega-3 and omega-6 fatty acids. Refrigerate all oils and dressings.

Estrogen Metabolism

The most active estrogen circulating in the body is estradiol (E2). It is a steroidal hormone that is metabolized in the liver. E2 has a half-life of approximately three hours. There are multiple pathways with widely different biological activities that convert E2 to metabolites.

The second most potent estrogen is estrone. Through enzymatic reactions, it is easily converted back and forth from estradiol. Estrone and estradiol are metabolized by a process called hydroxylation. The products from hydroxylation are converted into estriol (E3) or are processed and secreted out of the body and excreted in the urine.

Several hundred micrograms of estradiol is produced in normal pre-menopausal women every day. Some of this estradiol finds its way to binding with the nuclei in a wide variety of tissues, resulting in genetic transcription as well as cellular division. While the production of estrogen is going on, a similar amount of estradiol is removed from the body, primarily in the liver. Estradiol is continually balanced through a production and destruction process.

The metabolites are all part of the estrogen family because the metabolites are estrogen derivatives. They all possess estrogenic properties in varying degrees. An indication of the metabolites' estrogenic potency is the degree of the hydroxylation, either through the two-hydroxylation or sixteen alpha-hydroxylation process.

The most prevalent metabolites of estradiol and estrone are metabolites such as 2-(OH)-estrone or 2-(OH)-estradiol, and are considered good estrogen. They are derived from hydroxylation of estrone. People who are obese and women who consume a diet high in animal fat have been shown to have decreased levels of these good estrogens. Consistent moderate exercise, a diet high in protein and low in fat, and consumption of food containing indol-3-carbinol, such as cabbage and broccoli, will increase the levels of good estrogen.

Another metabolite of estrone is called the 16 alpha-(OH) estrone, which has been proven to be more potent than estradiol. This is called the genotoxic form of estrogen, or bad estrogen. The risk of breast cancer is increasing significantly due to its ability to combine with estrogen receptors and transform the nuclei to synthesize DNA. It is also called the transforming estrogen. Another bad metabolite is 4-(OH)-estrone, a free radical generator that is currently being tested as possibly being a bad estrogen.

It is obvious that there are good and bad estrogens. Two-(OH)-estrone is considered good, being that it is a potent antioxidant and has anti-cancer properties. Estrones that are considered bad are 4-(OH)-estrone and 16-alpha (OH) because they are free radical generators and at high levels, they are considered to be important indicators of cancer risk. The ideal ratio of 2-(OH)-estrone to 16-alpha-(OH)-estrone as measured in the urine is 2.0 or more.

Herbal Medicine Indicated for Estrogen Dominance

Milk Thistle *(Silymarin marianus)*

Much research has been done on a special extract of milk thistle known as Silymarin, a group of flavonoid compounds. These compounds protect the liver from damage and enhance the detoxification process. Silymarin prevents damage to the liver by acting as an antioxidant and is much more effective than vitamins E and C. Numerous studies have demonstrated its protective effect on the liver and it also works by preventing the depletion of glutathione. The higher the glutathione concentration, the greater the liver's capacity to detoxify harmful chemicals. Silymarin has been shown to increase the level of glutathione by up to 35%. In human studies, Silymarin has been shown to exhibit positive effects in treating liver diseases of various kinds, including cirrhosis, chronic hepatitis, fatty infiltration of the liver, and inflammation of the bile duct. Dosage: standardized extract 200 to 800 mg a day

Curcumin *(Curcuma longa)*

Several studies have illustrated curcumin's hepatoprotective effects. This has led researchers to suggest its use in protecting the liver from exogenous insults from environmental toxins, including carbon tetrachloride and acetaminophen. Curcumin also has the capacity to increase bile flow and solubility, making it of potential benefit for someone with a tendency to form gallstones. The hepatoprotective effects of curcumin may stem from its potent antioxidant activity. In addition to its antioxidant effects, curcumin has been shown to enhance liver detoxification by increasing the activity of glutathione S-transferase, an enzyme necessary to conjugate glutathione with a wide variety of toxins in order to facilitate their removal from the body. Dosage: 500mg-2000mg per day

Specific Nutrients for Estrogen Dominance

Diindolylmethane (DIM)

DIM is a powerful metabolizer of estrogen, assisting in removing excess estrogen and benefiting individuals with conditions associated with estrogen dominance. Supplementation with DIM can help promote proper estrogen levels in women through the pre- and perimenopausal years, and in men experiencing higher estrogen levels. These conditions include, but are not limited to, uterine fibroid tumors, fibrocystic breasts, and glandular dysfunction. DIM can also benefit men by improving estrogen dominance-related health issues such as hair loss, atherosclerosis, prostrate problems, lowered libido, and impotency. DIM promotes testosterone action, which improves mood, fights depression, boosts libido, improves cardiovascular health, improves memory, and supports muscular development. DIM is a balancer of estrogen metabolism. It increases 2-hydroxyestrone (2-OHE), which is also known as the good or protective estrogen. Dosage: 70 mg to 400 mg per day

N-acetylcysteine (NAC)

N-acetylcysteine (NAC) is the precursor of both the amino acid L-cysteine and reduced glutathione (GSH). Animal and human studies of NAC have shown it to be a powerful antioxidant and a therapeutic agent for heavy metal toxicity and other diseases characterized by free radical, oxidative damage. As a source of sulfhydryl groups, NAC stimulates glutathione synthesis, enhances glutathione- S-transferase activity, promotes liver detoxification by inhibiting xenobiotic biotransformation, and acts as a powerful nucleophile, capable of scavenging free radicals. Historically, the most prevalent and well-accepted use of NAC has been as an antidote for acetaminophen (Tylenol) poisoning. The resultant liver toxicity is due to an acetaminophen metabolite that depletes the hepatocytes of glutathione and causes hepatocellular damage and possibly even death. NAC administered intravenously or orally within twenty-four hours of overdose is effective at preventing liver toxicity; however, improvement is most notable if treatment is initiated within eight to ten hours of acetaminophen overdose. NAC has also been effective for poisoning by carbon tetrachloride, acrylonitriles, halothane, paraquat, acetaldehyde, coumarin, and interferon. In addition to its dramatic effects on liver poisoning, NAC is effective in promoting normal liver detoxification. Dosage: 350 mg to 2,000 mg a day

Calcium D-Glucarate

Calcium D-glucarate is a botanical extract found in grapefruit, apples, oranges, broccoli, spinach, and Brussels sprouts. It is also made naturally in small quantities by the body. Scientists are discovering that it appears to protect against cancer and other diseases via a different mechanism than antioxidants such as vitamin C, carotenoids, and folic acid. These vitamin antioxidants work by neutralizing toxic free radical damage in the body. However, there are other mechanisms by which the human body can detoxify itself, such as conjugation and glucuronidation.

Conjugation and glucuronidation are detoxification processes that occur when toxins, carcinogens, and used hormones are combined with and bound to water-soluble substances in the liver, thus making them easier to remove from the body. D-glucarate has been shown to support this vital process of removal by inhibiting an enzyme called beta-glucuronidase that can break bonds between toxins and used hormones, allowing them to be re-circulated into the bloodstream rather than excreted.

D-glucarate may directly detoxify any environmental agents responsible for cancer formation. It has been postulated that D-glucarate exerts some of its effects by equilibrium conversion to D-glucarolactone, which is a potent beta-glucuronidase inhibitor. This is one of the most important nutrients to enhance liver function. Dosage: 250 mg to 1,000 mg a day

Omega 3 Fatty Acids- Fish Oil

A diet low in fish oil has a decreased ratio of 2-(OH)-estrogen to 16-alpha-(OH)-estrogen and thereby, an increased cancer risk. Intake of fish oil also has been observed to inhibit the formation of human breast cancer cells in laboratory studies. Several theories have been proposed to explain the link between the high intake of fish oil and the low risk of cancer. Among the most important is the inhibition of eicosanoid production from arachodoinic acid and omega-6. Eicosanoids belong to a class of compounds that are derived from poly and saturated fatty acids including prostaglandins, hydroxyl, prostaglandins, and leukotrienes. Prostaglandins are unsaturated fats and are a group of lipids made at sites of tissue damage or infection that are involved in dealing with injury and illness. They control processes such as inflammation, blood flow, formation of blood clots and the induction of labour. Prostaglandin E2 (PGE2) has been linked to the formation of several types of breast and prostate cancer. Tumor cells generally produce a large amount of AA derived from PGE2, and fish oil inhibits the oxidation of AA to PGE2. Eicosanoids derived from AA are also related to the modulation of estrogen metabolism. DHA has been shown to improve the response of breast tumors to cytotoxic agents. Dosage: 500 mg to 10,000 mg a day

Bioidentical Progesterone Cream

The USP progesterone used for hormone replacement comes from plant fats and oils, usually from a substance called diosgenin that is extracted from a very specific type of wild yam that grows in Mexico, or from soybeans. In the laboratory, diosgenin is chemically synthesized into real human progesterone. The other human steroid hormones, including estrogen, testosterone, progesterone, and the cortisones, are also nearly always synthesized from diosgenin. Because progesterone is very fat-soluble, it is easily absorbed through the skin. Progesterone is absorbed into capillary blood from subcutaneous fat. Thus, absorption is best at skin sites where people blush: face, neck, chest, breasts, inner arms, and palms of the hands. Dosage: For premenopausal women, the usual dose is 15 mg to 24 mg per day for fourteen days before expected menses, stopping approximately one day before menses. For postmenopausal women, the dose that generally works best is 15 mg per day for twenty-five days of the calendar month. (Bioidentical progesterone cream should contain 450 mg to 500 mg of progesterone per ounce and 900 mg to 1000 mg per two ounce container.)

Top 5 Strategies for Estrogen Dominance

1. Complete Hormone testing
2. Reduce and eliminate exposure to xenoestrogens
3. Liver detoxification
4. Consume a nutrient dense, organic whole food diet
5. Supplement with DIM, Calcium D-glucarate, NAC, Vitamin D3, Zinc, Curcumin, Omega 3's and Bioidentical Progesterone when needed

Tina's Story- Estrogen Dominance

Tina is a thirty-seven-year-old female who presented with the main concern of weight gain. Tina stated that before she had children, she had no weight issues at all and could virtually eat anything she wanted without consequence. Tina stuck to a very strict eating plan that should have produced the desired effects of weight loss, but instead, she only lost a total of four pounds over the course of a six month period. Tina also enjoyed going to boot camp classes—intense workouts designed to achieve weight loss goals—four times per week.

Tina had been a hairdresser for fifteen years and recently made a career change into the field of customer management. She is the mother of three teenage children.

Although Tina slept an average of seven to nine hours per night, she still complained of fatigue and related it to performing intense physical exercise. Tina's cycles were regular but were consistently heavier in flow since having children and she also experienced breast tenderness, weight gain, mood swings, and cramping with each cycle.

Lab testing:

- Low progesterone levels
- High estrogen levels
- Low progesterone to estrogen ratio
- Poor hepatic conversion of T4 into T3

Management Plan

Tina was administered the following natural medicine therapies:

- Modified Mediterranean Lifestyle Nutrition Plan to balance hormones (See "Specific Guidelines for Nutritional Lifestyle Management in Weight Gain" section)
- Estrogen detoxification: DIM, calcium D-glucarate, SGS (standardized to contain 30mg glucoraphanin glucosinolate), hops extract (0.12% 8-prenylnaringenin) two capsules with breakfast
- Bioidentical progesterone cream one pump on days fourteen through twenty-eight of her menstrual cycle
- Thyroid support: iodine (as potassium iodide), zinc (as zinc picolinate), copper (as copper chelate), L-tyrosine, thyroid glandular- two capsules two times per day
- Medical food: a powdered medical food designed to nutritionally support the management of conditions associated with metabolic syndrome (including altered body composition)

Tina returned for a follow-up four weeks later to report that she had been feeling well with the plan but felt that it was too soon to tell. BIA testing revealed a two pound weight loss in fat.

Tina was recommended to stay on the same protocol.

Tina returned eight weeks later to report that her cycles were dramatically improved. In fact, she had experienced no symptoms in the previous two cycles was very happy about this. She continued to battle with fatigue but not as much as before. She was recommended to find an alternative form of exercise that was not so physically demanding to see if her energy improved. Tina had been battling with nutrition, as her children and career kept her too busy to prepare meals and snacks in advance. By the time she got home, there was no time left to prepare a healthy meal. Due to this situation, the choice would be something fast and not on her plan. She felt ashamed of this fact but was assured that it was normal for struggles like this to occur.

The following changes were made to Tina's protocol:

- Stay with the above recommendations
- Purchase a membership to www.eatcleanmenus.com, which is a clean eating menu planning website

Tina came for a follow-up twelve weeks later. She happily reported that she had lost seven pounds and BIA testing confirmed those findings. Tina also stated that she no longer had any hormonal issues with PMS. She was very thankful for Eat Clean Menus, as it gave her the tools she needed to have healthy meals all the time. Tina was recommended to stay with the current medical foods, thyroid support, and meal plan but to slowly decrease the progesterone cream to one-half of a pump for one month, to one-fourth of a pump for one month, and then to go completely off the progesterone cream. She was also advised to continue with the estrogen detoxification remedy but at half the dose for continual detoxification because of the years of accumulated endocrine disruptors to which she was exposed during her hairdressing career.

Premenstrual Syndrome (PMS)

Premenstrual syndrome (PMS) is a common disorder in women of reproductive age that is characterized by the cyclic recurrence of physical, affective, and cognitive (or performance) symptoms. The symptoms typically occur in the second half of the menstrual cycle, resolve after menses begins, and are often absent during the early phase of the menstrual cycle. As many as 85% of menstruating women experience one or more symptoms of PMS. Approximately 5% to 10% of women have symptoms severe enough to be debilitating.[134] PMS affects women of all cultures and socioeconomic levels but types of symptoms and levels of discomfort vary from woman to woman and may have cultural influences. More than three hundred symptoms have been associated with PMS.[135] Among the most prominent and consistently described symptoms are depression, anxiety, irritability, craving for sweet or salty foods, headaches, weight gain, fluid retention, breast pain and swelling, abdominal bloating, and acne flare-ups on the face and shoulders. Some of the other commonly associated symptoms include:

- Abdominal bloating
- Abdominal cramping
- Accident proneness, coordination difficulties
- Acne, hives
- Aggression, rage
- Alcohol intolerance

---

134 The American College of Obstetricians and Gynecologists. *ACOG News Release*. Accessed April 5, 2004 from http://www.acog.org/from_home/publications/press_releases/nr03-31-00-1.cfm.

135 Halbreich U. The etiology, biology, and evolving pathology of premenstrual syndromes. Psychoneuroendocrinology 2003; 28(3 Suppl):S55-S99.

- Anxiety, irritability, suicidal thoughts
- Asthma
- Back pain
- Breast swelling and pain
- Bruising
- Confusion
- Depression, withdrawal from others, emotional lability
- Edema
- Exacerbation of pre-existing conditions (e.g., lupus, arthritis, ulcers, herpes)
- Fatigue, lethargy
- Fainting (vasovagal syncope)
- Food binges, salt cravings, sweet cravings
- Headache, migraine
- Heart palpitations
- Insomnia
- Joint swelling and pain
- Nausea
- Seizures
- Sex drive changes
- Sinus problems
- Sore throat
- Urinary difficulties

Hormonal fluctuations during the menstrual cycle have been identified as possible underlying causes of menstrual complaints. A normal menstrual cycle in a woman of reproductive age can be divided into three distinct phases: follicular, ovulatory, and luteal.[136]

Follicular Phase—The follicular phase, which initiates the development of an ovarian follicle, is characterized by a rise in estrogen and follicle stimulating hormone (FSH). It begins when gonadotropin-releasing hormone (GnRH) is secreted from neurons in the hypothalamus and transported to the anterior pituitary, stimulating the anterior pituitary to release FSH. FSH stimulates the development of an ovarian follicle. The rising FSH levels also activate aromatase and FSH receptors, resulting in a higher ratio of estrogens to androgens within the follicle. The rising estrogen levels trigger a negative feedback mechanism on the pituitary—inhibiting the pituitary production of FSH—while a positive feedback mechanism stimulates the pituitary to begin secreting luteinizing hormone (LH).

Ovulatory Phase—A peak in LH and estrogen levels takes place in the middle of the menstrual cycle, predicting ovulation. At this point, the follicle has acquired LH receptors and is responsive to LH, which induces the secretion of enzymes to rupture the follicular wall, releasing the egg into a fallopian tube. The rise in LH also allows the remaining follicular cells, which organize on the corpus luteum (a process known as luteinization), to secrete small amounts of progesterone.

Luteal Phase—The shift from estrogen dominance to progesterone dominance and the gradual reduction in LH and FSH levels characterize the luteal phase. This is the last part of the menstrual cycle in which premenstrual symptoms can begin, followed by their remittance during the beginning of the subsequent follicular phase. In the luteal phase, the egg travels through the fallopian tube, wherein fertilization can occur. The ruptured follicle, which has formed

---

[136] Natural Interventions for Premenstrual Syndrome BY JOSEPH L. MAYO, MD, FACOG APPLIED NUTRITIONAL SCIENCE REPORTS 2004 by Advanced Nutrition Publications, Inc.

the corpus luteum, continues to release moderate amounts of estrogen and also starts to secrete progesterone. If the egg is fertilized, it will implant on the lining of the uterus; if it is not fertilized, the corpus luteum will disintegrate, stopping its production of estrogen and progesterone. This rapid fall in estrogen and progesterone causes the lining of the uterus to shed along with the unfertilized egg and blood, marking the beginning of menses and the end of the menstrual cycle.

Causes of PMS

The exact cause of PMS is not fully understood and may be related to a number of factors. The current theories on the underlying causes focus mostly on levels of sex hormones (e.g., estrogen, progesterone) and neurotransmitters (i.e., brain chemicals that control mood), dietary influences, and emotional factors.

Dietary Factors Influencing PMS

- Diets high in animal fats have been shown to increase prostaglandin (PGE2) production and aggravate PMS symptoms.
- Increased alcohol consumption during the premenstrual phase interferes with the liver's ability to detoxify excess circulating hormones.
- Nutritional deficiencies such as calcium, magnesium, zinc, vitamin B6, vitamin E, and essential fatty acids contribute to PMS.
- Increased caffeine consumption causes an imbalance of cortisol and blood sugar and further inhibits the liver's ability to balance serotonin, estrogen, and progesterone, leading to breast tenderness and swelling.

Many factors can contribute to or trigger PMS by causing hormonal changes in the body, including:

- High consumption of dairy products
- Excessive consumption of caffeine (soft drinks, coffee, chocolate)
- Excessive consumption of high glycemic foods
- A relatively high blood level of estrogen
- A relatively low blood level of progesterone
- Diet that leads to increased levels of the hormone prostaglandin F2
- Excess body weight
- Low levels of vitamins C and E and selenium
- Magnesium deficiency
- Lack of exercise

Other factors:

- Perimenopause
- Discontinuing birth control pills
- Childbirth or termination of pregnancy
- Tubal ligation
- Unusual trauma
- Decreased light associated with autumn and winter

PMS has been divided into four categories according to specific sets of symptoms.

PMS Symptoms and Imbalances

PMS-A ANXIETY *(affects 65% to 75% of PMS sufferers)*	PMS-A ANXIETY *(affects 65% to 75% of PMS sufferers)*
Symptoms	**Imbalances**
• Anxiety • Tension, feeling on edge • Irritability, anger • Finding fault with one's partner • Mood swings • Insomnia • Depression • Suicidal thoughts • Low self esteem • Sensitivity to rejection or criticism • Feeling overwhelmed	• Too much estrogen relative to progesterone in the latter half of the menstrual cycle (luteal phase) • Low serotonin • Drop in TSH and cortisol (thyroid and adrenal function) during luteal phase • High epinephrine/cortisol ratio • Increased testosterone

PMS-C CRAVINGS *(affects 33% of PMS sufferers)*	PMS-C CRAVINGS *(affects 33% of PMS sufferers)*
Symptoms	**Imbalances**
• Cravings (sweets, chocolate, carbohydrates) • Increased appetite • Headaches • Fatigue • Fainting spells, dizziness • Heart palpitations	• Drop in cortisol causes sugar cravings • Imbalance in body's regulation of insulin and cortisol • Low serotonin may cause CHO cravings—CHO ingestion can temporarily raise serotonin levels • Deficiency in PGEI (Prostaglandin E1), a beneficial prostaglandin can cause low blood sugar with sweet and food cravings

PMS-D DEPRESSION *(affects 25% to 35% of PMS sufferers)*	PMS-D DEPRESSION *(affects 25% to 35% of PMS sufferers)*
Symptoms	**Imbalances**
• Depression • Forgetfulness • Confusion • Lethargy, sluggishness, easily tired • Withdrawal, disinterest in usual activities • Insomnia	• Drop in thyroid hormones during the luteal phase may trigger symptoms • Low serotonin levels may cause low melatonin

PMS-H HYPERHYDRATION/WATER RETENTION *(affects over 50% of PMS sufferers)*	PMS-H HYPERHYDRATION/WATER RETENTION *(affects over 50% of PMS sufferers)*
Symptoms	**Imbalances**
• Breast swelling and tenderness • Abdominal bloating • Weight gain of over 3 lbs. (1.5 kg) • Swelling of the face, hands, fingers, and ankles	• Increased estrogen relative to progesterone (estrogen causes salt and water retention) • Increased aldosterone and adrenal elevation during stress, which causes water retention • Excess sugar intake causes insulin levels to rise quickly, triggering sodium and water retention • Elevated prolactin, which may be higher when the thyroid is underactive, when dopamine levels are lower, or there is excess estrogen

Laboratory Testing for PMS

The signs and symptoms of PMS are not unique, and there are currently no laboratory tests to confirm a definitive diagnosis. There are, however, many contributing factors that can be tested in laboratories to refine the treatment protocol. Uncovering hormonal imbalances is imperative to treating the underlying causes of PMS. The following lab panels have been proven effective in identifying any imbalances in regard to PMS:

Neurotransmitter Testing	Medical science has discovered that neurotransmitters are at the foundation of many psychiatric and neurological disorders. Imbalances in neurotransmission, due to excessive or deficient neurotransmitter levels at the synaptic cleft, are associated with depression, insomnia, anxiety, behavioural disorders, memory disorders, and a spectrum of other brain-related functions. Because neurotransmitters play an integral role in these disease states, they are prime targets for treating nervous system disorders and mental health concerns. Neurotransmitters are recognized as the primary biochemical messengers of the central and peripheral nervous systems. Studies have demonstrated that urinary neurotransmitter measures are reflective of circulating levels as evidenced by renal neurotransmitter clearance mechanisms. Laboratory methodology for the accurate assessment of urinary neurotransmitter levels has been established. Urinary measures are not recognized as a direct reflection of central activity, however, definite associations exist. The ability to measure neurotransmitters has led to the generation of scientific literature that demonstrates that urinary neurotransmitter measurements have clinical value as representative biomarkers of various neurological, immunological, and endocrinological conditions.
Adrenal Stress Index	The panel utilizes four saliva samples. Salivary cortisol measurement reflects the free (bioactive) fraction of serum cortisol. The test report shows the awake diurnal cortisol rhythm generated in response to real-life stress.

	The cortisol/DHEA relationship highlights the many facets of stress maladaptation. The cortisol/DHEA ratio helps determine the projected time for recovery, and the substances (hormones, supplements, and botanicals) that promote this recovery. The cortisol/DHEA ratio regulates a multitude of functions. The panel measures P17-OH levels in order to evaluate the efficiency of the conversion of adrenal precursors into cortisol. Certain adrenal fatigue patients who are genetically predisposed to low production of cortisol will not benefit from exogenous supplementation of pregnenolone or progesterone. The panel includes fasting and non-fasting insulin measurements. The insulin values are used to diagnose insulin resistance-functional insulin deficit (pre-diabetes), as well as to correlate elevated cortisol with insulin to help explain glycemic dysregulation problems.
Complete Female Hormone Panel	Estradiol and progesterone levels and their ratio are an index of estrogen/progesterone balance. An excess of estradiol, relative to progesterone, can explain many symptoms in reproductive agewomen. Testosterone levels can also be either too high or too low. Testosterone in excess, often caused by ovarian cysts, leads to conditions such as excessive facial and body hair, acne, and oily skin and hair. Polycystic ovarian syndrome (PCOS) is thought to be caused, in part, by insulin resistance. On the other hand, too little testosterone is often caused by excessive stress, medications, contraceptives, and surgical removal of the ovaries. This leads to symptoms of androgen deficiency including loss of libido, thinning skin, vaginal dryness, loss of bone and muscle mass, depression, and memory lapses. SHBG binds tightly to circulating estradiol and testosterone, preventing their rapid metabolism and clearance and limiting their bioavailability to tissues. SHBG gives a good index of the extent of the body's overall exposure to estrogens.
Thyroid Hormone Testing	A complete thyroid profile includes free T4, free T3, TSH, and TPO and can indicate the presence of an imbalance in thyroid function. Hypothyroidism includes feeling cold all the time, low stamina, fatigue (particularly in the evening), anxiety, depression, low sex drive, weight gain, and high cholesterol. Hyperthyroidism includes heat intolerance, anxiety, palpitations, weight loss, tired but wired feeling, visual disturbances, and insomnia.
Anemia	Low serum iron, hematocrit, and low blood hemoglobin levels can predispose a person to extreme fatigue, contributing to depression.

Conventional Pharmaceutical Medications Indicated for PMS

Conventional medicine is limited in therapeutic treatments for PMS. Typically, a patient is administered either the birth control pill (BCP) or an antidepressant (SSRI).

Selective Serotonin Reuptake Inhibitors (SSRIs)

SSRIs are believed to increase the extracellular level of the neurotransmitter serotonin by inhibiting its reuptake into the presynaptic cell, increasing the level of serotonin in the synaptic cleft available to bind to the postsynaptic receptor. They have varying degrees of selectivity for the other monoamine transporters, with pure SSRIs having only a weak affinity for the noradrenaline and dopamine transporter.[137] The antidepressants Prozac (fluoxetine) and sertraline are effective when taken for the two weeks preceding the menstrual period as they prolong serotonin activity. There are many side effects associated with this type of therapy such as stomach upset, anxiety, dizziness, sexual dysfunction, drowsiness, insomnia, weight gain or loss and headache.

Birth Control Pills (BCPs)

BCPs decrease estrogen, progesterone, and testosterone and provide temporary relief of symptoms that return once the BCP is discontinued. Typical side effects can include acne, breast tenderness and enlargement, spotting between periods, nausea, and vomiting. Additional side effects include changes in your eyes that make it more difficult to wear contact lenses, bloating, headaches, changes in sex drive (typically a decrease), and increased risk of blood clotting disorders.

Nutritional Factors Affecting PMS

Foods to Avoid	Foods to Eat
Sugar	Two to three servings of fruit daily plus four to six servings of vegetables daily
White flour products and baked goods	Whole grains: barley, rice, amaranth, quinoa, millet, and buckwheat
Caffeine	Herbal teas
Foods that contain PCBs, dioxin, and brominated fire retardants—these include non-organic fish, dairy, beef, pork, lamb, and eggs	Limited quantities of organic poultry and meats, tofu, beans, nuts, and seeds
Peanuts, which increase arachidonic acid production and aggravate PMS	Other raw nuts and seeds in moderation, especially sunflower, pumpkin, and almond
Fruits and vegetables sprayed with pesticides (which disrupt hormones and are estrogenic)	Organic fruits and vegetables
Animal-derived saturated fats and most vegetable oils	Extra-virgin olive oil—one tablespoon daily, flaxseed oil—two tablespoons daily, and pure fish oil—one to two tablespoons daily
Excessive amounts of raw brassicas (cabbage, cauliflower and broccoli)—only if there is a thyroid issue	Two tablespoons of seaweed daily to support thyroid function (Nori, dulse, hiziki) Use cooked Brassicas liberally
Excess salt if there is water retention	Two teaspoons of turmeric, two tablespoons of freshly ground flax seeds, and one tablespoon of psyllium daily to improve estrogen metabolism and elimination
Alcohol	Two liters of purified water daily

[137] http://en.wikipedia.org/wiki/Selective_serotonin_reuptake_inhibitor

Herbal Medicine Indicated for PMS

Chasteberry *(Vitex agnus castus)*

Native to the Mediterranean, chasteberry has been used for centuries in the management of gynecological complaints. The greatest use of chasteberry has been in disorders associated with hormone function, such as premenstrual distress and dysmenorrhea.[138] Evidence of its effectiveness has led to its approval by the German Commission E as an intervention for premenstrual complaints, cyclical breast tenderness, and menstrual cycle irregularities.[139] Today, chasteberry is among the most popular herbs to help relieve a broad spectrum of PMS symptoms, such as breast tenderness, weight gain, abdominal cramps, depression, and mood swings.

Various mechanisms related to the menstrual cycle have been demonstrated through chasteberry's properties. Chasteberry has the ability to decrease prolactin via binding at pituitary dopamine-D2 receptors and has therefore been shown to be a dopamine agonist.[140] Elevated prolactin levels are thought to be associated with PMS and may play a role in complaints of cyclical breast tenderness. Chasteberry also appears to contain constituents that influence mood by acting via opioid receptors or the GABA-system. Regardless of its mode of action, chasteberry's clinical efficacy and tolerability is well documented.

Any hepatoprotective herb is well-suited in the treatment of PMS. Liver detoxifying is central to the treatment of any hormonal condition, especially PMS.

Milk thistle *(Silymarin marianus)*

Much research has been done on a special extract of milk thistle known as silymarin, a group of flavonoid compounds. These compounds protect the liver from damage and enhance the detoxification process. Silymarin prevents damage to the liver by acting as an antioxidant and is much more effective than vitamin E and vitamin C. Numerous research studies have demonstrated its protective effect on the liver and it also works by preventing the depletion of glutathione. The higher the glutathione concentration, the greater the liver's capacity to detoxify harmful chemicals. Silymarin has been shown to increase the level of glutathione by up to 35%. In human studies, Silymarin is shown to exhibit positive effects in treating liver diseases of various kinds including cirrhosis, chronic hepatitis, fatty infiltration of the liver, and inflammation of the bile duct. Dosage: standardized extract 200 to 800 mg a day

Curcumin *(Curcuma longa)*

Several studies have illustrated curcumin's hepatoprotective effects. This has led researchers to suggest its use in protecting the liver from exogenous insults from environmental toxins, including carbon tetrachloride and acetaminophen. Curcumin also has the capacity to increase bile flow and solubility, making it of potential benefit for someone with a tendency to form gallstones. The hepatoprotective effects of turmeric may stem from its potent antioxidant activity. In addition to its antioxidant effects, curcumin has also been shown to enhance liver detoxification by increasing the activity of glutathione S-transferase, an enzyme necessary to conjugate glutathione with a wide variety of toxins in order to facilitate their removal from the body. Dosage: 500mg- 2000mg per day

St John's wort *(Hypericum perforatum)*

St. John's wort (*Hypericum perforatum*) has been popularly used for decades in the management of mild to moderate depression. With its extensive history, St. John's wort has been approved by the German Commission E health authorities for the management of depressive moods, anxiety, and nervous unrest. In a recent pilot study, St. John's wort was also shown to be effective in women with PMS. In this study, nineteen women with PMS given St. John's

---

[138] Snow JM. *Vitex agnus-castus* L. (*Verbenaceae*). *Protocol J Botanical Med* 1996; 1:20-23.

[139] Blumenthal M, Busse WR, Goldberg A, et al. *The complete German Commission E monographs*. Boston: Integrative Medicine Communications; 1998.

[140] Halaska M, Beles P, Gorkow C, Sieder C. Treatment of clyclical mastalgia with a solution containing a *Vitex* agnus castus extract: results of a placebo-controlled double-blind study. The Breast 1999; 8:175-81.

wort extract (300 mg per day) for two menstrual cycles reported significant improvements in overall symptoms. The greatest reductions in symptoms included depression, confusion, anxiety, and insomnia.[141] There are several factors involved in St John's wort anti-depressive abilities. It appears to inhibit serotonin, norepinephrine, and dopamine reuptake by postsynaptic receptors, increase the density of serotonin and dopamine receptors, elevate the affinity for GABA receptors, and inhibit monoamine concentrations in the synaptic cleft.[142] Caution: St John's wort should not be taken with conventional antidepressants. Dosage: 30mg-900mg per day

Specific Nutrients for PMS

Vitamin B6

Vitamin B6 can be used to increase levels of serotonin, dopamine, and progesterone, which are commonly deficient in PMS sufferers. Since these neurotransmitters are crucial for control of depression, pain perception, and anxiety, pyridoxine deficiency may exacerbate premenstrual dysphoria, whereas adequate pyridoxine status has a favorable impact. Typical symptoms that respond to B6 therapy include acne flares, depression, irritability, breast tenderness, headaches, edema, and bloating. In a study of thirty-two women with moderate to severe PMS, vitamin B6 given at a low dose of 50 mg per day for seven months was shown to provide a significant beneficial effect on symptoms—such as depression, irritability, and fatigue—during the premenstrual period. In fact, these symptoms were approximately halved in the treatment months when compared to the placebo months.[143] Dosage: 50 mg to 100 mg per day

Magnesium

PMS can present with a wide variety of neuropsychological symptoms, including depression, agitation, personality changes, and memory and concentration difficulties, as well as physical complaints surrounding fluid balance. Magnesium is an essential cofactor in over three hundred enzymatic actions and plays a role in the maintenance of cell membrane electrical potential and electrolyte balance. It has therefore been postulated that magnesium deficiency may exacerbate certain PMS symptoms. Magnesium also reduces water retention, weight gain, swollen limbs, and abdominal bloating. It assists vitamin B6 and essential fatty acid metabolism. Dosage: 200mg to 600mg per day

Vitamin E

Prostaglandin synthesis has been implicated in PMS, and a deficiency of prostaglandin PgEl has been proposed to be involved in PMS. Vitamin E inhibits the negative prostaglandin PgF2 and increases the anti-inflammatory prostaglandin PgE1, which helps to relieve premenstrual swelling and breast tenderness. Vitamin E reduces arachidonic acid levels which further helps to reduce inflammation. Dosage: 400 to 800 IU per day

Evening Primrose Oil (EPO)

A defect in the linoleic acid conversion to gamma linolenic acid (GLA) is common in PMS sufferers. EPO contains preformed GLA and therefore, ingestion of EPO can bypass the metabolic block in prostaglandin synthesis. Four double-blind, crossover, controlled trials of EPO have demonstrated a significant effect over the placebo group. EPO has been shown to be most effective for relieving clumsiness and headaches, although other symptoms including depression, irritability, bloating, and breast tenderness showed a marked improvement. Dosage: 1000 mg to 4000mg per day

---

141 Stevinson C, Ernst E. A pilot study of *Hypericum perforatum* for the treatment of premenstrual syndrome. BJOG 2000; 107(7):870-76.

142 Rodriguez-Landa JF, Contreras CM. A review of clinical and experimental observations about antidepressant actions and side effects produced by Hypericum perforatum extracts. Phytomedicine 2003;10:688-99

143 Doll H, Brown S, Thurston A, Vessey M. Pyridoxine (vitamin B6) and the premenstrual syndrome: a randomized crossover trial. J R Coll Gen Pract 1989; 39(326):364-68.

Diindolylmethane (DIM)

DIM is a powerful metabolizer of estrogen, assisting in removing excess estrogen and benefiting conditions associated with estrogen dominance. Supplementation with DIM can help promote proper estrogen levels in women through the pre- and perimenopausal years and in men experiencing higher estrogen levels. These conditions include uterine fibroid tumors, fibrocystic breasts, and glandular dysfunction. It can also benefit men by improving estrogen dominance-related health issues such as hair loss, atherosclerosis, prostrate problems, lowered libido, and impotency. DIM also promotes testosterone action, which improves mood, fights depression, boosts libido, improves cardiovascular health, improves memory, and supports muscular development. DIM is a balancer of estrogen metabolism. It increases 2-hydroxyestrone (2-OHE), which is also known as the good or protective estrogen. Dosage: 70 mg to 400 mg per day

5-Hydroxytryptophan (5-HTP)

5-HTP is extracted from the seeds of the African plant, Griffonia simplicifolia. It is the intermediate metabolite of the essential amino acid L-tryptophan in the biosynthesis of serotonin. Unlike L-tryptophan, 5-HTP cannot be shunted into niacin or protein production. Therapeutic use of 5-HTP bypasses the conversion of L-tryptophan into 5-HTP by the enzyme tryptophan hydroxylase. This is the rate-limiting step in the synthesis of serotonin but is inhibited by numerous factors, including stress, insulin resistance, vitamin B6 deficiency, magnesium deficiency, and increasing age. It easily crosses the blood-brain barrier and effectively increases central nervous system (CNS) synthesis of serotonin. This makes it an effective treatment in a wide variety of conditions, including depression, fibromyalgia, insomnia, binge eating associated with obesity, and chronic headaches. In combination with vitamin B6, it may improve PMS tension, mood swings, and irritability by increasing serotonin levels. Dosage: 50 mg to 600 mg per day with food. Dosage: 50mg-300mg per day with food

Bioidentical Progesterone Cream

For severe PMS symptoms that have not responded to nutritional, botanical, and lifestyle changes, especially symptoms starting a few days to one week before the menses, bioidentical progesterone cream can be of extreme benefit. The USP progesterone used for hormone replacement comes from plant fats and oils, usually from a substance called diosgenin, which is extracted from a very specific type of wild yam that grows in Mexico, or from soybeans. In the laboratory, diosgenin is chemically synthesized into real human progesterone. The other human steroid hormones, including estrogen, testosterone, progesterone, and the cortisones are also nearly always synthesized from diosgenin. Because progesterone is very fat-soluble, it is easily absorbed through the skin. Progesterone is absorbed into capillary blood from subcutaneous fat. Thus, absorption is best at all the skin sites where people blush: face, neck, chest, breasts, inner arms, and palms of the hands. Dosage: For premenopausal women, the usual dose is 15 mg to 24 mg per day for 1fourteen days before expected menses, stopping the day before menses. (Bioidentical Progesterone Cream should contain 450 mg to 500 mg of progesterone per ounce and 900 mg to 1000 mg per two ounce container.)

Exercise Indicated for PMS

Several studies have shown that regular exercise greatly diminishes PMS. Although the mechanisms of action remain elusive, the evidence is clear. Aerobic training (walking, jogging, swimming, and cycling) appears more effective at reducing PMS symptoms than strength training (weight lifting).[144] Frequency of exercise, but not intensity, seems to relate to decreased rating of selected menstrual distress symptoms. Regular exercisers show improvement in emotional PMS symptoms, including improved concentration and reduction in feelings of pain, hostility, fear, guilt, and sadness. Regularly exercising women report a significant decrease in anxiety.[145]

---

[144] Steege J Blumenthal J. "The Effects of Aerobic Exercise on Premenstrual Symptoms in Middle Aged Women: A Preliminary Study" J Psychosom Res 1993;37:127

[145] Choi P, Salmon P. "Stress responsivity in exercisers and non-exercisers during different phases of the menstrual cycle." Soc Sci Med 1995; 41:769.

Top 5 Strategies for PMS

1. Complete Hormone testing
2. Liver detoxification
3. Optimize nutrition through a whole food diet
4. Eliminate sugar and caffeine
5. Supplement with 5-HTP, Evening Primrose Oil, Vitamin E, Vitamin B6, Magnesium, Vitex, DIM and Bioidentical Progesterone days 14-28 when needed

Samantha's Story - PMS

Samantha is a thirty-five-year-old female who presented with complaints of PMS. Sam stated that although her cycles were regular in length, she experienced severe PMS symptoms, including mood swings, acne, weight gain, and breast tenderness. Sam noted that she had been dealing with these issues for years.

Sam is a busy, working mom with two young children. She runs her own business and has therefore increasing amounts of stress in her life. She also stated that she had a long history of "yo-yo" dieting and had a tendency to gain weight easily. She would skip meals in order to lose weight, which often worked in the past but had not been working for the past year. Sam worked out vigorously five days per week and had done so for years.

Lab testing:

- Low progesterone
- Low progesterone to estrogen ratio
- Low mid-day cortisol
- Elevated night time cortisol
- Low Free T3
- Elisa Multi food allergy testing revealed allergies to dairy and shellfish

Sam was administered the following natural medicine therapies:

- Estrogen detoxification: DIM, calcium D-glucarate, SGS (standardized to contain 30mg glucoraphanin glucosinolate), Hops extract (0.12% 8-prenylnaringenin) two capsules with breakfast
- Thyroid support: iodine (as potassium iodide), zinc (as zinc picolinate), copper (as copper chelate), L-tyrosine, thyroid glandular (thyroxine free) two capsules two times per day
- Medical food: a powdered medical food designed to nutritionally support the management of conditions associated with metabolic syndrome (including altered body composition)
- Modified Mediterranean Lifestyle Nutrition Plan to balance hormones (See "Specific Guidelines for Nutritional Lifestyle Management in Weight Gain" section)
- Cortisol Management: ashwagandha, L-theanine, phosphatidylserine one capsule before bed
- Blackcurrant oil one capsule two times per day
- Multi B-6: a B-complex with additional B6 one capsule two times per day

Sam came back for a follow-up eight weeks later because she had been out of town on business for much of the previous month. She noted that she was sleeping very well. She had not really noticed beforehand that her sleep was below average, as she always just felt wired. She was now experiencing eight hours of very good quality sleep per night. She did admit to have more difficulty sticking to the meal plan while travelling, but made the best choices that she could at the time. She had lost a total of six pounds, which BIA testing confirmed. Sam also stated that the previous two menstrual cycles had 50% less symptoms than before but she was still experiencing some less severe PMS symptoms.

The following modifications were made to the protocol:

- Continue with all previous remedies
- Bioidentical Progesterone Cream one pump on days fourteen through twenty-eight of the cycle

Sam returned eight weeks later to happily report that she had lost a total of twelve pounds, which was more than she had ever lost on any other plan. She stated that her previous two cycles were much less severe and that she thought the progesterone cream really made a difference. She was no longer experiencing any acne, breast tenderness, or pre-cycle weight gain. Sam noted that she had only had one half-day of irritability before her cycle, which was a marked improvement from previous cycles. She was recommended to stay on the protocol but to discontinue the estrogen detoxification formula.

Fibroids

Fibroids, also called leiomyomas or myomas, are the most common benign uterine tumors of smooth muscle origin. Fibroids are typically slow-growing, non-cancerous growths which occur on the inside or outside walls of the uterus. They are firm and round, are usually found in groups, and can vary in size from microscopic to larger than a grapefruit. They cause enlargement and distortion of the uterus in 20% to 25% of women by age forty and account for one-third of hysterectomies each year.

Fibroids are classified according to their location: submucosal (just under the endometrium), intamural (within the uterine wall), and subserosal (on the outer wall of uterus).

Symptoms of Fibroids

The majority of fibroids (an estimated 50% to 80%) are asymptomatic, but when symptoms do begin to occur, they often start as a vague feeling of pelvic discomfort. Whether or not fibroids cause symptoms depends on their size and location. The most common symptoms of fibroids are heavy and irregular menstruation with menstrual cramps and pelvic pain. Other symptoms associated with fibroids may include:

- Increased menstrual symptoms—pain, heavy bleeding, irregular periods, mid-cycle bleeding
- Feeling of pressure, congestion, or bloating
- Pain or bleeding with intercourse
- Urinary frequency and/or increasing irritation of the bladder
- Back pain
- Excessive vaginal discharge
- Abdominal enlargement
- Anemia (due to heavy blood loss during menstruation)
- Fatigue
- Infertility
- Miscarriage
- Compression of the ureter, resulting in kidney enlargement
- Obstruction of the bowel

The Cause of Fibroids

The cause of fibroids is uncertain but researchers have confirmed that fibroids have more estrogen receptors than normal uterine tissue and are stimulated by high estrogen levels. Fibroids will often experience a growth spurt during perimenopausal periods and pregnancy, when there are increased levels of estrogen. Conversely, fibroids tend to atrophy after menopause when estrogen levels drop. The presence and size of fibroids is greater in women who do not ovulate (i.e., ovaries fail to release eggs). Anything that interferes with ovulation will decrease the levels of progesterone in the body and increase the relative levels of estrogen. Several other factors may contribute to the development of fibroids:

Dietary Factors

- Excess consumption of dietary acids (animal proteins and grains) and a lack of alkaline-forming foods (fruits and vegetables)
- Pesticides and heavy metals are linked to the growth of fibroids as they increase estrogen dominance, which is the driving force behind fibroids
- Excess animal protein, which increase the inflammatory agent arachidonic acid and disrupt natural hormone rhythms
- Insufficient dietary fiber causes the buildup of harmful estrogens in the body leading to estrogen dominance

Bowel and Liver Toxicity

- Constipation increases levels of circulating estrogens
- An imbalance between the beneficial bacteria and pathogenic bacteria in the bowel can increase the risk factor for the development of fibroids
- If the liver is over-burdened with alcohol and other toxins, there will be a decrease in its ability to detoxify harmful estrogens

Other Predisposing Factors

- Birth control pills (increased estrogen; anovulatory)
- Hormone replacement therapy (increased estrogen)
- Pregnancy (increased blood supply and high estrogen levels)
- Perimenopause (anovulatory)
- Pituitary tumors, or tumors of the hypothalamus gland
- Ovarian cysts
- Polycystic ovary syndrome
- Thyroid dysfunction (hyper- or hypothyroid)
- Amenorrhea
- Anorexia or low BMI
- Function problems in ovaries
- Melatonin deficiency (as melatonin decreases the number of estrogen receptors in the body)

Laboratory Testing and Diagnosing Fibroids

If a fibroid tumor is present, it can often be felt during a pelvic examination. The uterus can be irregularly shaped or irregularly enlarged and often feels like it has protrusions. Upon discovery of a fibroid during a physical examination, a pelvic ultrasound is the most useful tool in diagnosis. An ultrasound can identify fibroids and delineate the size, and to some degree, the location. The ultrasound can also detect the contour of the uterus, compression of the ureters, potential enlargement of the kidneys, and the presence of an enlarged uterus.

Lab testing will help to determine the presence of estrogen dominance, which greatly contributes to fibroid presence. In addition, the thyroid should be evaluated to determine whether or not an imbalance is an underlying cause and anemia should be ruled out.

Complete Female Hormone Panel	Estradiol and progesterone levels and their ratio are an index of estrogen/progesterone balance. An excess of estradiol, relative to progesterone, can explain many symptoms in reproductive age-women. Testosterone levels can also be either too high or too low. Testosterone in excess, often caused by ovarian cysts, leads to conditions such as excessive facial and body hair, acne, and oily skin and hair. Polycystic ovarian syndrome (PCOS) is thought to be caused, in part, by insulin resistance. On the other hand, too little testosterone is often caused by excessive stress, medications, contraceptives, and surgical removal of the ovaries. This leads to symptoms of androgen deficiency including loss of libido, thinning skin, vaginal dryness, loss of bone and muscle mass, depression, and memory lapses. SHBG binds tightly to circulating estradiol and testosterone, preventing their rapid metabolism and clearance and limiting their bioavailability to tissues. SHBG gives a good index of the extent of the body's overall exposure to estrogens.
Thyroid Hormone Testing	A complete thyroid profile includes free T4, free T3, TSH, and TPO and can indicate the presence of an imbalance in thyroid function. Hypothyroidism includes feeling cold all the time, low stamina, fatigue (particularly in the evening), anxiety, depression, low sex drive, weight gain, and high cholesterol. Hyperthyroidism includes heat intolerance, anxiety, palpitations, weight loss, tired but wired feeling, visual disturbances, and insomnia.
Anemia	Low serum iron, hematocrit, and low blood hemoglobin levels can predispose a person to extreme fatigue, contributing to depression.

Conventional Medicine Indicated for Fibroids

Many fibroids require no treatment conventionally, only an observation of growth at annual pelvic exams. For fibroids that are manifesting negative symptoms, the following are treatment options:

- Myomectomy: removal of the fibroid, leaving the uterus in place
- Hysterectomy: removal of the uterus (this remains the only proven permanent solution for uterine fibroids)
- Myoma coagulation and reconstruction: elimination of the fibroids with the use of lasers that puncture the fibroids and deflate them
- Gonadotropin-releasing hormones (Gn-RH) agonists: produces opposite effects to those of the natural hormones, causing estrogen and progesterone levels to fall, menstruation to stop, fibroids to shrink, and anemia to improve

- Androgens: shrink fibroids, reduce uterine size, stop menstruation, and correct anemia
- Uterine artery embolization: small particles are injected into the arteries supplying the uterus and cutting off blood flow to the fibroids, causing them to shrink
- Endometrial ablation: can be used if the fibroids are only within the uterus and not intramural, and are relatively small. High failure and recurrence rates are expected in the presence of larger or intramural fibroids.

Nutritional Factors Affecting Fibroids

Although dietary changes will not "cure" fibroids, improving one's diet may help in small ways to decrease heavy bleeding and the pain and discomfort caused by the fibroids. Poor nutritional habits can lead to dysfunctional estrogen metabolism and inhibit the body's ability to break down and excrete excess estrogen. Estrogen is metabolized in the liver so it can be eliminated from the body by converting it to estrone and finally to estriol, a weaker form of estrogen that has very little ability to stimulate the uterus. If the liver cannot effectively metabolize estradiol, the uterus may become over-estrogenized and respond with fibroid growths.

Increase:

- **Complex carbohydrates:** whole grains such as brown rice, oats, buckwheat, millet, and rye are excellent sources of B vitamins. Whole grains also help the body to excrete estrogens through the bowel.
- **Fruits and vegetables**
- **Fiber**: low-fiber diets are associated with elevated estrogen levels and poor excretion of estrogen. A high-fiber diet may also help to relieve some of the bloating and congestion associated with fibroids. By bulking up the stool and regulating bowel movements, some of these symptoms may improve. Some women have a hard time tolerating increased fiber in their diet because of compromised digestive function. In these cases, it may be necessary to increase fiber slowly and include digestive support supplement, such as enzymes or acidophilus.
- **Increase legumes and flaxseeds:** these contain phytoestrogens, which bind with estrogen receptor sites in the body and stop the uptake of more harmful xenoestrogens (from chemicals) and stronger estrogens (e.g., estradiol) This decreases estrogen stimulation of the uterus.
- **Cruciferous vegetables:** such as broccoli, cabbage, cauliflower, kale, and Brussels sprouts. These contain a phytonutrient called diindolylmethane (DIM) that supports the activity of enzymes that improve estrogen metabolism.
- **Bitter greens:** such as dandelion greens, endive, and radicchio added to salad will help to stimulate the liver and other digestive enzymes.
- **Hot water and lemon juice:** will help to stimulate the liver and digestive enzymes.
- **Blackstrap molasses:** contains high levels of bioavailable iron (good for those who have heavy menstrual flow) and B-vitamins (used by the liver to metabolize estrogens).

Decrease:

- **Saturated fats**: diets high in saturated fats are associated with high blood levels of estrogen, potentially exacerbating the problem.
- **Caffeine and alcohol:** these interfere with the liver's ability to transform estrogen into safe metabolites.
- **Sugar**: this interferes with the body's ability to metabolize estradiol to estrone and estriol and is also deficient in B-vitamins and interferes with B-vitamin metabolism. If B-vitamins are lacking in the diet, the liver is missing some of the raw materials it needs to carry out its metabolic processes and regulate estrogen levels.
- **Red meats:** contribute to the production of inflammatory prostaglandins (hormone-like substances that can contribute to menstrual cramping and pain).

Herbal Medicine Indicated for Fibroids

Chasteberry *(Vitex agnus castus)*

Chasteberry regulates pituitary function, which in turn helps regulate ovulation and production of progesterone. It can help stabilize an irregular cycle and reduce many of the symptoms of fibroids (including heavy bleeding, menstrual cramps, and clotting). Chasteberry has dopaminergic action in that it inhibits the secretion of prolactin from the pituitary gland and normalizes pituitary gland function. This will, in turn, restore levels of progesterone, decreasing the prevalence of estrogen dominance. Chasteberry has the therapeutic effect of lowering harmful estrogen levels while also maintaining progesterone levels, taken at very small doses (5 mL per day).

Liver-stimulating herbs: these include dandelion root, milk thistle, burdock, artichoke, and turmeric. These can be taken in tincture, tea, juice or capsule form.

Specific Nutrients Indicated for Fibroids

The liver is responsible for the conversion of the most potent form of estrogen, estradiol, to a weaker form of estrogen, estriol, which can then be eliminated from the body. Therefore, the main treatment motivation is to detoxify and protect the liver.

Lipotropic Factors: Nutrients such as inositol and choline exert a lipotropic effect, meaning they promote the removal of fat from the liver. They are designed to support the liver's function in removing fat, detoxifying the body's wastes, detoxifying external harmful substances (e.g., pesticides and fossil fuels), and metabolizing and excreting estrogens. As a precursor to phosphatidylcholine and glycine and their derivatives–betaine, dimethylglycine, and serine–choline is a premier lipotrope. Choline deficiency is a well-documented cause of fatty liver. Choline emulsifies lipids, provides the substrate for phosphatidylcholine biosynthesis, and promotes repair of damaged hepatic cell membranes. Dosage: usually taken two times per day; dependent upon formulation

Calcium-d-glucarate: Supports estrogen metabolism in the liver and excretion out of the colon. Conjugation and glucuronidation are detoxification processes that occur when toxins, carcinogens, and used hormones are combined with and bound to water-soluble substances in the liver, thus making them more easily removed from the body. D-glucarate has been shown to support these vital processes by inhibiting an enzyme called beta-glucuronidase that can break bonds between toxins and used hormones, allowing them to be re-circulated into the bloodstream rather than excreted.

D-glucarate may directly detoxify any environmental agents responsible for cancer formation. It has been postulated that D-glucarate exerts some of its effects by equilibrium conversion to D-glucarolactone, which is a potent beta-glucuronidase inhibitor. This is one of the most important nutrients to enhance liver function. Dosage: 250 mg to 1,000 mg per day

B-Complex: B-vitamins are the raw materials needed for enzyme reactions carried out in the liver to metabolize estrogens. Vitamin B6, in particular, enhances the breakdown and removal of estrogen from the body. Dosage: 50 mg to 100 mg per day

Essential Fatty Acids (EFAs): These good fats are required for the production of hormones and the production of anti-inflammatory and anti-spasmodic prostaglandins (hormone-like substances). A combination of omega-6 fatty acids (e.g., evening primrose oil and borage oil) and omega-3 fatty acids (e.g., fish oils) has been found to be most beneficial in the treatment of fibroids. Dosage: 1000mg-3000mg per day

N-acetyl cysteine (NAC)

NAC is the precursor of both the amino acid L-cysteine and reduced glutathione (GSH). Animal and human studies of NAC have shown it to be a powerful antioxidant and a therapeutic agent for heavy metal toxicity and other diseases characterized by free radical, oxidative damage. As a source of sulfhydryl groups, NAC stimulates glutathione synthesis, enhances glutathione-S-transferase activity, promotes liver detoxification by inhibiting xenobiotic biotransformation, and is a powerful nucleophile capable of scavenging free radicals. Dosage: 500 mg to 1500 mg per day

Curcumin (*Curcuma longa*)

Several studies have illustrated curcumin's hepatoprotective effects. This has led researchers to suggest its use in protecting the liver from exogenous insults from environmental toxins, including carbon tetrachloride and acetaminophen. Curcumin also has the capacity to increase bile flow and solubility, making it of potential benefit for someone with a tendency to form gallstones. The hepatoprotective effects of turmeric may stem from its potent antioxidant activity. In addition to its antioxidant effects, curcumin has been shown to enhance liver detoxification by increasing the activity of glutathione S-transferase, which is an enzyme necessary to conjugate glutathione with a wide variety of toxins in order to facilitate their removal from the body. Dosage: 500mg-3000mg per day

Diindolylmethane (DIM)

DIM is a powerful metabolizer of estrogen, assisting in removing excess estrogen and benefiting conditions associated with estrogen dominance. Supplementation with DIM can help promote proper estrogen levels in women through the pre- and perimenopausal years and in men experiencing higher estrogen levels. These conditions include uterine fibroid tumors, fibrocystic breasts, and glandular dysfunction. It can also benefit men by improving estrogen-dominance related health issues such as hair loss, atherosclerosis, prostrate problems, lowered libido, and impotency. DIM promotes the action of testosterone, which improves mood, fights depression, boosts libido, improves cardiovascular health, improves memory, and supports muscular development. DIM is a balancer of estrogen metabolism. It increases 2-hydroxyestrone (2-OHE), which is also known as the good or protective estrogen. Dosage: 300 mg per day

Pancreatic Enzymes

Pancreatic enzymes taken between meals have been shown to aid in the breakdown of fibroid tumors. Dosage: two to four capsules three times per day in between meals

Bioidentical Progesterone

Historically, studies have shown that progesterone may inhibit the growth of uterine fibroids. The USP progesterone used for hormone replacement comes from plant fats and oils, usually from a substance called diosgenin, which is extracted from a very specific type of wild yam that grows in Mexico, or from soybeans. In the laboratory, diosgenin is chemically synthesized into real human progesterone. The other human steroid hormones, including estrogen, testosterone, progesterone, and the cortisones, are also nearly always synthesized from diosgenin. Because progesterone is very fat-soluble, it is easily absorbed through the skin. Progesterone is absorbed into capillary blood from subcutaneous fat. Thus, absorption is best at all the skin sites where people blush: face, neck, chest, breasts, inner arms, and palms of the hands. Dosage: For premenopausal women, the usual dose is 15 mg to 24 mg per day for fourteen14 days before expected menses, stopping the day before menses. (Bioidentical Progesterone Cream should contain 450 mg to 500 mg of progesterone per ounce and 900 mg to 1000 mg per two ounce container.)

Castor Oil Packs: Apply a castor oil pack to the lower abdomen three to five times per week. The skin absorbs the warm castor oil's active constituents, lectins, which stimulate the immune response to help shrink fibroids. Castor oil is extracted from the castor plant (*Ricinus communis*). It should not be taken internally, as it will act as a powerful laxative. But if applied externally or topically, it has unique medicinal actions on the body. It penetrates skin and muscle to reach right into underlying tissue and assists in the decongestion and the breakdown of inflammatory material through enhancing blood flow and lymphatic flow in the area. This also helps in the removal of toxins and the elimination of wastes. Castor oil is warming to the tissues, easing stiffness and pain.

Occasions to use a castor oil pack

- Lymphatic congestion
- Arthritis or Rheumatism
- Fibromyalgia
- Muscle spasms
- Abdominal inflammations
- Pelvic congestion
- Glandular swellings
- Deep infections
- Adhesions
- Fibroids
- Endometriosis
- Backache
- Muscle tension
- Local pain due to inflammation or spasm

How to make a castor oil pack

- Take a piece of flannel or towel. Fold it three to four times, so that it is large enough to entirely cover the area to be treated.
- Pour castor oil over it until thoroughly soaked.
- Place over the skin and cover with a large piece of saran wrap.
- Cover this with a heating pad or hot water bottle and leave in place for one to two hours.
- After use, the pack can be wrapped in plastic and stored in the refrigerator (bring back to room temperature before re-use). You may wish to add a little more castor oil with each use. The pack should be discarded after ten uses.

Exercise: Regular exercise can help to increase the circulation to the pelvic area, decrease the number of anovulatory cycles, and decrease menstrual cramping. Exercise will also help you to lose weight, which will decrease the estrogen load in your body.

Reduce Exposure to Environmental Estrogens

Xenoestrogens found in certain pesticides, plastics, fuels, and drugs are usually synthetic, difficult for the body to break down, and can amplify the effects of estrogen. These substances can increase the estrogen load in the body over time and are difficult to detoxify through the liver. Exposure to xenoestrogens is a concern for everyone. Those with estrogen dominance conditions such as fibroids should be particularly concerned with avoiding xenoestrogens.

Xenoestrogens can be found in many of our meats and dairy products in the form of chemicals and growth hormones that are given to the animals from which these products came. These can be quite powerful, and should be avoided whenever possible. Choosing meat and dairy items that are organic can help to decrease xenoestrogen exposure.

Sources of Xenoestrogens that should be avoided:

- Commercially raised meat
- Canned foods
- Plastics, plastic food wraps
- Styrofoam cups
- Industrial wastes
- Personal care products
- Pesticides and herbicides
- Paints, lacquers, and solvents
- Plant estrogens (soy, flaxseeds)
- Car exhaust and indoor toxins
- Cosmetics
- Birth control pills and spermicide
- Detergents
- All artificial scents
- Air fresheners, perfumes

Top 5 Strategies for Fibroids

1. Complete Hormone testing/Anemia evaluation
2. Reduce exposure to xenoestrogens
3. Liver detoxification
4. Consume a nutrient dense, high fiber, organic diet/Eliminate sugar, caffeine, alcohol and red meat
5. Supplement with DIM, Calcium D-glucarate, Lipotropic factors, Pancreatic enzymes, Curcumin, NAC, Vitex and Bioidentical Progesterone when needed/Apply castor oil packs regularly

Diana's Story - Fibroids

Diana is a forty-eight-year-old woman who had recently cancelled a scheduled surgery for fibroid removal. She had decided that she would seek alternative medicine in lieu of surgery and if it did not work, then she would go ahead with the surgery. Diana was extremely uncomfortable as the fibroid was sitting on her bladder, which caused pressure and frequency of urination. She was carrying approximately fifty extra pounds and stated that she would love to lose some weight. Diana had been suffering with a long-term thyroid dysfunction and despite the fact that she was on medication, her thyroid still remained unbalanced.

Diana was under an extreme amount of stress and described herself as a typical "Type A" personality. She was always rushing and rarely ate regular meals. She often drank pre-made meal replacement drinks and consumed large amounts of coffee with sugar. She had very sluggish bowels and relied heavily on a natural laxative remedy in order to have a bowel movement.

Medications:

- Levothyroxine (Synthroid) 100 mcg per day

Lab testing:

- Low progesterone levels
- Estrogen dominance
- Elevated TSH
- Low DHEA
- Low cortisol levels

Management Plan

Diana was administered the following natural medicine therapies:

- Modified Mediterranean Lifestyle Nutrition Plan to balance hormones (See "Specific Guidelines for Nutritional Lifestyle Management in Weight Gain" section)
- Liver detoxification formula: choline, betaine, methionine, taraxacum (dandelion), silymarin marianus, cynara scolymus (artichoke) and curcumin two tablets two times per day
- Adrenal Support: vitamins C, B5, and B6, magnesium, and citrus bioflavonoids two times per day
- Adrenal Support: licorice root and ashwagandha root two times per day
- Estrogen detoxification: DIM, calcium D-glucarate, SGS (standardized to contain 30 mg of glucoraphanin glucosinolate), hops extract (0.12% 8-prenylnaringenin) two capsules with breakfast
- Two tablespoons of ground flax seed per day
- Two tablespoons of multi-fiber formula: psyllium, prune powder, and apple pectin
- Calcium 250mg /Magnesium citrate 250mg one to one ratio three tablets before bed
- Decrease coffee consumption
- Daily exercise for thirty minutes (walking, biking, swimming, or dancing)

Diana returned four weeks later to report that the fibroid cramping and pain had decreased by about 35%. She also stated that she was no longer using her natural laxative formula and was having at least one proper bowel movement per day. She had been trying to stick to the eating plan as best she could and she felt much less stress when eating regularly, but admitted that her nutrition was still in progress.

The following modifications were made to the protocol:

- Castor oil packs three to four times per week at night
- Bioidentical progesterone cream one pump, twenty-five days on and five days off per month

Diana reported back eight weeks later to state that the pressure on her bladder had almost completely gone, she was still having regular bowel movements, her perception of stress was much less heightened, and she had much more energy. She also noted that she was much quicker to get out of bed in the morning instead of dragging herself out of bed. She had had her TSH levels testes four weeks previously and for the first time in years, her levels were stable and within the normal range. She was happy to continue with the protocol until her next ultrasound to determine the level of fibroid shrinkage.

Endometriosis

Endometriosis is a very common condition, affecting approximately 10% to 15% of women in their reproductive years from age twenty-five to forty-five. About 30% of affected women are infertile. In some cases, symptoms begin with the onset of menstruation and in others, symptoms begin later and progressively become worse until menopause.

Endometriosis is a condition where the endometrium (the lining of the uterus) is found in locations outside of the uterus. Locations can include the ovaries, fallopian tubes, vagina, abdomen, deep inside the uterine muscle, bowel, bladder, utero-sacral ligaments (ligaments that hold the uterus in place), peritoneum (covering lining of the pelvis and abdominal cavity), or other parts of the body. Endometriosis can grow between organs and cause adhesions. When the uterine endometrial lining is shed at the end of a menstrual period, the cells in the rampant tissue also bleed into surrounding tissue, forming blood blisters that become cysts. These cells can also run on their own monthly rhythm. This creates local inflammation and pain and the cysts form scars or adhesions. Scars or adhesions on the fallopian tubes can cause infertility.

Symptoms of Endometriosis

The most common symptoms of endometriosis are:

- Pain before and during periods
- Pain with intercourse
- General, chronic pelvic pain throughout the month
- Low back pain
- Heavy and/or irregular periods
- Painful bowel movements, especially during menstruation
- Painful urination during menstruation
- Fatigue
- Infertility
- Diarrhea or constipation

Other symptoms that are common with endometriosis include:

- Headaches
- Low-grade fevers
- Depression
- Hypoglycemia (low blood sugar)
- Anxiety
- Susceptibility to infections, allergies

In the later stages of endometriosis, adhesions usually develop in the pelvic cavity, which are caused by untreated cysts, which can 'glue' pelvic organs together. These adhesions seriously interfere with normal functions of organs in the pelvis, causing bowel obstructions, digestive problems, infertility, urinary problems, and agonizing pain when the adhesions are pulled.

As endometriosis develops, a woman's immune system becomes more and more impaired, leading to further health problems. Due to increased research, as well as surveys of endometriosis patients, it is now becoming clear that women with the disease are susceptible to other serious health problems including:

- Chronic fatigue syndrome (one hundred times more common in women with endometriosis)
- Hypothyroidism (seven times more common in women with endometriosis)
- Fibromyalgia
- Rheumatoid arthritis

Causes of Endometriosis

- **Retrograde menstruation:** This theory was postulated in the early 1920s by Dr. Sampson. He speculated that during menstruation, a certain amount of menstrual fluid flows backward from the uterus to "shower the pelvic organs and pelvis lining" with endometrium cells. However, studies have shown that many women experience retrograde menstruation but do not go on to develop endometriosis. In fact, it is thought that

90 % of women have retrograde menstruation. This theory also fails to explain why endometriosis can be found in remote areas such as the lungs, breasts, lymph nodes, and even the eyes.

- **Altered Immune Function:** The endometrial tissue survives and responds to the hormone estrogen.
- **Free Radical Production:** Increased free radical production promotes the growth of endometrial tissue.
- **The transplantation theory:** This theory states that endometriosis spreads via the circulatory and lymphatic systems.
- **Coelomic Metaplasia:** This theory holds that certain cells, when stimulated, can transform themselves into a different kind of cells, as occurs in women taking estrogen replacement therapy.
- **The hereditary theory:** Women with family members who have endometriosis are more susceptible to developing the disease. Similar to this theory is the idea that women can be born with migrant endometrial cells in the pelvic cavity, which later in life can develop into endometriosis.
- **Environmental factors:** A great deal of research clearly highlights that women who are exposed to environmental toxins are at much greater risk of developing endometriosis along with other serious health disorders. These toxins include PCBs, DDT, and dioxin, all of which are widely spread throughout the world today. The other major environmental toxins are collectively known as xenoestrogens. These are compounds and chemicals found in the environment and food chain that react negatively with the natural balance of the body, both male and female, causing a damaging imbalance in the system.
- **Liver disorders:** The liver regulates and removes estrogen from the body. If the function of the liver is compromised, then serious health problems can emerge, including endometriosis.
- **Autoimmune disorder:** Of all the theories postulated for the cause of endometriosis, the idea that this disease is an autoimmune disease seems the most likely, credible and feasible. Autoimmune diseases are now widely believed to occur based on genetic predisposition that may be triggered by environmental and other external factors.

Risk Factors for Endometriosis

- Family history of endometriosis, especially mother or sister
- Late childbearing (after age thirty)
- History of long menstrual cycles (longer than seven days) with a shorter than normal time between cycles (shorter than twenty-five days)
- Abnormal uterus structure
- Diet high in hydrogenated fat (trans fat) and animal fats
- Higher stress levels and poor adaptation to stress
- Estrogen dominance
- Hormone replacement therapy
- Environmental estrogen exposure
- Increased body fat
- Lack of exercise from an early age
- Use of an intrauterine device (IUD)
- Being a redhead
- Childhood sexual abuse
- Alcohol use
- Prenatal exposure to high estrogen levels
- Poor liver function
- Bowel toxicity and constipation
- Dysbiosis, or imbalance in the bowel flora

Protective Factors

- Vegetarian diet that restricts dairy and sugar
- Avoidance of animal fat to reduce arachidonic acid, which causes inflammation and pain
- Increased dietary fiber
- Balanced bowel flora
- Optimal bowel function—three bowel movements daily reduces estrogen
- High intake of antioxidants, which reduces adhesions
- Optimal liver function
- Regular exercise

Laboratory Testing and Diagnosis of Endometriosis

Diagnosis methods of endometriosis can include:

Physical examination

A pelvic examination involves the physician manually assessing and looking for abnormalities that are associated with endometriosis in the pelvic area. Physical findings depend on the severity and location of the disease. There may be palpable nodules or tenderness in the pelvic region, enlarged ovaries, a tipped-back (retro-displaced) uterus, or lesions on the vagina or on surgical scars.

Laparoscopy

A laparoscopy is an exploratory procedure that allows the physician to see inside the pelvic region to observe and check for endometrial growths. The procedure involves making a small incision near the navel and inserting a laparoscope (a long, thin, lighted instrument) into the abdomen. The abdomen is distended with carbon dioxide gas to make it easier to see the abdominal organs. Usually, the endometrial growths can easily be seen. Because endometriosis implants or growths vary in appearance and can be mistaken for other conditions, the lesions should be surgically removed and examined under a microscope to confirm the presence of the disease.

Imaging tests

Imaging tests (e.g., pelvic ultrasound, magnetic resonance imaging) may be used to identify individual endometrial lesions, but they are not used to determine the extent of the disease. The implants are not easily identified using this method.

Biochemical markers

There has been extensive investigation of a membrane antigen called CA-125 in women with endometriosis. Several reports suggest that levels of CA-125 are elevated in women with endometriosis, particularly those in the advanced stages of the disease. A recent study of this antigen level showed it to be high in 90% of women with endometriosis. Possible diagnosis with a blood test to check levels of CA-125 could be used to check for endometriosis.

In addition, lab tests to determine if estrogen dominance is a factor should be administered.

Complete Female Hormone Panel	Estradiol and progesterone levels and their ratio are an index of estrogen/ progesterone balance. An excess of estradiol, relative to progesterone, can explain many symptoms in reproductive age-women. Testosterone levels can also be either too high or too low. Testosterone in excess, often caused by ovarian cysts, leads to conditions such as excessive facial and body hair,

	acne, and oily skin and hair. Polycystic ovarian syndrome (PCOS) is thought to be caused, in part, by insulin resistance. On the other hand, too little testosterone is often caused by excessive stress, medications, contraceptives, and surgical removal of the ovaries. This leads to symptoms of androgen deficiency including loss of libido, thinning skin, vaginal dryness, loss of bone and muscle mass, depression, and memory lapses. SHBG binds tightly to circulating estradiol and testosterone, preventing their rapid metabolism and clearance and limiting their bioavailability to tissues. SHBG gives a good index of the extent of the body's overall exposure to estrogens.

Conventional Medicine Treatments Indicated for Endometriosis[146]

Drug Therapy

- Non-steroidal anti-inflammatory drugs, such as ibuprofen, naproxen, and mefenamic acid, relieve mild to moderate pain in about 80% of women
- Drug treatments are geared toward manipulating hormone levels, either through oral contraceptive use, progestins, or gonadotrophin releasing hormone (GnRH) analogs, which cause a decline in FSH and LH and inhibit ovulation and menstruation, putting women in a menopausal state
- It is usually recommended to take oral contraceptives continuously so there is no menstrual bleeding, and this prevents implanted endometrial tissue from enlarging, bleeding, and causing pain. Oral contraceptives must be continued long-term to be effective.

Surgery

- Surgery can bring long-lasting pain relief to some women
- Adhesions may be removed so pregnancy becomes possible. Surgical techniques include laser surgery, electro cautery (burning), knife excision and scraping, and a partial or full hysterectomy

Nutritional Factors Affecting Endometriosis

Populations from certain countries show a much higher incidence of hormonal symptoms, especially in the Western hemisphere, where they derive a large part of their dietary calories from fat. Women who switched from a typical high-fat, refined-carbohydrate diet to a low-fat, high-fiber, plant-based diet have shown to have decreasing estrogen levels even though they did not adjust their total calorie intake. Plants contain over five thousand known sterols that have progestogenic effects. Cultures whose eating habits are more wholesome and who exercise more have a far lower incidence of hormonal symptoms because their pre- and postmenopausal levels of estrogen do not drop as significantly due to healthier lifetime nutrition.

The following recommendations are specifically indicated for endometriosis:

- Eat a high fiber diet: Use two tablespoons per day of ground flax seed to displace strong estrogens and cleanse the bowel. Use 45 mg of fiber daily by taking two tablespoons of wheat bran (if not allergic). Take

[146] Complete Natural Medicine Guide to Women's Health Sat Dharam Kaur, ND pg. 366

one tablespoon of psyllium, two tablespoons of freshly ground flax seed, and one cup of beans daily to improve elimination of estrogen

- Add two tablespoons of unheated flax seed oil to your food to decrease inflammation
- Use two tablespoons or more of turmeric daily to inactivate environmental estrogens, cleanse your liver and decrease inflammation
- Eat a high protein vegetarian diet
- Increase intake of vegetable, nuts, and seeds
- Eat cold water fish (salmon, tuna, sardines, mackerel, or herring) two to three times per week
- Eat organic foods
- Omit alcohol, dairy, red meat, sugar, and caffeine
- Studies have shown that drinking more than two cups of coffee per day may increase estrogen levels in women. It could also lead to problems such as endometriosis and breast pain. An average cup of coffee (four ounces) contains about 100 mg of caffeine and an average cup of tea (eight ounces) contains about a third to half the caffeine content of coffee.

Herbal Medicine Indicated for Endometriosis

Estrogen is metabolized in the liver. Herbs that fortify the liver will speed up estrogen clearance from the body. Estrogen that is not metabolized by the liver will continue to circulate and exert its effect on the body, worsening any developing endometriosis.

Milk Thistle *(Silymarin marianus)*

Much research has been done on a special extract of milk thistle known as silymarin, a group of flavonoid compounds. These compounds protect the liver from damage and enhance the detoxification process. Silymarin prevents damage to the liver by acting as an antioxidant and is much more effective than vitamin E and vitamin C. Numerous research studies have demonstrated its protective effect on the liver and it also works by preventing the depletion of glutathione. The higher the glutathione concentration, the greater the liver's capacity to detoxify harmful chemicals. Silymarin has been shown to increase the level of glutathione by up to 35%. In human studies, silymarin is shown to exhibit positive effects in treating liver diseases of various kinds, including cirrhosis, chronic hepatitis, fatty infiltration of the liver, and inflammation of the bile duct. Dosage: standardized extract 200 mg to 800 mg a day

Dandelion Root *(Taraxacum officinalis)*

Dandelion root works on the liver and gallbladder to help remove waste products and has been deemed one of nature's most detoxifying herbs. By supporting the liver, excessive estrogens and toxins can be deactivated. In addition, dandelion leaf contains vitamins A, C, and K, potassium, calcium, and choline.

Prickly Ash *(Xanthoxylum americanum)*

Through its stimulation of blood flow throughout the body, prickly ash helps enhance the transport of oxygen and nutrients and the removal of cellular waste products. Prickly ash is known for its specific action on capillary engorgement and sluggish circulation. For women with pelvic congestion, this herb enhances circulation throughout the pelvis.

Motherwort *(Leonorus cardiaca)*

Motherwort is a mild sedative and a well-known anti-spasmodic. Women with endometriosis generally experience uterine cramps and pain; motherwort is useful in promoting relaxing during times of extreme bearing-down pain in the uterus and other regions. The alkaloids stachydrine, betonicine, and leonurine are responsible for these anti-spasmodic effects. Motherwort promotes blood flow to reproductive organs, balances hormones, affecting the menstrual cycle, and is of specific use in conditions with associated nervous origin, such as anxiety or tension.

Chasteberry *(Vitex agnus castus)*

Chasteberry regulates pituitary function, which in turn helps to regulate ovulation and production of progesterone. It can help stabilize an irregular cycle and reduce many of the symptoms of fibroids (including heavy bleeding, menstrual cramps, and clotting). Chasteberry has dopaminergic action in that it inhibits the secretion of prolactin from the pituitary gland and normalizes pituitary gland function. This will in turn restore levels of progesterone, decreasing the prevalence of estrogen dominance. Chasteberry has the therapeutic effect of lowering harmful estrogen levels while also maintaining progesterone levels at very small doses (5 mL per day).

Specific Nutrients Indicated for Endometriosis

Magnesium

Magnesium is a mineral believed to ease cramping with menstruation. Low levels in the diet and in our bodies increase susceptibility to diseases, including heart disease, high blood pressure, kidney stones, cancer, insomnia, PMS, and menstrual cramps. Dosage: 200 mg to 600 mg per day

Zinc

Zinc is essential for enzyme activity, helping cells to reproduce, which helps with healing. Zinc is also reported to improve the immune system and help to create an emotional sense of well-being. Zinc lowers estrogen production in endometrial cells by inhibiting aromatase enzyme. Thirty-three percent of healthy adults over age fifty have zinc deficiency and are unaware of it. The percentage increases to 90% for those older than 70 years of age. Dosage: 50 mg per day with food

Calcium

Levels of calcium in menstruating women decrease ten to fourteen days before the onset of menstruation. Deficiency may lead to muscle cramps, headache, or pelvic pain. Dosage: 500 mg to 1500 mg per day

Beta Carotene

Beta carotene (or pro vitamin A) is the compound that colors vegetables yellow or orange. Beta carotene, one of over four hundred identified carotenes, protects plants from oxidative damage during photosynthesis. Beta carotene consists of two molecules of vitamin A linked to each other; the body converts beta carotene into vitamin A as needed. Beta carotene acts as an antioxidant, trapping and neutralizing single oxygen molecules and other free radicals, which can damage the body's cellular membranes, lipids, proteins, and vitamins. In addition, beta carotene enhances the immune system by stimulating the activity of interferon. Dosage: 15 mg to 45 mg of beta carotene per day (25,000 to 75,000 IU)

B vitamins

B vitamins are important for the breakdown of proteins, carbohydrates, and fats in the body. B vitamins are reported to improve the emotional symptoms of endometriosis. They act by enabling the liver to inactivate estrogen. Studies have shown that supplementation of B vitamins may cause the liver to become more efficient in processing estrogen. Dosage: 50 mg to 100 mg per day

Vitamin C

Vitamin C is well-known for helping to boost the immune system and helping to provide resistance to disease. It is also used in the body to build and maintain collagen. Studies using vitamin C show an increase in cellular immunity and decreases in autoimmune progression and fatigue. Vitamin C also enhances immunity and decreases capillary fragility and tumor growth, all of which are involved in various levels in endometriosis. Dosage: six grams to ten grams per day in divided doses, starting at one gram and increasing every four days

Vitamin E

Vitamin E plays an important role by increasing oxygen-carrying capacities and strengthening the immune system. Vitamin E helps to correct abnormal progesterone/estradiol ratios through the inhibition of the arachidonic lipid pathway, which helps to prevent the release of chemicals that would normally cause edema, inflammation, and smooth muscle contraction. Dosage: 400 to 800 IU per day

Omega-3 Fatty Acids-Fish Oils

Fish oils increase anti-inflammatory prostaglandins and decrease inflammatory prostaglandins (PGE2, PGF2-alpha). Fish oils have also been shown to decrease endometrial growth and pain. Recent research demonstrates that a higher omega-3 to omega-6 fatty acid ratio may have a suppressive effect on the *in vitro* survival of endometrial cells. The obvious conclusion is that omega-3 fatty acids may be useful in the management of endometriosis by decreasing inflammation. Dosage: 1000 mg to 6000 mg per day

Bioidentical Progesterone

Natural progesterone helps to reduce the risk of ovarian, endometrial, and breast cancers. Unopposed estradiol causes are frequently associated with fibrocystic breast disease, endometriosis, PMS, fibroids, and breast cancer. Specific dosage varies depending on the condition. For endometriosis, apply 20 mg of natural progesterone cream starting on day eight and continue until day twenty-six of a usual twenty-eight-day menstrual cycle. It can take up to six months to notice the effect, and if no results are seen within two months, the dosage may have to be increased up to 40 mg per day. As the desired results are obtained, the dosage can be decreased until the lowest effective dose is found. Continue until menopause, and if flare-ups occur, increase the dosage to reduce symptoms.

Castor Oil Packs

Apply a castor oil pack to the lower abdomen three to five times per week. The skin absorbs the warm castor oil's active constituents, lectins, which stimulate the immune response to help shrink fibroids. Castor oil is extracted from the castor plant (*Ricinus communis*). It should not be taken internally, as it will act as a powerful laxative. But if applied externally or topically it has unique medicinal actions on the body. It penetrates skin and muscle to reach right into underlying tissue and assists in decongestion and breakdown of inflammatory material through enhancing blood flow and lymphatic flow in the area. This also helps in the removal of toxins and the elimination of wastes. Castor oil is warming to the tissues, easing stiffness and pain.

Occasions to use a castor oil pack

- Lymphatic congestion
- Arthritis or rheumatism
- Fibromyalgia
- Muscle spasms
- Abdominal inflammations
- Pelvic congestion
- Glandular swellings
- Deep infections
- Adhesions
- Fibroids
- Endometriosis
- Back ache
- Muscle tension
- Local pain due to inflammation or spasm

How to make a castor oil pack

- Take a piece of flannel or towel and fold it three or four times, so that it is large enough to entirely cover the area to be treated.
- Pour castor oil all over until thoroughly soaked.
- Place over the skin and cover with a large piece of saran wrap.
- Cover with a heating pad or hot water bottle and leave in place for one to two hours.
- After use, the pack can be wrapped in plastic and stored in the refrigerator (bring back to room temperature before re-use). You may wish to add a little more castor oil with each use. The pack should be discarded after ten uses.

Exercise

Properly performed exercises have been shown to modulate hormonal imbalances. Moderate exercise also increases the body's production of endorphins, which are natural pain relievers. Those who exercise regularly are generally happier, less depressed, and have a more optimistic outlook on life. This results in increased life expectancy.

Precision anti-aging exercises must incorporate flexibility, cardiovascular, and strength-training exercises: five minutes of flexibility training every day, twenty to thirty minutes of cardiovascular training three times a week, and fifteen to twenty minutes of strength training two times a week. A properly structured program takes an average of thirty, minutes a day which is less than 2% of the entire day.

Reduce Exposure to Environmental Estrogens

Xenoestrogens found in certain pesticides, plastics, fuels, and drugs are difficult for the body to break down, and can amplify the effects of estrogen. These substances can increase the estrogen load in the body over time and are difficult to detoxify through the liver. Exposure to xenoestrogens is a concern for everyone. Those with estrogen dominance conditions, such as fibroids, should be particularly concerned with avoiding xenoestrogens.

Xenoestrogens can be found in many of our meats and dairy products in the form of chemicals and growth hormones that are given to the animals from which these products come. These can be quite powerful and should be avoided whenever possible. Choosing meat and dairy items that do not contain Rbst can help decrease xen-oestrogen exposure.

Sources of xenoestrogens that should be avoided:

- Commercially raised meat
- Canned foods
- Plastics, plastic food wraps
- Styrofoam cups
- Industrial wastes
- Personal care products
- Pesticides and herbicides
- Paints, lacquers, and solvents
- Plant estrogens (soy, flaxseeds)
- Car exhaust and indoor toxins
- Cosmetics
- Birth control pills and spermicide
- Detergents
- All artificial scents
- Air fresheners and perfumes

Top 5 Strategies for Endometriosis

1. Complete Hormone testing
2. Reduce exposure to xenoestrogens
3. Liver detoxification
4. Consume a nutrient dense, high fiber, organic vegetarian diet/ Eliminate sugar, caffeine and alcohol
5. Supplement with DIM, Calcium D-glucarate, B-Complex vitamins, Magnesium, Zinc, Omega 3's and a combination of Prickly Ash, Motherwort, Ginger, Cramp bark and Vitex as well as Bioidentical Progesterone when needed/Apply castor oil packs regularly

Polycystic Ovarian Syndrome (PCOS)

PCOS is a common condition that affects 4% to 10% of North American women of reproductive age and accounts for approximately 8% of all anovulation cases. PCOS is a syndrome rather than a disease because it is not a specific and constant set of symptoms and physical characteristics. PCOS is rather used to describe a group of clinical presentations characterized by bilateral polycystic ovaries, potentially combined with amenorrhea, anovulation, infertility, insulin resistance, truncal obesity, and hirsuitism. Hormonal imbalances can range from the hypothalamus, pituitary gland, ovaries, and adrenal glands to insulin excess, androgen excess, and prolactin excess.[147] Polycystic ovaries are defined as twelve or more follicles in at least one ovary as seen by an ultrasound. Follicles are small, fluid-filled sacs containing eggs. In PCOS, the follicles bunch together to form cysts. Note that not every woman with PCOS has polycystic ovaries.

Symptoms of PCOS

- **Weight gain or inability to lose weight.** Weight accumulation is particularly found around the waist (waste: hip ratio is greater than 0.85) and this weight gain is linked with imbalances of glucose and insulin in the body.
- **Absent or Irregular Periods** (amenorrhea or oligomenorrhea). Nine or fewer menstrual cycles per year may be a sign of PCOS. Bleeding may be heavier than normal. These conditions are caused because the ovaries are not producing hormones that keep the menstrual cycle regular. Irregular or absent menses indicates that a woman is likely not ovulating.
- **Infertility**. The high levels of excess insulin seen with PCOS can stimulate the ovaries to produce large amounts of the male hormone (androgens), which can possibly prevent the ovaries from releasing an egg each month, thus causing infertility.
- **Excess hair growth** (Hirsuitism). High levels of circulating testosterone cause excess hair in the facial area and on the arms, legs, abdomen, chest, and back.
- **Thinning hair.** This is caused by higher levels of androgens in women.
- **Acne.** Due to the higher levels of androgens, the acne is usually found around the face (especially along the jaw line), chest, and back.

---

[147] Fundamentals of Naturopathic Endocrinology Michael Friedman, MD pg. 151

- **Ovarian Cysts.** The elevation in insulin levels contributes to the formation of cysts in the ovaries, in part due to the hormonal imbalances, and also because the ovaries are highly sensitive to the influence of insulin.
- **Recurrent miscarriage**. Forty-five percent of women with PCOS miscarry in the first trimester.
- **Fatigue**. Fatigue is a common symptom that may be related to PCOS in that insulin resistance and the possibility of hypothyroidism can cause reduced energy levels.
- **Other Skin Problems.** Skin tags-thick lumps of skin sometimes as large as raisins—can form as a result of PCOS. They are usually found in the armpits, at the bra line, or on the neck. Darkening and thickening of the skin can also occur around the neck, groin, underarms, or skin folds. This condition, called Acanthosis Nigricans, is a sign of insulin resistance. Other women with PCOS note an increase in dandruff.
- **Mood Swings**. Many women with PCOS may find themselves more anxious or depressed by their appearance or their inability to become pregnant.
- **High cholesterol** (Hyperlipidemia) **and high blood pressure** (Hypertension).
- **Sleep Apnea.** Women with PCOS have a high risk for sleep apnea. This may be due to the increased BMI (Body Mass Index) in about half of women with PCOS. Another possible reason for the increased prevalence of sleep apnea in people with PCOS is the effect of testosterone on the blood vessels.

Current studies clearly link polycystic ovarian syndrome to insulin resistance. A report released in the British Journal of Obstetrics and Gynecology in 2000 indicated that up to 40% of women with PCOS have either impaired glucose tolerance or Type 2 Diabetes by age forty. In addition, with polycystic ovarian syndrome, high levels of insulin stimulate the ovaries to produce large amounts of testosterone, which can possibly prevent the ovaries from releasing an egg each month, thus causing infertility. High testosterone levels can also cause excessive hair growth, male pattern baldness, and acne. Researchers have found a link between polycystic ovarian syndrome and other metabolic conditions such as high levels of obesity, LDL (the "bad" cholesterol), and high blood pressure. These are all risk factors for coronary heart disease, as well as symptoms of metabolic syndrome. Also known as Syndrome X, this disorder substantially increases your chances of developing cardiovascular disease.

The underlying cause of PCOS is varied and still evolving. Some of the most current findings include:

- Elevated secretions of androgens from the ovaries and/or adrenal glands that overwhelm the body's ability to convert these androgens into estrogen
- Abnormal ratios of the pituitary hormones—luteinizing hormone (LH) to follicle stimulating hormone (FSH)
- Failure of the monthly maturing of a follicle in the ovaries
- Resistance to insulin
- Likely a genetically-driven defect in the action of insulin

Laboratory Testing and Diagnosis of PCOS

Women with PCOS are at high risk for diabetes, high blood pressure, heart disease, and cancer. Findings substantially raised the bar on the seriousness of the condition and made it even more important that physicians correctly diagnose PCOS and recommend appropriate therapy. Specific hormonal imbalances are typically seen in patients with PCOS and testing should therefore include the following:

- Elevated fasting insulin levels
- Elevated LH, which causes the ovaries to produce more androgens
- Elevated androstenedione and testosterone
- Elevated prolactin (in 25% of cases)
- Elevated estrogen, specifically estrone
- Decreased levels of SHBG (sex hormone binding globulin)
- Increased levels of growth hormone

- Increased levels of IGF-1
- Elevated triglycerides
- Elevated LDL; lowered HDL
- Elevated cortisol

The following lab panels are indicated:

Adrenal Stress Index	The panel utilizes four saliva samples. Salivary cortisol measurement reflects the free (bioactive) fraction of serum cortisol. The test report shows the awake diurnal cortisol rhythm generated in response to real-life stress. The cortisol/DHEA relationship highlights the many facets of stress maladaptation. The cortisol/DHEA ratio helps determine the projected time for recovery, and the substances (hormones, supplements, and botanicals) that promote this recovery. The cortisol/DHEA ratio regulates a multitude of functions. The panel measures P17-OH levels in order to evaluate the efficiency of the conversion of adrenal precursors into cortisol. Certain adrenal fatigue patients who are genetically predisposed to low production of cortisol will not benefit from exogenous supplementation of pregnenolone or progesterone. The panel includes fasting and non-fasting insulin measurements. The insulin values are used to diagnose insulin resistance-functional insulin deficit (pre-diabetes), as well as to correlate elevated cortisol with insulin to help explain glycemic dysregulation problems.
Complete Female Hormone Panel	Estradiol and progesterone levels and their ratio are an index of estrogen/progesterone balance. An excess of estradiol, relative to progesterone, can explain many symptoms in reproductive age-women. Testosterone levels can also be either too high or too low. Testosterone in excess, often caused by ovarian cysts, leads to conditions such as excessive facial and body hair, acne, and oily skin and hair. Polycystic ovarian syndrome (PCOS) is thought to be caused, in part, by insulin resistance. On the other hand, too little testosterone is often caused by excessive stress, medications, contraceptives, and surgical removal of the ovaries. This leads to symptoms of androgen deficiency including loss of libido, thinning skin, vaginal dryness, loss of bone and muscle mass, depression, and memory lapses. SHBG binds tightly to circulating estradiol and testosterone, preventing their rapid metabolism and clearance and limiting their bioavailability to tissues. SHBG gives a good index of the extent of the body's overall exposure to estrogens.
Thyroid Hormone Testing	A complete thyroid profile includes free T4, free T3, TSH, and TPO and can indicate the presence of an imbalance in thyroid function. Hypothyroidism includes feeling cold all the time, low stamina, fatigue (particularly in the evening), anxiety, depression, low sex drive, weight gain, and high cholesterol. Hyperthyroidism includes heat intolerance, anxiety, palpitations, weight loss, tired but wired feeling, visual disturbances, and insomnia.

Cardiometabolic Profile (hs-CRP), Fasting Insulin, Hemoglobin A1c (HbA1c), Fasting Triglycerides, Total Cholesterol, LDL Cholesterol, VLDL Cholesterol, and HDL Cholesterol	High Sensitivity C-Reactive Protein (hs-CRP) Hs-CRP is an established marker of inflammation and has recently been suggested to be an important contributor to pro-inflammatory and prothrombic elements of cardiovascular disease risk. Increased CRP levels, which correlate inversely with insulin sensitivity, have been found in individuals with polycystic ovarian syndrome and may be a marker of early cardiovascular risk in these patients. Fasting Insulin High fasting insulin levels are a good indicator of insulin resistance, which occurs when the cellular response to the presence of insulin is impaired, resulting in a reduced ability of tissues to take up glucose for energy production. Chronically high insulin levels are seen as the body attempts to normalize blood sugar levels. HbA1c HbA1c levels above 6% can predict CVD and DM2 in high-risk individuals. Fasting Triglycerides Hypertriglyceridemia, a triglyceride level greater than 150 mg/ld., is an established indicator of atherogenic dyslipidemia and is often found in untreated DM2 and obesity. Total Cholesterol, LDL Cholesterol, VLDL Cholesterol, and HDL Cholesterol Abnormalities in the lipid profile, including high total cholesterol, high LDL cholesterol, high VLDL cholesterol, and low HDL cholesterol, are a significant component of coronary heart disease risk because of their contribution to the development of atherosclerosis.

Conventional Pharmaceutical Indications for PCOS

- Oral Contraceptives: These artificially regulate the menstrual cycle and prevent excess hair growth but will cause insulin levels to become higher and increase long-term risk of heart disease and breast cancer
- Ovulation induction: Drugs such as Clomid are used to induce ovulation in women who are attempting to conceive and more than six cycles increase the risk of ovarian cancer
- Metformin: This is the most commonly prescribed medication for PCOS. It increases body cell sensitivity to insulin so that less needs to be secreted. By lowering insulin levels, Metformin lowers testosterone, androstenedione, and LH levels, increases SHBG, and enhances ovulation
- Spironolactone: This is a drug that inhibits the binding of testosterone to receptors in hair follicles and therefore decreases abnormal hair growth. Side effects include excess urination, weight gain, breast tenderness, and dizziness

Nutritional Factors Affecting PCOS

- Avoid all sugars and sweeteners other than stevia and consume moderate amounts of whole fruit
- Avoid carbohydrates that have a high glycemic index, such as white rice, corn, millet, and white flour
- Avoid all refined and processed foods

- Consume low glycemic carbohydrates such as pearl barley and beans (legumes)
- Avoid red meat and dairy as they increase the risk factors for heart disease and cancer
- Eat small, frequent meals throughout the day rather than the typical two to three large meals
- Combine protein with every meal or snack to lower insulin resistance
- Eat high-fiber foods that are low in glycemic load, such as apples, cabbage, raw carrots, oatmeal, oat bran, sesame seeds, flax seeds, psyllium seed powder, and beans
- Consume three to four cups of organic green tea daily to lower testosterone and insulin
- Consume complex carbohydrates at breakfast, such as steel cut oatmeal, buckwheat (which contains D-chiro-Inositol), or oat bran with sliced organic apple and cinnamon (to lower blood sugar) and unsweetened soy, almond, or hemp milk

Herbal Medicine Indicated for PCOS

Saw palmetto *(Seronoa serrulata)*

Saw palmetto reduces the conversion of testosterone to dihydrotestosterone, which is the more potent form, by inhibiting the activity of the enzyme 5-alpha reductase. This reduction of testosterone aids in decreasing the PCOS symptoms of acne, excess facial and body hair, and hair loss from the scalp. Saw palmetto's actions are mainly due to its content of polysaccharides, steroids, and fixed oils, including free fatty acids. These constituents inhibit androgen binding action and are estrogenic in nature.

Gymnema *(Gymnema sylvestre)*

Gymnema is a plant that has been used for over two thousand years in Ayurvedic medicine in India to treat diabetes and to improve the blood glucose lowering effects of insulin. Gymnema is often given clinically to women with polycystic ovarian syndrome because it acts in a very similar manner to metformin. One study of lab animals showed that gymnema suppresses the elevation of blood glucose levels by inhibiting glucose uptake in the intestine.[148] Gymnema regenerates the cells in the islets of Langerhans, which are specialized cells in the pancreas which produce insulin. Gymnema also stimulates the pancreas to produce more insulin and increases the activity of certain enzymes that help the cells to utilize glucose therefore increasing their sensitivity. In addition, gymnema increases the uptake of glucose into the muscles and cells of the body where it can be used for energy and it reverses damage done to the liver by high blood sugar.

Licorice Root *(Glycyrrhiza glabra)*

In a 1982 trial, eight anovulatory infertile women with elevated testosterone were investigated for lowering serum testosterone levels and inducing regular ovulation by a formula containing equal parts of peony root (Paeonia lactiflora) and licorice root (Glycyrrhiza glabra). Serum testosterone levels were significantly lowered in seven patients by doses of five to ten grams of the combination daily for two to eight weeks. Six of eight patients ovulated regularly and two of eight patients conceived (Yaginuma et al.)[149] In a similar trial in 1988, a significant reduction of circulating testosterone occurred in eighteen of twenty female subjects with PCOS (Takahashi et al.). Five of the eighteen became pregnant. The mechanisms of action of licorice root are partly due to its content of glycyrrhetic acid, a metabolite of glycyrrhizin that inhibits the conversion of androstenedione to testosterone. Armanini et al. suggested that glycyrrhizin, or its metabolites, act on the enzymes that convert 17-hydroxy-progesterone to androstenedione, effectively lowering testosterone.

---

[148] http://www.ovarian-cysts-pcos.com/gymnema.html

[149] http://www.digitalnaturopath.com/cond/C485625.html

Chasteberry *(Vitex agnus castus)*

Chasteberry acts on the hypothalamus and pituitary glands by increasing luteinizing hormone (LH) production and mildly inhibiting the release of follicle stimulating hormone (FSH). The result is a shift in the ratio of estrogen to progesterone, in favor of progesterone. Chasteberry may be helpful for women with PCOS who do not have a normal menstrual cycle and thus don't ovulate or menstruate. A large percentage of these menstrual problems are related to insufficient progesterone during the luteal phase of the menstrual cycle, which is called a luteal phase defect or corpus luteum insufficiency. A corpus luteum insufficiency is defined as an abnormally low progesterone levels three weeks after the onset of menstruation. Insufficient levels of progesterone may result in the formation of ovarian cysts

Specific Nutrients Indicated for PCOS

D-chiro-inositol

D-chiro-inositol is a relative of common inositol (a B vitamin) and is found in small concentrations in the human body and in some foods. It is a compound that has been reported to affect the action of insulin. There is evidence that the insulin resistance seen in women with PCOS is due in part to a deficiency of D-chiro-inositol or to a defect in its utilization in the tissues. If these abnormalities can be reversed by supplementation with D-chiro-inositol, then this compound might be beneficial for women with PCOS. To test that possibility, forty-four obese women with PCOS were randomly assigned to receive, in double-blind fashion, D-chiro-inositol (1,200 mg once a day) or placebo for eight weeks. Supplementation with D-chiro-inositol resulted in an improvement in insulin resistance and a 55% reduction in testosterone levels compared to the placebo group. Significantly more women ovulated in the D-chiro-inositol group than in the placebo group (86% vs. 27%). D-chiro-inositol supplementation decreased testosterone levels and improved ovulatory function, presumably by enhancing the action of insulin.[150] Dosage: 1200mg per day

Vitamin D

Vitamin D plays a role in glucose metabolism and is commonly deficient in individuals with Type 2 diabetes, a common complication of PCOS. Supplementing with vitamin D has been shown to improve glucose tolerance, insulin secretion, and insulin sensitivity in those with diabetes. A deficiency of vitamin D may be more frequent in women with PCOS and in a small study, five of thirteen women had an overt vitamin D deficiency. Seven of the nine women with no menses or infrequent menses had a return to a normal menstrual cycle within two months of being given 50,000 IU once or twice per week of vitamin D and 1,500 mg per day of calcium.[151] Dosage: 1000 IU to 10,000 IU

Chromium

Chromium potentiates the action of insulin, probably by facilitating the binding of insulin to its receptor, by enhancing insulin-dependent functions, or both.[152] Supplementation with chromium has been shown in some studies to improve the blood sugar control in those with type 2 diabetes. Giving women with PCOS 1,000 mcg per day of chromium for as little as two months was able to improve insulin sensitivity by 30% and by 38% in obese women with PCOS.[153] Dosage: 600 to 1000mcg per day

---

[150] Diabetes Care 2006;29: pp.300-305] [Engl J Med. 1999 Apr 29;340(17): pp.1314-20]Specific Nutrients Indicated for PCOS

[151] Prager N, Bicket K, French N, Marovici G. A randomized, double-blind, placebo-controlled trial to determine the effectiveness of botanically derived inhibitors of 5-alpha-reductase in the treatment of androgenetic alopecia. JAH and Comple Med 2002; 8(2): 143-152.

[152] Mertz W. Chromium and it relation to carbohydrate metabolism. Med Clin North Am 1976;60:739-744

[153] Lydic L, McNurlan M. Komaroff E, et al. Effects of chromium supplementation on insulin sensitivity and reproductive function in PCOS: a pilot study. Fertil Steril 2003;80 (Suppl 3):S45-S46

Omega 3 Fatty Acids- Fish Oils

Fish oil supplements rich in the omega-3 fatty acids EPA and DHA can decrease insulin resistance and aid in the treatment of PCOS. In addition to being characterized by insulin resistance as well as hyperinsulinemia, or high blood insulin levels, the hormonal imbalance underlying PCOS also includes high androgen levels. A study published in the March 2011 issue of the *American Journal of Clinical Nutrition* showed that omega-3 fat supplementation in young women with PCOS resulted in improved androgen levels. [154]. In addition, it improves glucose metabolism and promotes healthy prostaglandin production. Dosage: 2000 to 4000mg per day

N-acetyl-cysteine (NAC)

NAC is a derivative of the amino acid cysteine, which has antioxidant properties and is required for the body's production of glutathione. Glutathione, along with NAC, is a powerful antioxidant that is needed in the treatment of PCOS. NAC is not found in the diet but is available as a nutritional supplement. It has been shown to be incredibly beneficial in controlling PCOS. A recent study evaluated the effect of NAC on insulin secretion and insulin resistance in six lean and thirty-one obese women with polycystic ovary syndrome. The lean women took 1.8 grams of NAC daily for five to six weeks. Six of the thirty-one obese patients were treated with placebo. Those treated with NAC had a reduction of their insulin resistance and a significant fall in testosterone levels. [155] Dosage: 1800mg to 3000mg per day

Alpha Lipoic Acid (ALA)

ALA is one of the most potent antioxidants, with the unique ability to cross the blood-brain barrier and work as a free radical scavenger in the brain. ALA is both water- and fat-soluble and is therefore capable of providing antioxidant benefits to both the inside and outside of the cells. ALA helps the body to re-use other antioxidants such as vitamins C and E, the amino acid glutathione, and substances such as coenzyme Q10, which is very important in glucose metabolism and regulation of blood sugar levels. Of particular relevance to women with PCOS, ALA has been shown to greatly increase insulin sensitivity. It has also been proven to increase the rate of glucose transportation from the blood into the cells where it can provide energy to the muscles and brain, increasing muscle performance (under exercise conditions) and providing increased brain energy availability. Dosage: 600mg per day in divided doses

Bioidentical Progesterone Cream

Women with PCOS always have low progesterone levels and therefore one of the core treatments is correcting these levels by supplementing with bioidentical progesterone. Bioidentical progesterone is progesterone which is derived from a natural plant source, such as yams, and then converted to progesterone. Bioidentical progesterone has the same molecular configuration as the progesterone produced by the body and can be used to supplement the progesterone produced by the body and to balance estrogen, testosterone, and progesterone levels. Bioidentical progesterone has no side effects when 20 mg to 40 mg per day is used. Dosage: In early PCOS, use 32 mg from days twelve to twenty-six of the menstrual cycle; in advanced PCOS, use 54 mg from days twelve to twenty-six of the cycle; in severe PCOS with pain, use 64 mg from days five to twenty-six.

Exercise and PCOS

By exercising four to eight hours per week, muscle mass can be increased, fat mass can be decreased, and hormones can be balanced. A number of studies have demonstrated that women with PCOS or insulin resistance can greatly benefit from regular exercise. For example, a study conducted at the University of Adelaide in Australia showed that a six month program of diet and exercise helped eighteen overweight women with PCOS normalize their hormones. They experienced an 11% reduction in central fat, 71% improvement in insulin sensitivity, 33% fall in insulin levels, and 39% reduction in LH (luteinizing hormone) levels. The women in this study achieved surprising results with a combination of diet and exercise in just six months. This study is relevant because insulin resistance and chronically

---

[154] http://www.todaysdietitian.com/newarchives/td_1004p14.shtml

[155] http://pcosinfo.com/nac-pcos/

high insulin and LH are reasons why women with PCOS don't ovulate and why they have a number of other troubling symptoms.[156]

Top 5 Strategies for PCOS

1. Complete Hormone testing/Cardio Metabolic testing
2. Strict reduction of starchy high glycemic carbohydrates and sugar for weight loss
3. Consume a nutrient dense, high fiber, organic diet
4. Implement exercise regime
5. Supplement with Saw Palmetto, Gymnema, Vitex, Paeonia root Extract, Fenugreek, Fennel, Biotin,
6. D-chiro Inositol, Chromium, ALA, NAC and Omega 3's and Bioidentical Progesterone cream when needed

Kristi's Story - PCOS

Kristi is a thirty-year-old female who presented with hormonal imbalances and migraine headaches. Kristi had been on the birth control pill for fifteen years to regulate her period. Although she had ceased using the BCP over one year ago, she had still not had a period. Kristi was concerned that she might not be able to conceive when the time was right. Kristi also had weight issues: she was five feet two inches tall and weighed 214 pounds. Kristi attributed her weight issues to her poor nutritional choices-it was common for Kristi to go without eating for an entire day and have her first meal at dinnertime. She consumed large amounts of coffee throughout the day.

Kristi wanted to know the underlying cause of her hormonal issues and also wanted her thyroid tested, as she had a strong family history of hypothyroidism.

Lab Testing:

- Elevated testosterone levels
- Very low progesterone levels
- Estrogen dominance
- Elevated androstenedione levels
- Elevated TSH levels
- Elisa multi-food allergy testing revealed severe allergies to dairy, eggs, wheat, and sugar

Management Plan

Kristi was administered the following natural medicine remedies:

- Detoxification diet and cleanse for twenty-one days; elimination of allergenic foods as well as inflammatory foods including dairy, wheat, eggs, soy, beef, pork, shellfish, peanuts, corn, sugar, processed foods and alcohol

156 http://www.ovarian-cysts-pcos.com/exercise.html

- Thyroid support: iodine (as potassium iodide), zinc (as zinc picolinate), copper (as copper chelate), L-tyrosine, thyroid glandular (thyroxine free) two capsules two times per day
- Estrogen detoxification: DIM (Diindolymethane), calcium D-glucarate, SGS (sulforaphane glucosinolate) (standardized to contain 30 mg glucoraphanin glucosinolate), hops extract (0.12% 8-prenylnaringenin) two capsules with breakfast

Kristi returned three weeks later to report that she felt much better overall from the cleanse. She reported more energy, better digestion, clearer thinking, and improved sleep. She did not, however, experience any hormonal improvements.

The following modifications were made to the protocol:

- Continue with the thyroid support and estrogen detoxification
- Medical food: a powdered medical food designed to nutritionally support the management of conditions associated with metabolic syndrome (including altered body composition)
- Modified Mediterranean Lifestyle Nutrition Plan to balance hormones (see "Specific Guidelines for Nutritional Lifestyle Management Plan in Weight Gain" section)
- Bioidentical progesterone cream half a pump on days fourteen to twenty-eight of the menstrual cycle
- Testosterone lowering formula: saw palmetto (berry, standardized to 25% fatty acids), fennel (*Foeniculum vulgare*, seed), urtica dioica (leaf, standardized to 1% plant silica), ocimum sanctum (leaf), trigonella foenum-graecum (seed), and pygeum africanum (bark, standardized to 12% phytosterols)
- Vitex agnus castus 5 mL per day

Kristi reported back eight weeks later. She was thrilled that she had lost eleven pounds and she was really being diligent with her meal plan and avoidance of allergenic foods. Kristi stated that she did not have any migraines in the past two months, which was a marked improvement. Kristi had not yet had any signs of a cycle but was happy to continue with the regime.

The following modifications were made to the protocol:

- Increase bioidentical progesterone cream to one full pump on days fourteen to twenty-eight of the menstrual cycle
- Blood sugar management: A multi-nutrient formulated product containing a full range of multi vitamins as well as chromium, alpha lipoic acid, cinnamon, taurine, L-carnosine, and catechins one tablet before each meal

Kristi reported back eight weeks later and stated that she had now lost a total of twenty-three pounds and she was really feeling great. Over the last two cycles, she had noticed signs of menstruation starting, including mild pelvic cramping.

The following modifications were made to the protocol:

- Increase bioidentical progesterone cream to one full pump on twenty-five days of the month with a five-day break
- Increase testosterone-lowering product to two capsules two times per day
- Myo-inositol one scoop two times per day

Kristi returned twelve weeks later and was very happy to report that she had experienced two normal menstrual cycles. She continued to lose weight and was recommended to stay on her current protocol.

Ovarian Cysts

Ovarian cysts are a common gynecological problem that can affect any woman at any stage of life. This chronic disease is difficult to diagnose at times, as the symptoms are not always apparent, but can be the cause of vague feelings of heaviness or pressure in the lower abdomen. Ovarian cysts are fluid-filled sacs that are formed within the ovary. Ovarian cysts may form when ovulation fails to occur (the eggs are not released from the follicle), leaving the developing follicle to grow beyond its normal time. Cysts may also form after ovulation if the corpus luteum persists. Cysts that are bigger than two centimeters are formally diagnosed as ovarian cysts. Many ovarian cysts are functional in nature in that they rarely ever cause complications. However, in some cases, the cysts may develop certain complications such as rupturing, bleeding, or becoming twisted. Risks and complications of ovarian cysts depend on the type of cyst and the stage of treatment.

Symptoms of Ovarian Cysts

Often, ovarian cysts cause no issues and may resolve on their own. However, certain symptoms may occur in some women, including the following:

- Pain in the pelvic area
- Severe sudden pain, which is a symptom of ruptured ovarian cysts
- A sensation of pressure or fullness in the lower abdomen or pelvis
- Irregular or absent menstrual periods
- Pelvic pain during menstrual periods
- Pain in the pelvic area after exercise
- Pelvic pain following sexual intercourse
- Vaginal discharge
- Pressure or pain when urinating or having a bowel movement
- Nausea and vomiting
- Breast tenderness
- Weight gain
- Aches in the thighs and lower back
- Infertility

Causes of Ovarian Cysts

There are many primary factors leading to ovarian cysts. These factors should not be isolated, because the combination can lead to ovarian cysts. These factors may include the following:

- **Genetic predisposition:** Research has shown that genetic predisposition is often considered to be the primary cause of ovarian cysts.
- **Poor nutritional habits:** Diets high in refined, processed foods that are also high in sugar have been linked to hormonal imbalances that can weaken the immune system.
- **Poor immune function:** Decreased immune function inhibits the body's ability to fight off and eliminate harmful toxins that can contribute to the development of ovarian cysts.
- **Insulin resistance:** High level of insulin can stimulate ovarian androgen production. This reduces the serum sex-hormone binding globulin, or SHGB, which can in turn aggravate ovarian cysts.
- **Anovulation:** When the ovaries fail to release an egg on a monthly basis, progesterone production is inhibited, leading to hormonal imbalances such as estrogen dominance. This can then lead to the formation of ovarian cysts.

- **Accumulation of xenoestrogens:** Accumulation of xenoestrogens along with liver and bowel toxicity can lead to ovarian cysts.
- **Hormonal imbalances:** Hormonal imbalances such as adrenal fatigue, hypothyroidism, or a melatonin deficiency can be underlying factors in ovarian cyst formation.
- **Emotional factors:** Emotional factors relating to sexuality, reproduction, and creativity can trigger the onset of ovarian cysts. Some holistic practitioners believe that the ovaries are a common place for women to store tension, anger, or jealousy.

Complications of Ovarian Cysts

- **Ruptured ovarian cyst:** This is one the most serious complications that can lead to internal bleeding. Ruptured ovarian cysts can cause hemorrhages, which require immediate medical attention.
- **Ovarian torsion:** There can be twisting of the ovary, which can lead to infertility. Ovarian torsion may disturb blood supply to the ovary, as well, which can lead to ovarian necrosis, inflammation, and septic shock.
- **Peritonitis:** Inflammation of the mucus membrane that lines the abdominal cavity can cause excruciating pain and in some cases, the resulting complications can be life-threatening.
- **Infertility:** Infertility caused by ovarian cysts can be temporary or permanent, depending upon the extent of the damage.
- **Cancer:** In rare but significant instances, ovarian cysts may turn cancerous.

Lab Testing

A pelvic exam and ultrasound will confirm the presence of a cyst but additional lab testing is required to rule out hormonal imbalances as a cause.

Adrenal Stress Index	The panel utilizes four saliva samples. Salivary cortisol measurement reflects the free (bioactive) fraction of serum cortisol. The test report shows the awake diurnal cortisol rhythm generated in response to real-life stress. The cortisol/DHEA relationship highlights the many facets of stress maladaptation. The cortisol/DHEA ratio helps determine the projected time for recovery, and the substances (hormones, supplements, and botanicals) that promote this recovery. The cortisol/DHEA ratio regulates a multitude of functions. The panel measures P17-OH levels in order to evaluate the efficiency of the conversion of adrenal precursors into cortisol. Certain adrenal fatigue patients who are genetically predisposed to low production of cortisol will not benefit from exogenous supplementation of pregnenolone or progesterone. The panel includes fasting and non-fasting insulin measurements. The insulin values are used to diagnose insulin resistance-functional insulin deficit (pre-diabetes), as well as to correlate elevated cortisol with insulin to help explain glycemic dysregulation problems.
Complete Female Hormone Panel	Estradiol and progesterone levels and their ratio are an index of estrogen/progesterone balance. An excess of estradiol, relative to progesterone, can explain many symptoms in reproductive age-women. Testosterone levels can also be either too high or too low. Testosterone in excess, often caused by ovarian cysts, leads to conditions such as excessive facial and body hair, acne, and oily skin and hair.

	Polycystic ovarian syndrome (PCOS) is thought to be caused, in part, by insulin resistance. On the other hand, too little testosterone is often caused by excessive stress, medications, contraceptives, and surgical removal of the ovaries. This leads to symptoms of androgen deficiency including loss of libido, thinning skin, vaginal dryness, loss of bone and muscle mass, depression, and memory lapses. SHBG binds tightly to circulating estradiol and testosterone, preventing their rapid metabolism and clearance and limiting their bioavailability to tissues. SHBG gives a good index of the extent of the body's overall exposure to estrogens.
Thyroid Hormone Testing	A complete thyroid profile includes free T4, free T3, TSH, and TPO and can indicate the presence of an imbalance in thyroid function. Hypothyroidism includes feeling cold all the time, low stamina, fatigue (particularly in the evening), anxiety, depression, low sex drive, weight gain, and high cholesterol. Hyperthyroidism includes heat intolerance, anxiety, palpitations, weight loss, tired but wired feeling, visual disturbances, and insomnia.
Melatonin	Salivary hormone testing for melatonin will determine a deficiency in this hormone.

Conventional Pharmaceutical Medicine and Treatments Indicated for Ovarian Cysts

- Ultrasound monitoring using transvaginal ultrasound to monitor the size of the cysts
- Oral contraceptives can hasten the regression of ovarian cysts
- Surgery is required for cysts larger than 6 cm (2.5 in) to rule out ovarian cancer

Nutritional Factors Affecting Ovarian Cysts

- Avoid chocolate, alcohol, and coffee, as these interfere with the liver's ability to transform estrogen into safe metabolites
- Use olive oil for cooking and use flaxseed oil on your food after it has been cooked—avoid butter, margarine, and all other oils
- Use two teaspoons or more of turmeric daily
- Use two tablespoons of ground flax seed daily
- Avoid all sugars and sweeteners other than stevia and moderate amounts of whole fruit
- Avoid carbohydrates that have a high glycemic index such as white rice, corn, millet, and white flour
- Avoid all refined and processed foods
- Consume low glycemic carbohydrates such as pearl barley and beans (legumes)
- Avoid red meat and dairy, as they increase the risk factors for heart disease and cancer
- Eat small, frequent meals throughout the day rather than the typical two to three large meals
- Combine protein with every meal or snack to lower insulin resistance
- Eat high fiber foods that are low in glycemic load such as apples, cabbage, raw carrots, oatmeal, oat bran, sesame seeds, flax seeds, psyllium seed powder, and beans

Herbal Medicine Indicated for Ovarian Cysts

Maca *(Lepidium meyenii)*

Maca is an herbal remedy that assists the body in increasing the production of progesterone to normal levels. This herb increases fertility in women and has no hormonal effect, which makes it effective in shrinking overgrowth of tissues that respond to hormonal stimulation. These tissues include endometrium, fibroids, and cysts in breasts and ovaries. It is recommended to take 1,000 mg of maca daily to balance progesterone, to establish regular menstrual cycles, and to reduce the size of the cysts. Dosage: 750mg-1500mg per day

Chasteberry *(Vitex agnus castus)*

Chasteberry acts on the hypothalamus and pituitary glands by increasing luteinizing hormone (LH) production and mildly inhibiting the release of follicle stimulating hormone (FSH). The result is a shift in the ratio of estrogen to progesterone, in favor of progesterone. The ability of chasteberry to raise progesterone levels in the body is an indirect effect, so the herb itself is not a hormone. A large percentage of hormonal problems in ovarian cysts are related to insufficient progesterone during the luteal phase of the menstrual cycle, which is called a luteal phase defect or corpus luteum insufficiency. A corpus luteum insufficiency is defined as an abnormally low progesterone level three weeks after the onset of menstruation. Insufficient levels of progesterone may result in the formation of ovarian cysts. Dosage: 225mg-450mg per day

Hepatotropic and hepatoprotective herbs are useful in the treatment of ovarian cysts to improve the ability of the liver to detoxify harmful estrogens.

Milk Thistle *(Silymarin marianus)*

Much research has been done on a special extract of milk thistle known as silymarin, a group of flavonoid compounds. These compounds protect the liver from damage and enhance the detoxification process. Silymarin prevents damage to the liver by acting as an antioxidant and is much more effective than vitamins E and C. Numerous research studies have demonstrated its protective effect on the liver and it also works by preventing the depletion of glutathione. The higher the glutathione concentration, the greater the liver's capacity to detoxify harmful chemicals. Silymarin has been shown to increase the level of glutathione by up to 35%. In human studies, silymarin has been shown to exhibit positive effects in treating liver diseases of various kinds, including cirrhosis, chronic hepatitis, fatty infiltration of the liver, and inflammation of the bile duct. Dosage: standardized extract 200 mg to 800 mg per day

Curcumin *(Curcuma longa)*

Several studies have illustrated curcumin's hepatoprotective effects. This has led researchers to suggest its use in protecting the liver from exogenous insults from environmental toxins, including carbon tetrachloride and acetaminophen. Curcumin also has the capacity to increase bile flow and solubility, making it of potential benefit for individuals with tendencies to form gallstones. The hepatoprotective effects of turmeric may stem from its potent antioxidant activity. In addition to its antioxidant effects, curcumin has been shown to enhance liver detoxification by increasing the activity of glutathione S-transferase, an enzyme necessary to conjugate glutathione with a wide variety of toxins in order to facilitate their removal from the body. Dosage: 500mg-3000mg per day

Burdock Root *(Arctium lappa)*

Burdock root is one of the foremost cleansing herbs, providing nourishing support for the blood, the liver, and the natural defense system. It is rich in vitamins B-1, B-6, B-12, and E, plus manganese, copper, iron, zinc, and sulfur. Burdock root contains inulin along with bitter compounds and mucilage, which provides its ability to control liver damage and protect the liver from further burdens. Burdock root also promotes the flow and release of bile, which not only helps in cleansing the liver but also aids the digestive process. Dosage: can be taken in the capsule, tea or tincture form

Dandelion Root *(Taraxacum officinalis)*

The *Australian Journal of Medicinal Herbalism* has cited two studies that show the liver-regenerating properties of dandelion in cases of jaundice, liver swelling, hepatitis, and indigestion. The root of the dandelion plant is effective as a detoxifying agent, acting especially on the liver and gallbladder, and it helps to remove toxins and waste products. It stimulates and tonifies the digestive system. Its cholagogue, or bile secreting effect, creates a mild laxative effect which allows for expulsion of toxins. Dandelion root is therefore useful in the treatment of liver conditions such as jaundice, metabolic toxicity, hepatitis, and cholelithiasis (gallstones), as well as chronic conditions of the digestive system, conditions of the skin such as acne and eczema, and joint problems such as arthritis. Dosage: can be taken in the capsule, tea or tincture form

Globe Artichoke *(Cynara scolymus)*

Globe artichoke contains a powerful compound called cynaropicrin which is a sesquiterpene lactone that stimulates the flow of bile from the liver and makes it a useful liver detoxifier and protector. Due to its ability to promote detoxification and improve bile flow, globe artichoke is useful in all cases of insufficient liver production and digestion. Dosage: can be taken in the capsule, tea or tincture form

Specific Nutrients Indicated in Ovarian Cysts

Bioidentical Progesterone Cream

Natural progesterone, according to Dr. John Lee, is one of the most important natural ovarian cyst treatment methods available to women. It nourishes the endocrine system, leading to the shrinkage of the functional cyst and to more regular cycles, healthy ovulation, and increased fertility. Natural progesterone cream should be applied from day ten until day twenty-eight of the menstrual cycle. This type of treatment suppresses ovulation, preventing the formation of new follicles and allowing the body to naturally re-absorb the cyst. This form of natural hormone therapy should be followed for at least three months in order to give the body enough time to shrink the cyst. If you are trying to conceive, you should use natural progesterone cream only from day fourteen (or after ovulation) until day twenty-eight or as soon as the cycle starts.

Diindolylmethane (DIM)

DIM is a powerful metabolizer of estrogen, assisting in removing excess estrogen and benefiting conditions associated with estrogen dominance. Supplementation with DIM can help promote proper estrogen levels through the pre and perimenopausal years and in men experiencing higher estrogen levels. These conditions include uterine fibroid tumors, fibrocystic breasts, and glandular dysfunction. It can also benefit men by improving estrogen dominance-related health issues such as hair loss, atherosclerosis, prostrate problems, lowered libido, and impotency. DIM promotes testosterone action, which improves mood, fights depression, boosts libido, improves cardiovascular health, improves memory, and supports muscular development. DIM is a balancer of estrogen metabolism. It increases 2-hydroxyestrone (2-OHE), which is also known as the good or protective estrogen. Dosage: 70 mg to 400 mg

Alpha Lipoic Acid (ALA)

ALA is the remarkable "universal antioxidant" as it is both water and fat-soluble, proving to have antioxidant effects on the inside and outside of the cells. ALA helps to neutralize the effects of all free radicals and enhances the antioxidant functions of vitamins C and E and glutathione. Research shows that ALA is effective in neutralizing toxins from over-the-counter and prescription drugs before they can cause liver damage.

Glutathione

Glutathione is one of the molecules used in Phase 2 detoxification and is produced in the body by the liver and evels of glutathione naturally decrease with the aging process. Glutathione is made up of cysteine, glutamic acid, and glycine. The amount of cysteine in the body will determine how much glutathione is produced. Glutathione has tremendous liver-protecting effects which block the effects of environmental pollution, medications, radiation, mercury, and other heavy metals. Glutathione aids in detoxification by removing fungicides, herbicides, carbamate, organophosphates, pesticides, nitrates, notrosamines, flavorings, plastics, steroids, phenolic compounds, and certain medications from the body.

Vitamin C

Vitamin C is a water-soluble antioxidant vitamin which is not produced within the body and therefore must be replenished through dietary means on a daily basis. Deficiencies in vitamin C have been shown to decrease the metabolism of xenobiotics by lowering the level of cytochrome P450. Vitamin C aids in detoxification by combating free radicals. Vitamin C also prevents damage from exposure to numerous hepato-toxic agents including pollutants, carbon monoxide, heavy metals, sulfur dioxide, carcinogens, stored lipophilic chemicals, medications, anesthetics, radiation, bacterial toxins, and poisons.

N-Acetyl Cysteine (NAC)

NAC is thought to be an intermediate compound in cysteine metabolism, which makes it a derivative of cysteine. NAC has the ability to boost glutathione levels, which is critical to Phase 2 detoxification. NAC protects the liver from toxic compounds, has tremendous chemo-protectant effects, and protects the body from radiation. NAC is a potent liver vasodilator, which increases the blood flow to the liver and thereby enhances its detoxification abilities.

Methionine

Due to methionine's sulfur content, it is a powerful antioxidant that has the ability to inactivate free radicals, support liver detoxification, protect cell membranes against lipid peroxidation, and protect glutathione levels in the body. Methionine, when at sufficient levels, has the added effect of preventing the accumulation of fat in the liver.

Coenzyme Q10

COQ10 is the most powerful antioxidant in the body. COQ10, also called ubiquinone, is a potent free radical scavenger, which protects the cellular membranes against damage caused by toxins and is a crucial co-factor for energy production within the body.

Vitamin B5

Vitamin B5, also known as pantothenic acid, is part of the B-complex family of vitamins. B5 is the main vitamin that is used in times of stress as it stimulates adrenal hormone production and supports adrenal function, preventing adrenal exhaustion during prolonged stress. B5 is a critical nutrient involved in Phase 1 detoxification. It aids the body in its detoxification efforts by protecting against harmful radiation. It also counters the effects and toxicity of antibiotics, aids in the production of hydrochloric acid in the stomach, and stimulates the synthesis of cholesterol.

Vitamin B6

Vitamin B6, or pyridoxine, is involved in more bodily processes than any other single nutrient and has an effect on both physical and mental health. B6 is needed for the metabolism of methionine, aids in the transport of amino acids across the cellular membrane, and supports liver detoxification. B6 is also needed for the proper metabolism and use of protein, fats, carbohydrates, and hormones.

Castor Oil Packs for Ovarian Cysts

Castor Oil Packs: Apply a castor oil pack to the lower abdomen three to five times per week. The skin absorbs the warm castor oil's active constituents, lectins, which stimulate the immune response to help shrink fibroids. Castor oil is extracted from the castor plant (Ricinus communis). It should not be taken internally, as it will act as a powerful laxative. But if applied externally or topically, it has unique medicinal actions on the body. It penetrates skin and muscle to reach into underlying tissue and assists in decongestion and breakdown of inflammatory material through enhancing blood flow and lymphatic flow in the area. This also helps in the removal of toxins and the elimination of wastes. Castor oil is warming to the tissues and this eases stiffness and pain.

Occasions to use a castor oil pack

- Lymphatic congestion
- Arthritis
- Rheumatism
- Fibromyalgia
- Muscle spasms
- Abdominal inflammations
- Pelvic congestion
- Glandular swellings
- Deep infections
- Adhesions Fibroids
- Endometriosis
- Back ache
- Muscle tension
- Local pain due to inflammation or spasm

How to make a castor oil pack

- Take a piece of flannel or towel and fold it three or four times, so that it is large enough to entirely cover the area to be treated.
- Pour castor oil all over it until thoroughly soaked.
- Place over the skin and cover with a large piece of saran wrap.
- Cover with a heating pad or hot water bottle and leave in place for one to two hours.
- After use, the pack can be wrapped in plastic and stored in the refrigerator (bring back to room temperature before re-use). You may wish to add a little more castor oil with each use. The pack should be discarded after ten uses.

Top 5 Strategies for Ovarian Cysts

1. Complete Hormone testing
2. Consume a nutrient dense, high fiber, organic diet/Eliminate sugar, caffeine and alcohol
3. Liver detoxification
4. Reduce exposure to xenoestrogens
5. Supplement with Vitex, B-Complex vitamins, MACA, DIM, NAC, Vitamin C, Bioidentical Progesterone from day 10-28 and apply castor oil packs regularly

Denise's Story-Ovarian Cysts

Denise is a forty-two-year-old female who is the single mother of three teenage daughters. Denise presented with a long-standing history of monthly ovarian cyst ruptures. Denise stated that each month during ovulation, she would experience severe and debilitating pain as the cyst would rupture and this would be followed by two to three days of moderate cramping. Denise's cycles were regular in occurrence but extremely heavy in flow. She also experienced intolerable sugar cravings, which often led to binge eating and consequently, unwanted weight gain.

Denise's diet was very high in dairy products, red meat, and refined sugar. She reported that she felt the need to eat every two to three hours or she would feel anxious and shaky.

Denise had lost her father one year ago and was still grieving the loss. She was under the guidance of a grief counselor but admitted that she was moderately depressed.

Lab testing:

- Elevated testosterone levels
- Low progesterone levels
- Elevated estrogen levels
- Elevated fasting insulin levels
- High levels of circulating candida (a common yeast overgrowth)

Management Plan

Denise was administered the following natural medicine therapies:

- Liver detoxification formula: choline, betaine, methionine, taraxacum (dandelion), silymarin marianus, cynara scolymus (artichoke) and curcumin two tablets two times per day
- Testosterone lowering formula: saw palmetto (berry, standardized to 25% fatty acids), fennel (foeniculum vulgare, seed), urtica dioica (leaf, standardized to 1% plant silica), ocimum sanctum (leaf), trigonella foenum-graecum (seed), and pygeum africanum (bark, standardized to 12% phytosterols)
- Estrogen detoxification: DIM, calcium D-glucarate, SGS (standardized to contain 30mg glucoraphanin glucosinolate), hops extract (0.12% 8-prenylnaringenin) two capsules with breakfast
- Candida lowering agent: calcium-magnesium-caprylate complex (Caprylic acid)- two tablets daily on an empty stomach
- High potency probiotics two capsules before bed away from caprylic acid
- Candida cleansing nutritional regime—Avoid the following sugars and all of its forms, including fruit, yeast, alcohol, the flour of any grain, dairy except for yogurt, processed foods, red meat, pork, vinegar, and any fermented foods

Denise retuned four weeks later to report that she had had a very difficult time with the Candida diet at first and experienced severe sugar cravings. After three weeks, the cravings started to subside and she persisted. She noticed that her digestion had a marked improvement but she still had had an ovarian cyst rupture during her previous menstrual cycle. She also mentioned that her depression was becoming worse.

The following modifications were made to the protocol:

- Keep the previous recommendations the same
- Castor oil packs nightly for the first fourteen days of the menstrual cycle or until ovulation occurs
- Mood stabilizing support: 5-HTP, St John's wort, vitamins B3, B5, and B6, folic acid

Denise reported back eight weeks later. She had lost a marked amount of weight—BIA testing revealed that her total loss was twenty-one pounds. She was very happy with these results. Denise stated that although she still experienced the ovarian cysts each month, they were much less severe. She also noted that her mood had greatly improved about two weeks after starting the mood stabilizing formula.

The following modifications were made to the protocol:

- Keep the previous recommendations the same
- Bioidentical progesterone cream one pump on days fourteen to twenty-eight of the menstrual cycle
- Ovarian cyst pain formula—Viburnum opulus, Valeriana officinalis, Piscidia erythrina, Zingiber officinalis 5 mL as needed for ovarian cyst pain—not to exceed a daily maximum of 20 mL

Denise returned twelve weeks later. She was happy to report that she had not had any ovarian cyst issues over the past three cycles. In fact, she had not even opened the ovarian cyst pain formula. She had now lost a total of thirty-two pounds. She was feeling much more energy and her mood was stable.

Denise was advised to go off the Candida lowering agent, the testosterone lowering formula, and the liver detoxification. She was also told to decrease the probiotics to one capsule before bed and otherwise stay with the same protocol.

Menopause

The word "menopause" literally means "cessation of the monthly cycle." It is derived from the Greek words "*meno*" (month, menses) and "*pausis*" (cessation). When the ovaries no longer respond to stimulation from the pituitary gland to secrete estrogen and progesterone, menopause naturally occurs. Between the ages of forty-five and fifty-five, with the average age being fifty-two, the menses usually becomes irregular and stops. Menopause can last from six to thirteen years. Menopause is strictly defined as the point after twelve consecutive months of no menses following the final menstrual period. Despite our aging population and greater life expectancy, the age of menopause has not changed in the last few centuries. Three important factors that influence the age of onset of menopause are current smoking habits, familial factors, and genetic factors involving the estrogen receptors. Other influences that may affect the onset of menopause are increasing BMI, more than one pregnancy, history of no pregnancy, toxic chemical exposures, treatment of childhood cancers, and radiation, epilepsy and cognitive scores in childhood (the higher the score, the later the menopause). There appears to be no link between the age of onset of menopause and the history of hormonal contraception, socioeconomic or marital status, race, or age at the first menstrual cycle.

3 Types of Menopause

1. **Natural Menopause:** Between the ages of forty-five and fifty-five, a woman who has at least one of her ovaries generally enters into a five to ten year process that can sometimes take up to thirteen years. Periods are intermittent in duration, intensity, and flow.
2. **Premature Menopause:** This occurs in women in their thirties or early forties who have at least one ovary. Premature menopause is characterized by an earlier, faster, and shorter journey through menopause, which can last for one to three years. Approximately one in one hundred women completes this menopausal transition by age forty or younger. Illness or stress can affect the hormone-related reproductive function.
3. **Surgical Menopause:** This is induced by the surgical removal or disruption of the reproductive tract (including removal of ovaries or surgical disruption of the blood supply to the ovaries). This can also be

caused by radiation, chemotherapy, or the administration of certain medications that mimic menopause for medical reasons such as to shrink uterine fibroids.

Primer on Sex Hormones

Estrogen and progesterone are the two primary hormones secreted by the ovaries. The properties of one offset the other and together they are maintained in optimal opposing balance in our body at all times. An excess or deficiency of either hormone leads to significant medical problems.

Estrogen is not a single hormone but rather a trio of hormones working together. The three components of estrogen are estrone, estradiol, and estriol. In healthy young women, the typical mix approximates 15%, 15%, and 70%, respectively. Out of the three components of estrogen, estrone and estradiol are pro-cancer, while estriol is anti-cancer. Synthetic estrogen such as Premarin contains the pro-cancer components of estrogen (estrone and estradiol) in higher proportions compared to estriol. After menopause, estrogen levels drop to 40% to 60% of pre-menopausal levels.

Progesterone is made from pregnenolone, which in turn comes from cholesterol. Production occurs at several places, including the ovaries in females (production occurs just before ovulation and increases rapidly after ovulation), the adrenal glands in both sexes, and the testes in males. Its level is highest in women during the ovulation period (days thirteen to fifteen of the menstrual cycle) and if fertilization does not take place, the secretion of progesterone decreases and menstruation occurs. If fertilization does occur, progesterone is secreted during pregnancy by the placenta and acts to prevent spontaneous abortion. About 20 mg to 25 mg of progesterone are produced per day during a woman's monthly cycle. Up to 300 mg to 400 mg are produced daily during pregnancy. During menopause, the total amount of progesterone produced declines to a startling less than 1% of the pre-menopausal level.

Functionally, progesterone acts as an antagonist (opposite) to estrogen. For example, estrogen stimulates breast cysts while progesterone protects against breast cysts. Estrogen enhances salt and water retention while progesterone is a natural diuretic. Estrogen has been associated with breast and endometrial cancer, while progesterone has cancer preventive effects. Most significantly, it is known that high amounts of estrogen can induce a host of metabolic disturbances, and the body's way of counterbalancing estrogen naturally is with progesterone. When this balancing mechanism is dysfunctional, a multitude of health-related problems arise.

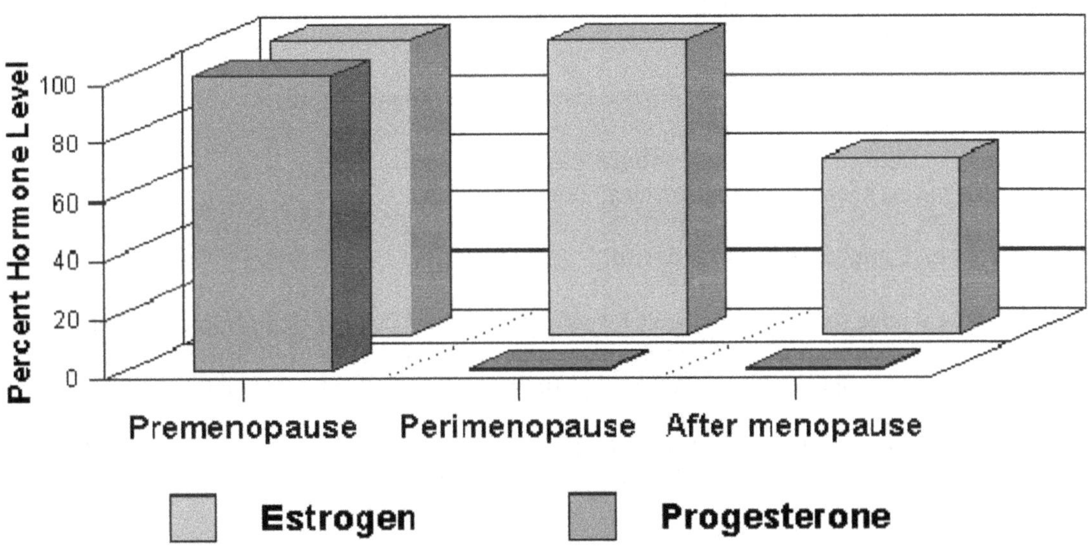

Symptoms of Menopause

The Most Common Symptoms of Menopause are:

- Hot flashes, flushes, night sweats and/or cold flashes, clammy feeling
- Irregular heart beat
- Irritability
- Mood swings, sudden tears
- Trouble sleeping through the night (with or without night sweats)
- Irregular periods, shorter, lighter periods, heavier periods, flooding, phantom periods, shorter cycles, longer cycles
- Loss of libido
- Dry vagina
- Crashing fatigue
- Anxiety, feeling ill at ease
- Feelings of dread, apprehension, and doom
- Difficulty concentrating, disorientation, mental confusion
- Disturbing memory lapses
- Incontinence, especially upon sneezing or laughing
- Itchy, crawly skin
- Aching, sore joints, muscles, and tendons
- Breast tenderness
- Headache change: increase or decrease
- Gastrointestinal distress, indigestion, flatulence, gas pain, nausea
- Increase in allergies
- Weight gain
- Hair loss or thinning (head, pubic, or whole body), increase in facial hair
- Dizziness, light-headedness, episodes of loss of balance
- Changes in body odor
- Electric shock sensation under the skin and in the head
- Tingling in the extremities
- Gum problems, increased bleeding
- Burning tongue, burning roof of mouth, bad taste in mouth, change in breath odor
- Osteoporosis (after several years)
- Changes in fingernails—softer, crack or break easier
- Tinnitus—ringing in ears, bells, "whooshing," buzzing

Additional Notes on Symptoms of Menopause:

- Hot flashes are due to the hypothalamic response to declining ovarian estrogen production. The declining estrogen state induces hypophysiotropic neurons in the arcuate nucleus of the hypothalamus to release gonadotropin-releasing hormone (GnRH) in a pulsatile fashion. This, in turn, stimulates the release of luteinizing hormone (LH). Extremely high pulses of LH occur during the period of declining estrogen production. The LH has vasodilator effects that lead to flushing.
- For some women, the libido loss is so great that they actually find sex repulsive in much the same way they felt before puberty.
- Dry vagina results in painful intercourse.
- Doom thoughts, include thoughts of death and picturing one's own death, may occur.

- Incontinence reflects a general loss of smooth muscle tone.
- Itchy, crawly skin feeling like ants crawling under the skin—not just dry itchy skin.
- Aching, sore joints may include such problems as carpal tunnel syndrome.
- Severe depression—the inability to cope is overwhelming. There is a feeling of loss of self. Hormone therapy ameliorates the depression dramatically.
- Weight gain often around the waist and thighs.
- Shock sensation such as "the feeling of a rubber band snapping in the layer of tissue between the skin and muscle." It is a precursor to a "hot flash."
- Tingling in extremities can also be a symptom of B-12 deficiency, diabetes, alterations in the flexibility of blood vessels, or a depletion of potassium or calcium.
- Tinnitus is a condition that seems to manifest in some women at the same time as menopause. It can be associated with health conditions such as hypothyroidism and heart disease. It is also a known side effect of many medications, including aspirin (salicylates) and Prozac.

Hot flashes are the most common symptom of menopause. They are characterized by episodes of flushing lasting a few seconds to a few minutes with increased heart rate, palpitations, skin blood flow, and skin temperature, accompanied by a sensation of heat and sometimes dizziness. Hot flashes occur for one to five years.

Causes of Hot Flashes[157]

- The hypothalamus is the part of the brain that regulates temperature. An imbalance in the hypothalamus causes hot flashes. Hot flashes coincide with ultradian surges in LH, which is secreted in bursts every thirty to sixty minutes or longer. Each hot flash begins as an LH level spike.
- Dilation of blood vessels, flushing, and sweating occur when a drop in estrogen levels activates the sympathetic nervous system to release higher amounts of the stimulating brain neurotransmitter norepinephrine.
- Neurotransmitters such as GABA, serotonin, and endorphins modulate the hypothalamic release of a hormone that causes LH to be released. A disturbance in their actions on the hypothalamus may also cause the LH rise, and this disturbance is magnified by stress.
- Specific prostaglandins stimulate the hypothalamus. These prostaglandins are increased by a diet containing red meat, dairy fat, peanuts, sugar, and shellfish. The prostaglandins are inhibited by bromelain, fish oil, antioxidants, and curcumin.

Factors that Aggravate Hot Flashes

- Alcohol
- Food containing histamine (cheese and red wine)
- Spicy foods
- Hot drinks
- Chocolate
- Caffeine
- Smoking
- Stress and overwork
- Exhaustion
- Physical inactivity
- Hot weather or very cold weather
- Maternal history of hot flashes

[157] Complete Natural Medicine Guide to Women's Health Sat Dharam Kaur, ND pg. 275

- Early onset menopause
- Early onset of menses
- History of irregular periods
- Hypothyroidism
- Red meat, dairy fat, peanuts, and shellfish
- Pharmaceuticals (Tamoxifen and aromatase inhibitors)

Menopause and Thyroid Imbalances

- Twenty-six percent of women in or near perimenopause are diagnosed with hypothyroidism, likely due to a cause and effect relationship between hypothyroidism and estrogen dominance
- When estrogen is not properly counterbalanced with progesterone, the action of thyroid hormone can be blocked and rendered ineffective, leading to symptoms of hypothyroidism
- Lab tests may show normal thyroid hormone levels because the thyroid gland itself is not malfunctioning

Menopause and Adrenal Imbalances

- As a woman reaches perimenopause or menopause and her adrenal glands are in a state of exhaustion, the journey through menopause is much more difficult
- Perimenopause and menopause other forms of stress when the adrenals are already exhausted
- DHEA, cortisol, and adrenalin levels begin to fluctuate as the adrenal glands attempt to take over the role of the once-fully functioning ovaries
- Common signs of adrenal exhaustion are exacerbated as a woman enters into menopause (fatigue, depression, irritability, loss of interest in life, anxiety, weight gain, and insomnia)
- Symptoms often experienced in menopause mirror those common to adrenal fatigue

Laboratory Testing for Menopause

It is usually very obvious when menopause is reached, as there is a complete cessation of the menstrual cycle. However, in cases of surgical menopause, drug-induced menopause, or even early onset menopause, testing becomes of the upmost importance. Determining the levels of all hormones involved in menopause, including the sex hormones, adrenal hormones, and thyroid hormones will help to bring clarity to the underlying causes of symptoms that occur in menopause. Lab tests can include the following:

Neurotransmitter Testing	Medical science has discovered that neurotransmitters are at the foundation of many psychiatric and neurological disorders. Imbalances in neurotransmission, due to excessive or deficient neurotransmitter levels at the synaptic cleft, are associated with depression, insomnia, anxiety, behavioural disorders, memory disorders, and a spectrum of other brain-related functions. Because neurotransmitters play an integral role in these disease states, they are prime targets for treating nervous system disorders and mental health concerns. Neurotransmitters are recognized as the primary biochemical messengers of the central and peripheral nervous systems. Studies have demonstrated that urinary neurotransmitter measures are reflective of circulating levels, as evidenced by renal neurotransmitter clearance mechanisms. Laboratory methodology for the accurate assessment of urinary neurotransmitter

	levels has been established. Urinary measures are not recognized as a direct reflection of central activity, however, definite associations exist. The ability to measure neurotransmitters has led to the generation of scientific literature that demonstrates that urinary neurotransmitter measurements have clinical value as representative biomarkers of various neurological, immunological, and endocrinological conditions.
Adrenal Stress Index	The panel utilizes four saliva samples. Salivary cortisol measurement reflects the free (bioactive) fraction of serum cortisol. The test report shows the awake diurnal cortisol rhythm generated in response to real-life stress. The cortisol/DHEA relationship highlights the many facets of stress maladaptation. The cortisol/DHEA ratio helps determine the projected time for recovery, and the substances (hormones, supplements, and botanicals) that promote this recovery. The cortisol/DHEA ratio regulates a multitude of functions. The panel measures P17-OH levels in order to evaluate the efficiency of the conversion of adrenal precursors into cortisol. Certain adrenal fatigue patients who are genetically predisposed to low production of cortisol will not benefit from exogenous supplementation of pregnenolone or progesterone. The panel includes fasting and non-fasting insulin measurements. The insulin values are used to diagnose insulin resistance-functional insulin deficit (pre-diabetes), as well as to correlate elevated cortisol with insulin to help explain glycemic dysregulation problems.
Complete Female Hormone Panel	Estradiol and progesterone levels and their ratio are an index of estrogen/progesterone balance. An excess of estradiol, relative to progesterone, can explain many symptoms in reproductive age-women. Testosterone levels can also be either too high or too low. Testosterone in excess, often caused by ovarian cysts, leads to conditions such as excessive facial and body hair, acne, and oily skin and hair. Polycystic ovarian syndrome (PCOS) is thought to be caused, in part, by insulin resistance. On the other hand, too little testosterone is often caused by excessive stress, medications, contraceptives, and surgical removal of the ovaries. This leads to symptoms of androgen deficiency including loss of libido, thinning skin, vaginal dryness, loss of bone and muscle mass, depression, and memory lapses. SHBG binds tightly to circulating estradiol and testosterone, preventing their rapid metabolism and clearance and limiting their bioavailability to tissues. SHBG gives a good index of the extent of the body's overall exposure to estrogens.
Thyroid Hormone Testing	A complete thyroid profile includes free T4, free T3, TSH, and TPO and can indicate the presence of an imbalance in thyroid function. Hypothyroidism includes feeling cold all the time, low stamina, fatigue (particularly in the evening), anxiety, depression, low sex drive, weight gain, and high cholesterol. Hyperthyroidism includes heat intolerance, anxiety, palpitations, weight loss tired but wired feeling, visual disturbances, and insomnia.

Conventional Pharmaceutical Treatments Indicated for Menopause

Hormone Replacement Therapy

Hormone replacement therapy (HRT) is a system of medical treatments for surgically menopausal, perimenopausal and, to a lesser extent, postmenopausal women. It is based on the idea that the treatment may prevent discomfort caused by diminished circulating estrogen and progesterone hormones. In the case of surgically or prematurely menopausal women, it may prolong life and may reduce the incidence of dementia.[158] HRT involves the use of one or more of a group of medications designed to artificially boost hormone levels. The main types of hormones involved are estrogens, progesterone, or progestins, and sometimes testosterone.[159]

Attitudes toward HRT changed in 2002 following the announcement by the Women's Health Initiative (WHI) of the National Institutes of Health that those receiving the treatment (Prempro®) in the main part of their study had a larger incidence of breast cancer, heart attacks, and strokes.[160] The WHI findings were reconfirmed in a larger national study done in the UK, known as The Million Women Study. As a result of these findings, the number of women taking hormone treatment dropped precipitously.[161] The Women's Health Initiative recommended that women with normal rather than surgical menopause should take the lowest feasible dose of HRT for the shortest possible time to avoid these risks.

Type of hormone replacement therapy

If, after weighing all the evidence with a physician, HRT is chosen–either for short-term relief or for long-term use because of a high risk for osteoporosis–natural hormone replacement using hormones identical to human estrogen and progesterone is recommended.

Conjugated estrogens (e.g., Premarin, Genisis), which are derived from pregnant mares' urine, progestins (synthetic progesterone formulations), and medroxyprogesterone products (e.g., Provera, Cycrin, Amen) are not biochemically identical and do not produce effects identical to human hormones.

Human estrogen is actually composed of three estrogens: estriol, estrone, and estradiol. Tri-Est, a formulation containing these three natural forms of human estrogen in a ratio equivalent to that found in the human body, along with natural progesterone, derived from wild yam but biochemically identical to human progesterone, is preferred.

Nutritional Factors Affecting Menopause

Soy Protein and Soy Isoflavones

Phytoestrogens such as genestein and diadzen are isoflavones that have weak estrogenic activity. Phytoestrogens are a diverse group of plant-derived substances that have estrogenic properties. The structures of these compounds are very close to that of estrogen, but their actions are much less powerful (about one one-thousandth as potent). Consequently, when estrogen levels are high, phytoestrogens compete for estrogen receptors, reducing the number of estrogen receptor sites and thus decreasing the effects of excessive estrogen. The

[158] Lynne T. Shuster, Deborah J. Rhodes, Bobbie S. Gostout, Brandon R. Grossardt, and Walter A. Rocca (2010). "Premature menopause or early menopause: long-term health consequences." Maturitas 65 (2): 161–6. doi:10.10.16/maturitas.2009.08.003. PMC 2815011. PMID 19733988.

[159] http://en.wikipedia.org/wiki/Hormone_replacement_therapy_(menopause)

[160] Writing Group for the Women's Health Initiative Investigators (2002). "Risks and Benefits of Estrogen Plus Progestin in Healthy Postmenopausal Women: Principal Results From the Women's Health Initiative Randomized Controlled Trial." JAMA 288 (3): 321–333. doi:10.1001/jama.288.3.321. PMID 12117397.

[161] Chlebowski, RT; Kuller LH; Prentice RL; Stefanick ML; Manson JE; Gass M; et al. (2009). "Breast cancer after use of estrogen plus progestin in postmenopausal women." NEJM 360 (6): 573–87. doi: 10.1056/NEJMoa0807684. PMID 19196674.

excess estrogens, in this case, are safely metabolized (broken down) by the liver. When estrogen levels are low, as in peri- and post-menopause states, phytoestrogens act as estrogen supplements. Phytoestrogens therefore help balance both excess and insufficient estrogen by acting both as anti-estrogens as well as weak estrogens, respectively.

It has been suggested that one of the reasons that hot flashes and other menopausal symptoms are much less common in Japanese women is that they consume large amounts of soy foods. Asians also depend on soy (such as tofu) as a source of protein (rather than red meat). The active ingredient in tofu is genestein. Studies have shown that genestein may reduce the symptoms of menopause, prevent bone loss, and possibly provide a safe alternative for prescription estrogens.

A reasonable approach to isoflavone consumption would be to ingest a daily level of isoflavones that does not exceed the amount typically consumed in ethnic diets that contain high amounts of isoflavones. The amount should be approximately 50 mg to 150 mg of isoflavones per day. The isoflavone content of soy foods varies with the form and therefore the following list will help to determine the daily amount. All soy should be consumed in organic non-genetically modified forms.

Soy Food	**Amount**	**Isoflavones (mg)**
Textured soy protein granules	one quarter of a cup	62
Roasted soy nuts	one-quarter cup	60
Tofu, low fat and regular	one-half cup	35
Tempeh	one-half cup	35
Soy beverage powders	one to two scoops	20 to 50
Regular soy milk	one cup	30
Low fat soy milk	one cup	20
Roasted soy butter	two tablespoons	17
Cooked soybeans	one-half cup	35

Flaxseed

Flaxseed contains two important lignans, matairesinol and secoisolariciresinol, which are known to have estrogenic activity. Other lignans are modified by intestinal bacteria to form estrogenic compounds. Lignans from plants such as flaxseed are absorbed in the circulation and have both estrogenic and anti-estrogenic activity, much like soy but to a lesser degree. Flaxseed flour and its defatted meal (flaxseed meal) are the highest plant producers of lignans.

The following table illustrates the specific dietary recommendations to reduce estrogen dominance, which is the main therapeutic dietary approach for balancing the hormones of menopause:

Food Group	**Foods To Include**	**Foods to Exclude**
Legumes	All legumes and legume products, especially organic non-genetically modified soy products	None
Vegetables	All, especially cruciferous (see note #1) and sea vegetables (various seaweeds)	None
Fruits	All whole and dry fruits, especially lemon and limes	None

Grains	All whole grains and whole-grain products, especially rye	Non-whole grains, refined flours, and refined flour products
Nuts/Seeds	All nuts and seeds and their butters, especially flaxseeds, walnuts, and pumpkin seeds (in their raw form only) (see note #2)	None
Fish	All, especially cold water fish: salmon, sardines, tuna, and halibut are excellent sources of omega-3 fatty acids	Salted or cured fish
Eggs	From organically raised hens	Non-organic eggs
Poultry/Meat	Organic meats and poultry (see note #3)	Non-organic meats and poultry, salted and cured meats
Dairy	Organic dairy products and soy, nut, and grain dairy substitutes	Non-organic dairy products
Oils	Organic cold-pressed, unrefined seed and nut oils, especially flaxseed, walnut, sesame, canola, and olive oil (See note #4)	Refined vegetable oils, butter, lard, margarine, shortening, and saturated or hydrogenated fats
Beverages	Mineral or filtered water, herbal tea, fresh fruit juice	Alcohol, coffee
Sweeteners	Brown rice syrup, fruit sweetener, molasses, stevia	Chocolate, refined or artificial sweeteners
Spices and Herbs	Especially nutmeg, anise, thyme, sage, fennel, caraway, turmeric, and fresh lemon and lime juice	High sodium foods, and salt

Additional Notes:

1. Cruciferous vegetables include: broccoli, cauliflower, all cabbages, Brussels sprouts, kale, bok choy, arugula, mustard greens, and watercress.
2. Omega-3 and some omega-6 fatty acids help to counteract symptoms associated with hormonal imbalance and should be consumed daily.
3. Non-organically raised livestock are often given hormones to improve their growth; unfortunately, these hormones can be passed on to the consumer and negatively influence hormone balance.
4. Important: Do not cook with oils that are not specified for cooking or baking, such as flaxseed or walnut oils. Olive, canola, and sesame oils are good choices for cooking or baking. Use flaxseed, olive, sesame, or walnut oils for homemade salad dressings. These provide valuable omega-3 and omega-6 fatty acids. Refrigerate all oils and dressings.

Herbal Medicine Indicated for Menopause

Licorice Root *(Glycyrrhiza glabra)*

During perimenopause, estrogen levels fluctuate widely while progesterone levels consistently drop. Licorice increases the estrogen-to-progesterone ratio by lowering estrogen levels while simultaneously raising progesterone levels, thus restoring hormonal balance. Licorice's phytoestrogenic properties are from its formononetin, coumarin and beta-sitosterol, which are one four-hundredth as active as estradiol.[162] Dosage: 300mg-600mg per day

Chasteberry *(Vitex agnus-castus)*

Chasteberry's therapeutic effects on pituitary function, specifically altering LH and FSH secretion, are likely the cause of its beneficial effects on menopausal symptoms. It has been shown to have a profound effect on pituitary function, increasing the secretion of LH and decreasing the production of FSH, which in turn shifts the production of hormones toward more progesterone and less estrogen. Although traditionally used in countries around the Mediterranean to suppress libido of women of childbearing age, chasteberry does not reduce libido during menopause. Dosage: 225mg-450mg per day

Black Cohosh *(Cimicifuga racemosa)*

A specific extract of black cohosh standardized to contain 1 mg of triterpenes calculated as 27-deoxyactein per tablet (trade name Remifemin) is the most widely used and thoroughly studied natural alternative to HRT. In 1997, ten million monthly units of this extract were sold in Germany, the US, and Australia. A large open study involving 131 doctors and 629 patients found that black cohosh extract produced clear improvement in menopausal symptoms (hot flashes, depression, and vaginal atrophy) in over 80% of patients within six to eight weeks. Additional studies that have compared black cohosh to conjugated estrogens (0.625 mg q.d.) or diazepam (a Valium-like drug) (2 mg q.d.) indicate that black cohosh extract is far more effective than either drug in relieving hot flashes, vaginal atrophy, and the depressive mood and anxiety associated with menopause. Black cohosh not only does not stimulate breast tumor cells but even inhibits their growth. When combined with Tamoxifen (an anti-estrogen drug often used to prevent a recurrence of breast cancer), black cohosh improves Tamoxifen's effectiveness. Detailed toxicology studies have shown no mutagenic or carcinogenic effects, indicating that even long-term use is safe. One of black cohosh's most important effects is that it inhibits the pituitary's release of LH without affecting the release of prolactin and FSH. FSH is responsible for stimulating estrogen, so further balancing FSH will only help the process. Dosage: 20mg-150mg per day

Maidenhair Tree *(Ginkgo biloba)*

Ginkgo's effects of improving blood flow throughout the vascular system make it especially useful for the cold hands and feet and the forgetfulness that often accompanies menopause. In human clinical trials, ginkgo extract has been shown to be effective in the treatment of Raynaud's disease, which is a peripheral vascular disease of the extremities characterized by very cold fingers and toes. Ginkgo is also very effective in improving mental health in patients with cerebral vascular insufficiency. It works not only by increasing blood flow to the brain but also by enhancing energy production within the brain. It increases the uptake of glucose by brain cells and even improves the transmission of nerve signals (memory is directly related to the speed at which the nerve impulse can be transmitted). The two groups of active compounds-terpene lactones and ginkgo flavone glycosides—are responsible in part for many of Ginkgo's therapeutic actions. Although most people report benefits within two to three weeks, ginkgo should be taken for at least twelve weeks in order to determine effectiveness. Dosage: 80mg-240mg per day

Dong quai *(Angelica sinensis)*

Dong quai is the predominant "female" remedy in Asia and is used to treat menopausal symptoms, especially hot flashes, as well as menstrual difficulties such as painful menstruation. Dong quai's active components are coumarins, which have both mild estrogenic effects and a stabilizing action on blood vessels—all of this contributes to its effectiveness in relieving hot flashes. Dosage: 200mg-600mg per day

---

[162] Zayed S, Hassan A, Elghamry M. "Estrogenic substances from Egyptian glyccyrrhiza glabra. Beta-sitosterol as an estrogenic principle." Zenralbi Veterinarmed 1964; 11(5):476-82

St John's wort *(Hypericum perforatum)*

St. John's wort acts pharmacologically to alter brain chemistry in ways similar to antidepressant drugs. "Hypericin, hyperforin, and other components (flavonoids) of the plant have been shown to inhibit the breakdown of several neurotransmitters within the brain that maintain normal mood and emotional stability." It appears to improve the signal produced by serotonin after it binds to its receptor sites on the brain cell. St John's wort is of specific benefit in menopause for the associated depression and mood fluctuations that may occur. Dosage: 300 mg to 900 mg per day

Maca *(Lepidium peruvium chacon)*

Maca, a plant native to Peru, is a cruciferous plant whose roots are eaten as a vegetable by the native people. Along with a rich mineral content, maca contains four alkaloids called macainas which clinical and anecdotal experience suggests may nourish the endocrine glands in an adaptogenic fashion. By balancing the effects of major steroid hormones such as estrogen, progesterone, and testosterone, maca may create effects that are specific to the age and neuroendocrine condition of the individual, elevating low levels of some hormones as well as lowering the levels of hormones present in excess. The scientist responsible for much of the current knowledge of the maca root is Dr. Gloria Chacon de Popivici, a biologist trained at the University of San Marcos in Lima, Peru. Dr. Chacon says that maca root works in a fundamentally different way than HRT, promoting optimal functioning of the hypothalamus as well as the pituitary, and consequently improving the functioning of all the endocrine glands. Dosage 750mg-1500mg per day

Specific Nutrient Therapies Indicated for Menopause

Vitamin E

Vitamin E is found primarily in the lipid (fatty) membrane of cells that it protects from free radical damage. Vitamin E is the main antioxidant in all fat-soluble areas of the body. A healthy cell membrane is essential for the passage of nutrients into and wastes out of cells and so an adequate supply of vitamin E is essential for healthy cellular metabolism. Vitamin E is particularly important during menopause, as it not only relieves menopausal symptoms but also protects against cancer and heart disease. In several clinical studies, vitamin E has been found to improve blood supply to the vaginal wall and to relieve atrophic vaginitis and hot flashes. In premenstrual syndrome and fibrocystic breast disease, two other female complaints related to hormonal imbalances, vitamin E has been shown to normalize circulating hormone levels and thus relieve many symptoms. Of all the antioxidants, vitamin E may offer the most protection against cardiovascular disease. Vitamin E reduces LDL (bad) cholesterol peroxidation, improves plasma LDL breakdown, inhibits excessive platelet aggregation, increases HDL (good) cholesterol levels, and increases the breakdown of fibrin, which is a clot-forming protein. Vitamin E significantly enhances both types of immune defense: non-specific, or cell-mediated, immunity and specific, or humoral, immunity. Cell-mediated immunity is the body's primary mode of protection against cancer. Dosage: oral use–800 IU (mixed tocopherols) per day until symptoms have improved, then 400 IU per day; topical us –vitamin E oil, creams, ointments, or suppositories can be used topically for symptomatic relief of vaginal dryness and irritation. Dosage: 400 IU-800 IU per day

Hesperidin

Like many other flavonoids, hesperidin improves vascular integrity and lessens excessive capillary permeability, which are primary factors in hot flashes. Hesperidin is one of the bioflavonoids and is a naturally occurring nutrient usually found in association with vitamin C. Hesperidin is a flavone glycoside (glucoside) comprised of the flavone hesperidin and the disaccharide rutinose. Hesperidin is the predominant flavonoid in lemons and oranges and when used in combination with a flavone glycoside called diosmin, is used in the treatment of venous insufficiency and hemorrhoids. Hesperidin is useful in treating the complaints of menopause. After supplementation of hesperidin for one month in combination with vitamin C, symptoms of hot flashes were relieved in 53% of patients and reduced in 34%. Nocturnal leg cramps, nosebleeds, and easy bruising were also lessened. The only side effects were a slight body odor and a tendency for perspiration to discolor clothing. Dosage: 900 mg per day in combination with at least 1,200 mg of vitamin C

Vitamin C

Vitamin C, the body's primary antioxidant in all water-soluble areas inside and outside cells, works synergistically with vitamin E and carotenes (its fat-soluble partners). As noted under hesperidin, vitamin C helps to alleviate hot flashes by strengthening the collagen structures of the vascular system, thus preventing excessive capillary permeability. Vitamin C regenerates oxidized vitamin E and enables it to resume its many beneficial activities. Vitamin C is also effective in reducing harmful prostaglandins that contribute to hot flashes. Vitamin C is extremely effective in its own right in protecting against cardiovascular disease by preventing oxidation of LDL cholesterol. Vitamin C also raises HDL cholesterol levels, lowers the total cholesterol level and blood pressure, and inhibits platelet aggregation. Dosage: 1,200 mg per day

Gamma-oryzanol (ferulic acid)

Gamma-oryzanol or ferulic acid is a growth promoting substance found in grains and isolated from rice bran oil. It is also commonly found in wheat, barley, oats, tomatoes, asparagus, olives, berries, peas, and citrus fruits. It has been shown to be effective in alleviating menopausal symptoms including hot flashes. Gamma-oryzanol also lowers blood cholesterol and triglyceride levels. In treating hot flashes, gamma-oryzanol's primary action is to enhance pituitary function and promote the release of endorphins by the hypothalamus. An extremely safe, natural substance, gamma-oryzanol has produced no significant side effects in experimental or clinical studies. Dosage: 300 mg per day

Vitamin B6

Vitamin B6 plays a critical role in the manufacture of serotonin as well as other neurotransmitters and provides support to the adrenal glands. Vitamin B6 is therefore beneficial in the treatment of depression, which is a common symptom of menopause. B6 levels decline as menopause sets in and mood swings become evident, so supplementation becomes necessary. Dosage: 50 mg to 200 mg per day

Calcium

The majority of the body's calcium is found in the skeletal system. Because of this, there is a constant exchange mechanism between the calcium which is held in the bones and the calcium which is in the bloodstream. As long as there is adequate calcium in the bloodstream from dietary sources, bone calcium can remain fairly consistent, with calcium being reabsorbed from the bone and deposited at similar rates. However, when blood serum calcium levels are constantly low, the body reabsorbs calcium into the blood from the bone faster than it can be deposited back, resulting in a loss of bone mass.

Magnesium and calcium appear to work in tandem in the body and both are necessary for many functions including maintaining normal blood pressure and preventing muscle spasms and dysmenorrhea. In addition to calcium, magnesium is essential for helping maintain bone density. Magnesium depletion impairs mineral homeostasis by reducing skeletal and renal sensitivity to parathyroid hormone and by reducing the activation of vitamin D. Dosage: 1000 mg of calcium citrate; 500 mg of magnesium citrate; 1000 IU of vitamin D3

Bioidentical Progesterone Cream

Menopausal women often have low progesterone levels and therefore one of the core treatments is correcting these levels by supplementing with bioidentical progesterone. Bioidentical progesterone is progesterone which is derived from a natural plant source, such as yams, and then converted to progesterone. Bioidentical progesterone has the same molecular configuration as the progesterone produced by the body and can be used to supplement the progesterone produced by the body and to balance estrogen, testosterone, and progesterone levels. Bioidentical progesterone has no side effects when 20 mg to 40 mg per day is used. Dosage: 20-40mg applied 1-2 times per day topically for a period of 25 days and then breaking for 5 days.

Bioidentical Estrogen

Bioidentical Estrogen cream contains an 80/20 combination of two bioidentical estrogens intended to help support women's optimal balance naturally, including the physiological changes of menopause and perimenopause. Estrogen (Estriol or E3 and Estradiol or E2) have been found to be effective at controlling symptoms of menopause, including hot flashes, insomnia, and vaginal dryness. Estrogen helps maintain bones, increases "good" cholesterol, decreases "bad" and total cholesterol, helps maintain memory, and has many other healthy functions in the body. Dosage: 1 mg of natural Estriol USP and 0.25 mg natural Estradiol USP applied topically for a period of 25 days and then breaking for days. (Caution- Bioidentical estrogen should always be combined with Bioidentical Progesterone and is contraindicated in those with a history or family history of estrogen related cancers).

Exercise and Menopause

A minimum of thirty minutes of exercise done four times a week is recommended for women in menopause. Impaired endorphin activity within the hypothalamus is a major factor in provoking hot flashes. Regular exercise increases the production and secretion of endorphins and thus reduces the frequency and severity of hot flashes. Endorphins are the body's internally-produced mood-elevating and pain-relieving compounds which reduce hot flashes via their effects on the functioning of the hypothalamus. Located in the center of the brain, the hypothalamus serves as the bridge between the nervous system and the endocrine system and controls many bodily functions. The hypothalamus regulates body temperature, metabolic rate, sleep patterns, libido, reactions to stress, and mood. It is also responsible for the release of pituitary hormones, including FSH, which is the hormone whose excessive secretion results in hot flashes. In a study in Sweden of seventy-nine postmenopausal women who took part in a regular exercise program, those who exercised an average of three and a half hours per week experienced no hot flashes. Similar results have been reported in other studies of women both on and off HRT. Regular exercise provides numerous other benefits, including decreased blood cholesterol levels, decreased bone loss, and an improved ability to deal with stress. Regular exercise also improves circulation, heart function, and oxygen and nutrient utilization in all tissues. It increases endurance and energy levels as well as increasing self-esteem, mood, and frame of mind and reducing blood pressure.

Top 5 Strategies for Menopause

1. Complete Hormone testing
2. Stress reduction and management when needed/Adrenal support
3. Consume a nutrient dense, organic, high fiber whole food diet/ Eliminate exposure to xenoestrogens
4. Implement exercise program
5. Supplement with Bioidentical hormones when needed, MACA, Black Cohosh, Hesperidin, DIM, Don quai, Vitex, Wild yam, Hops extract, Calcium and Magnesium, Vitamin D3, Vitamin E and B-complex vitamins

Susan's Story - Menopause

Susan is a fifty-three-year-old female who presented with increasing menopausal symptoms and pain. Susan had not had a menstrual cycle in fifteen months. Over the past year, she began to experience increasing hot flashes, night sweats, vaginal dryness and weight gain. Susan had also been experiencing body pain for almost 20 years but it had greatly increased over the past year. At times the pain was so debilitating that it prevented Susan from carrying on normal daily activities. She stated that she felt like her hormones were "a mess." She had continual mood swings, on which her husband often commented. Previous to menopause, Susan did not experience these issues at all. She had, however, been struggling with her weight issues for several years. She was noticeably obese; Susan was five feet eight inches in height and weighed 267 pounds.

Lab testing:

- Elisa multi-food allergy testing revealed allergies to eggs and shellfish
- Low progesterone
- Low estrogen
- Low progesterone to estrogen ratio
- Low morning and daytime cortisol
- Elevated fasting insulin
- Elevated LDL
- Elevated triglycerides
- Low HDL

Management Plan

Susan was administered the following natural medicine therapies:

- Wobenzyme Professional Strength three capsules two times per day without food
- Modified Mediterranean Lifestyle Nutrition Plan to balance hormones and correct hyperglycemia (see "Specific Dietary Modifications for Nutritional Lifestyle Management Plan" in the "Weight Gain" Section)
- Medical food: a powdered medical food designed to nutritionally support the management of conditions associated with metabolic syndrome (including altered body composition) two scoops two times per day
- Estrogen detoxification: DIM, calcium D-glucarate, SGS (standardized to contain 30 mg glucoraphanin glucosinolate), hops extract (0.12% 8-prenylnaringenin-) two capsules with breakfast
- Thyroid support: iodine (as potassium iodide), zinc (as zinc picolinate), copper (as copper chelate), L-tyrosine, thyroid glandular (thyroxine free) two capsules two times per day
- Adrenal support: L-histidine, N-acetyl-tyrosine, rhodiola rosea two capsules two times per day
- Blood sugar management: A multi-nutrient formulate product containing a full range of multivitamins as well as chromium, alpha lipoic acid, cinnamon, taurine, L-carnosine and catechins one tablet before each meal

Susan reported back four weeks later with absolutely no pain. She was very surprised that the pain had completely disappeared so quickly after she had been suffering with it for so many years. She had had years of testing from her medical doctor, who had only ever recommended antidepressants. BIA testing revealed that Susan had lost thirteen pounds so far. She was thrilled with the meal plan and found it very easy to follow. She stated that even her husband had lost weight as well. Susan reported that her menopausal symptoms had already improved by about 40% and she was very hopeful for a complete resolution.

There were no modifications made to the plan.

Susan returned eight weeks later to report that she had experienced very few night sweats and virtually no hot flashes. She also said she had a massive improvement in energy and focus. She still had no pain in her body and this allowed her to begin a walking program. BIA testing revealed a total weight loss of twenty-one pounds.

There were no modifications made to the plan.

Susan returned eight weeks later and reported that she felt great. She had now lost a total of thirty-three pounds and was experiencing absolutely no symptoms of menopause. Susan was advised to taper off of the estrogen detoxification and adrenal support. The other therapies remained the same.

In total, Susan lost seventy-four pounds.

Andropause

Andropause describes an emotional and physical change that many men experience as they age, due to falling testosterone levels. Although the manifestations of andropause are generally related to aging, they are also associated with significant hormonal alterations in the endocrine system. Researchers have known for years that the production of hormones by the testes slowly decreases as men age. Only recently has interest developed in the clinical implications of andropause. This stage in a male's life has several names including male climacteric andropause, late onset hypogonadism, irritable male syndrome (IMS), and androgen decline in the aging male (ADAM).

The process of andropause is much more subtle than that of female menopause. Male hormone production slowly falls over a period of years and thus the symptoms can often be mistaken for stress, aging, or depression. Andropause is unlike menopause where the production of ovarian estrogen and progesterone suddenly declines, making the onset of menopause unmistakably clear.

As one ages, there is an increase in fat cells, which in turn causes an elevation in an enzyme called aromatase. This enzyme transforms testosterone to estrogen in the body. Estrogen can indirectly cause an increase in a protein called sex-hormone-binding-globulin (SHBG), which binds to free testosterone and prevents its action. This protein will ultimately cause a decrease in testosterone.

In obese patients, there is excess aromatase enzyme activity, causing testosterone to convert to estradiol, leading to estrogen overload and testosterone deficiency. Poor liver function is another entity that causes excess estrogen because the liver then cannot detoxify even the small amounts of estrogen that men have. In this case, total testosterone levels are normal, free or usable testosterone levels are low, and estrogen levels are high, as much of the testosterone is being changed into estradiol. This often occurs with excess alcohol consumption.

Andropause is a fairly common condition and the incidence of it increases with age.

The occurrence of andropause occurs in the following ages:

- Forty to forty-nine years of age—2% to5%
- Fifty to fifty-nine years of age—30%
- Sixty to sixty-nine year of age—20% to 45%;
- Seventy to seventy-nine years of age—34% to 70%
- Eighty years of age—91%

The "spread" of normal ranges is fairly large because different specialists use different ways to measure androgens and use different levels to define andropause.

Common Symptoms of Andropause

- Mood changes including depression, anger, and irritability
- A decrease in intellectual activity
- Fatigue, loss of a sense of well being
- Changes in hair growth and skin quality
- A decrease in bone density, resulting in osteoporosis

- A decrease in lean body mass, along with decreases in muscle mass and strength
- An increase in fat surrounding the internal organs
- Diminished sexual desire and erectile quality. In particular, a decrease in nocturnal erections is a significant sign of decreased androgens
- Joint aches and stiffness of hands
- Night sweats
- Sleep disturbances
- Premature aging

Diagnosing Andropause

The following questionnaire will help to determine a male's hormonal status. Answer each question according to the scale below:[163]

SCALE

1 = None
2 = Mild
3 = Moderate
4 = Severe
5 = Extremely Severe

1. **Decline in feeling of general well-being** (general state of health, subjective feeling)
2. **Joint pain and muscular ache** (lower back pain, joint pain, pain in a limb, general back ache)
3. **Excessive sweating** (unexpected/sudden episodes of sweating, hot flushes independent of strain)
4. **Sleep problems** (difficulty in falling asleep, difficulty in sleeping through, waking up early and feeling tired, poor sleep, sleeplessness)
5. **Increased need for sleep, often feeling tired**
6. **Irritability** (feeling aggressive, easily upset about little things, moody)
7. **Nervousness** (inner tension, restlessness, feeling fidgety)
8. **Anxiety** (feeling panicky)

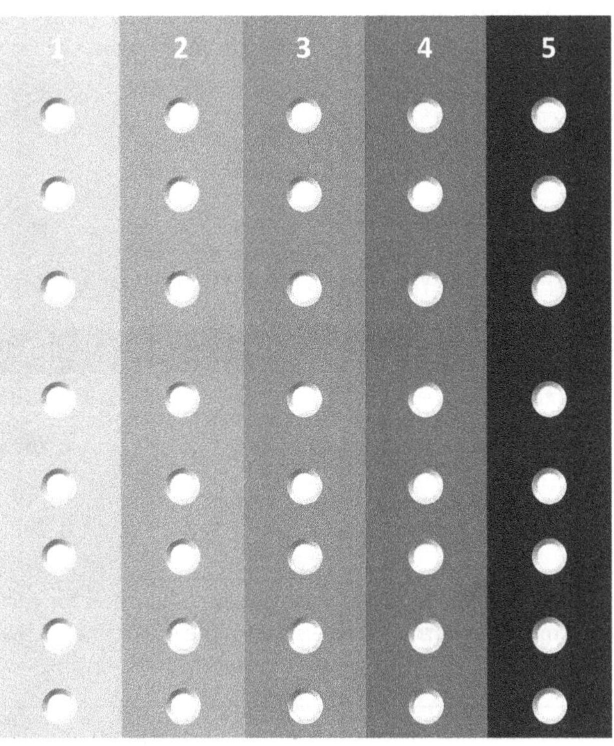

[163] http://www.allsaintsclinic.org/andropause-male-menopause-test.shtml

9. **Physical exhaustion/lacking vitality** (general decrease in performance, reduced activity, lacking interest in leisure activities, feeling of getting less done, of achieving less; of having to force oneself to undertake activities)
10. **Decrease in muscular strength** (feeling of weakness)
11. **Depressive mood** (feeling down, sad, on the verge of tears, lack of drive, mood swings, feeling nothing is of any use)
12. **Feeling that you have passed your peak**
13. **Feeling burnt out, having hit rock-bottom**
14. **Decrease in beard growth**
15. **Decrease in ability/frequency to perform sexually**
16. **Decrease in the number of morning erections**
17. **Decrease in sexual desire/libido** (lacking pleasure in sex, lacking desire for sexual intercourse)

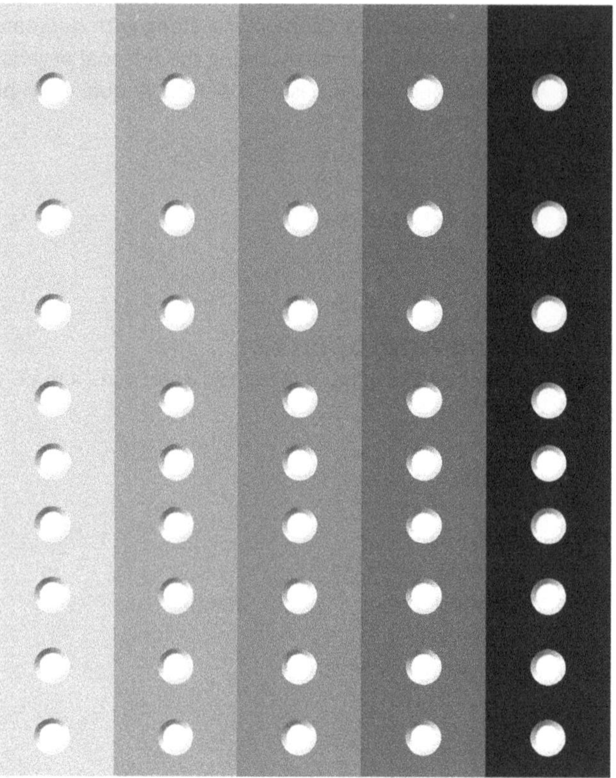

Final score:

Interpreting the results

- How did you score? Cross reference your score with the table below.

Final Score	Likelihood of Male Menopause
Less than 40	**You probably don't need Testosterone Replacement Therapy**
40 - 54	**You might benefit from Testosterone Replacement Therapy**
Greater than 54	**You almost certainly would benefit from Testosterone Replacement Therapy**

A score greater than forty indicates the need for further laboratory testing. The following lab tests will help determine the hormonal levels within the endocrine system:

Specific Lab Test	Description
Male Hormone Panel	Progesterone is a precursor to all androgens and is a physiologic modulator of DHT production.

	DHEA/DHEA-S, the main adrenal androgens, are the precursors to both testosterone and estradiol and are the limiting factor in their production, especially when the patient is under stress. 3Androstenedione, another adrenal androgen and precursor to estrone, is freely inter-convertible with testosterone. Estrone is the major estrogen in men and is the product of the peripheral aromatization of androstenedione in fat and muscle tissue. Estradiol is an estrogen with more proliferative properties. It is formed partially in the testes, but mostly by aromatase enzyme action in peripheral tissues from both testicular and adrenal androgens. Testosterone, the dominant testicular androgen, is the precursor to 5-dihydrotestosterone (DHT). The androgenic effect in various tissues is not exerted by testosterone but by the locally produced DHT. Dihydrotestosterone is the most potent androgen; it is three to five times more potent than testosterone. DHT is derived primarily from conversion of testosterone and other androgens in target tissues (scalp, skin, prostate, liver and others) from five alpha reductase enzyme activities, and derived partially from direct secretion of the testes. FSH and LH. Early detection of an increase in FSH and LH levels is indicative of a progressive decline in male sexuality and functionality. The pituitary neurohormones FSH and LH stimulate and regulate spermatogenesis and testosterone production, respectively.
Adrenal Stress Index	The panel utilizes four saliva samples. Salivary cortisol measurement reflects the free (bioactive) fraction of serum cortisol. The test report shows the awake diurnal cortisol rhythm generated in response to real-life stress. The cortisol/DHEA relationship highlights the many facets of stress maladaptation. The cortisol/DHEA ratio helps determine the projected time for recovery, and the substances (hormones, supplements, botanicals) that promote this recovery. The cortisol/DHEA ratio regulates a multitude of functions. The panel measures P17-OH levels in order to evaluate the efficiency of the conversion of adrenal precursors into cortisol. Certain adrenal fatigue patients who are genetically predisposed to low production of cortisol will not benefit from exogenous supplementation of pregnenolone or progesterone. The panel includes fasting and non-fasting insulin measurements. The insulin values are used to diagnose insulin resistance-functional insulin deficit (pre-diabetes), as well as to correlate elevated cortisol with insulin to help explain glycemic dysregulation problems.
Thyroid Hormone Panel	A complete thyroid profile includes free T4, free T3, TSH, and TPO and can indicate the presence of an imbalance in thyroid function. Hypothyroidism includes feeling cold all the time, low stamina, fatigue (particularly in the evening), anxiety, depression, low sex drive, weight gain, and high cholesterol. Hyperthyroidism includes heat intolerance, anxiety, palpitations, weight loss tired but wired feeling, visual disturbances, and insomnia.

The Male Hormone Panel is helpful for the following clinical uses:

- Measuring baseline hormones.
- Diagnosing andropause and hypogonadism.
- Therapeutic monitoring of HRT.
- Balancing hormones.
- Investigating prostate hypertrophy, hair thinning, and hirsutism.
- Evaluating low libido in both sexes.

Stress plays a major contributing role in the development of andropause. Evaluating stress hormone levels and their subsequent manifestations will enable the treatment protocol to be all-encompassing.

Conventional Pharmaceutical Treatments Indicated for Andropause

Testosterone Replacement Therapy

The treatment goals of conventional therapy for andropause include restoration of sexual functioning, increased libido, increased sense of well-being, and prevention of osteoporosis by optimizing bone density, restoration of muscle strength, and improved mental functioning. In the process of normalizing testosterone levels, current treatment options include oral tablets or capsules, injections, plantable long-acting slow release pellets, and transdermal (through the skin) patches and gels.

Efficacy[164]

Several studies have been conducted involving hormone replacement therapy in men. Unfortunately, at this point, we are approximately twenty years behind the studies of hormone replacement therapy of postmenopausal women, and many of these studies are preliminary. However, they do point to a number of definite benefits of testosterone replacement:

Improved sexual function: In general, testosterone has proved relatively effective for men who have low libido (desire levels). Libido is believed to be significantly hormone-dependent.

Improved erectile function: Erectile function is a more complicated phenomenon. There is a proven significant interaction between the hormone level and sexual functioning, but many other factors are also involved. Newer studies seem to show that men and women will respond more effectively to traditional treatments for sexual dysfunction (including oral medications and injections) if they have adequate testosterone levels.

Improved mood: In recent studies, older men on testosterone reported an improved sense of well-being and an overall improvement in mood when compared with similar men who had received a placebo. Energy levels often also improve.

Improved body composition and strength: Studies evaluating body composition have consistently shown that with testosterone therapy, there is a decline in body fat, an increase in lean body mass (largely muscle mass), or an improvement in both. Several studies also indicate that muscle strength improves, affecting the upper and lower extremities such as that hands, arms, and legs.

Increased bone density: Low bone density or osteoporosis is an increasing problem in men. Men with osteoporosis have a relatively high incidence of bone fractures and, most significantly, hip fractures. Hip fractures in older men are closely associated with disability and death. Testosterone therapy has been shown to increase bone mineral density, especially in the spine. It has also been shown to decrease the rate at which bone is lost.

Improved cardiovascular system: Men overall have a higher incidence of cardiovascular disease and cardiovascular-related deaths than women. It is not known whether this is due to the beneficial effects of female hormones

[164] http://www.wernermd.com/Andropause.html

(estrogen) or lifestyle patterns of women, or whether male hormones play a negative role in the cardiovascular system. However, it is believed that androgens may help lower the risk factors for cardiovascular disease, including serum lipoprotein profiles, vascular tone, platelet and red blood cell clotting parameters, and the process of atherosclerosis.

Early studies have shown that testosterone therapy may decrease platelet aggregation (clumping) and dilate blood vessels. This would have a positive effect on the cardiovascular system. Interestingly, and very importantly, testosterone therapy in older men has led to a decrease in total cholesterol levels. It has also led to a decrease in low-density lipoprotein cholesterol (bad cholesterol levels). These changes, however, have been modest. There has been no significant change in high-density lipoprotein cholesterol levels (HDL or good cholesterol levels) as a result of testosterone therapy.

Negative Effects[165]

Men with a history of prostate cancer or breast cancer are absolutely not candidates for testosterone therapy. The testosterone can make both of these hormone-sensitive cancers grow more rapidly.

Other negative effects may include:

Fluid retention: It is possible, especially within the first few months of treatment, for a man to retain fluid. Studies of healthy older men have shown problems with fluid retention leading to ankle or leg swelling, worsening of high blood pressure, or congestive heart failure. It is unclear whether there would be an effect in men who are ill, for example, those with congestive heart failure.

Liver toxicity: There have been no reports of liver toxicity from transdermal testosterone replacement. However, oral testosterone replacement can cause significant liver problems. Interestingly, every manufacturer (even those producing transdermal testosterone) mentions the possibility of liver problems. This should be taken into account.

Problems with fertility: Spermatogenesis (the production of sperm) in all men is dependent on production of testosterone by the testes. If testosterone is given from outside the testes (exogenous testosterone), as in testosterone replacement therapy, the testes will then stop producing their own testosterone. This will significantly decrease sperm production or shut down production completely in almost all men. This may be a temporary or permanent effect. It is very important that younger men who still plan to have a family take this into account. Some men have "banked" their sperm (for more information on this subject, visit www.SpermBankDirectory.com). Other men have delayed testosterone replacement until they have finished having children. It is important that any man considering a family be very careful in starting testosterone treatment of any kind.

Sleep apnea: Sleep apnea is a condition in which an individual stops breathing for periods of time while sleeping. This can have significant medical effects. There have been reports that increased testosterone levels exacerbate pre-existing sleep apnea. However, a recent thirty-six-month trial of testosterone therapy in older men reported no effect of treatment on apneic or hypoapneic episodes.

Tender breasts or enlargement of the breasts: This may occur in some older men who are on testosterone therapy. This may be due to the conversion of testosterone to estrogen, as breast tissue in both men and women is very estrogen-sensitive. Sometimes, this side effect can be overcome by decreasing the testosterone dose.

Increased red blood cell concentration (polycythemia): One of the most important side effects of testosterone replacement therapy can be an increase in the red blood cell mass and hemoglobin levels. This is particularly true in older men. Increased blood cell mass may increase thromboembolic events (heart attacks, strokes, or peripheral clotting in the veins). Men who develop increased hematocrit can decrease testosterone replacement or donate blood to decrease their blood cell mass.

Prostate growth: The growth of the prostate can have a negative effect on men in two ways. First, the prostate may increase in size (benign prostatic hyperplasia, or BPH). This may cause problems with urination. Second, it may promote the growth of cancerous prostate cells. It is important to remember that prostate cancer is a common cancer for older men and is the second most common cause of cancer deaths in older men.

[165] http://www.wernermd.com/Andropause.html

Nutritional Factors Affecting Andropause

The following table illustrates the specific dietary recommendations to reduce estrogen dominance and balance the endocrine system, which is the main therapeutic dietary approach for restoring the hormones of andropause:

Food Group	Foods To Include	Foods to Exclude
Legumes	All legumes and legume products	None
Vegetables	All, especially cruciferous (see note #1) and sea vegetables (various seaweeds)	None
Fruits	All whole and dry fruits, especially lemon and limes	None
Grains	All whole grains and whole-grain products, especially rye	Non-whole grains, refined flours, refined flour products
Nuts/Seeds	All nuts and seeds and their butters, especially flaxseeds, walnuts, and pumpkin seeds (in their raw form only) (see note #2)	None
Fish	All, especially cold water fish: salmon, sardines, tuna, and halibut are excellent sources of omega-3 fatty acids	Salted or cured fish
Eggs	From organically raised hens	Non-organic eggs
Poultry/Meat	Organic meats and poultry (see note #3)	Non-organic meats and poultry, salted and cured meats
Dairy	Organic dairy products and soy, nut, and grain dairy substitutes	Non-organic dairy products
Oils	Organic cold-pressed, unrefined seed and nut oils, especially flax seed, walnut, sesame, canola, and olive oil (see note #4)	Refined vegetable oils, butter, lard, margarine, shortening, and saturated or hydrogenated fats
Beverages	Mineral or filtered water, herbal tea, fresh fruit juice	Alcohol (see note #5), coffee
Sweeteners	Brown rice syrup, fruit sweetener, molasses, stevia	Chocolate, refined or artificial sweeteners
Spices and Herbs	Especially nutmeg, anise, thyme, sage, fennel, caraway, turmeric	High sodium foods, and salt

Additional Notes:

1. Cruciferous vegetables include: broccoli, cauliflower, all cabbages, Brussels sprouts, kale, bok choy, arugula, mustard greens, and watercress.
2. Omega-3 and some omega-6 fatty acids help to counteract symptoms associated with hormonal imbalance and should be consumed daily.
3. Non-organically raised livestock are often given hormones to improve their growth; unfortunately, these hormones can be passed on to the consumer and negatively influence hormone balance.

4. Important: Do not cook with oils that are not specified for cooking or baking, such as flaxseed or walnut oils. Olive, canola, and sesame oils are good choices for cooking or baking. Use flaxseed, olive, sesame, or walnut oils for homemade salad dressings. These provide valuable omega-3 and omega-6 fatty acids. Refrigerate all oils and dressings.
5. Alcohol should be avoided, as it causes the liver to be unable to detoxify the harmful buildup of estrogen that contributes to the decline of testosterone.

Weight Loss and Andropause

Increasing adipose levels results in accumulating levels of the enzyme aromatase, which converts testosterone into estrogen. The excessive estrogen causes an increase in SHBG which then binds to free testosterone, resulting in an end deficiency of testosterone. Weight loss should be considered a major part of the prescription in the treatment of andropause.

The following list of foods should be decreased or avoided at all times as they disrupt hormones and cause weight gain.

Foods that cause allergies

Food sensitivities cause inflammation, faulty digestion, and a compromised immune system and therefore should be detected through food allergy testing and eliminated.

Refined sugars

Refined white sugar and its products can trigger inflammation by raising blood sugar and insulin. One gram of sugar is equal to four teaspoons of white sugar in any ingredient list and is automatically stored as fat. Each year, the average person consumes forty-five kg (one hundred pounds) of sweetener. The average adult consumes ten to fourteen teaspoons of sugar daily.

Refined grains

White flour, white rice, and other refined grains all spike insulin levels and contribute to insulin resistance. Refined grains are blamed for the obesity epidemic in our nation.

Saturated Fats

Excess saturated fats naturally found in meats, shellfish, egg yolks and dairy products can promote inflammation as they contain arachidonic acid, which contributes to the inflammatory process.

Excess omega-6 fatty acid

Omega-6 and omega-3 fatty acids cannot be produced in the body and therefore need to be consumed through the diet. Omega-6 fatty acids are found in abundance in today's diet in foods such as corn, safflower, and sunflower oils, which are used in processed and packaged food items in place of trans fatty acids. Sixty years ago, the average American diet included a one to two ratio of omega-6 to omega-3; today, the ratio is estimated at approximately twenty-five to one. The optimal ratio is one to one.

Trans Fats

Foods that contain trans fats, including margarine and partially hydrogenated oils, greatly contribute to the free radical process in the body and stimulate weight gain.

Processed Meats

Processed meats containing nitrates and sulfites, including hot dogs, sausages, and deli meats, are all associated with increased inflammation.

Artificial Sweeteners

Artificial sweeteners such as aspartame have been shown to cause consumers to gain weight. People who consume artificial sweeteners are 65% more likely to gain weight than those who do not consume them.

High Fructose Corn Syrup

High fructose corn syrup (HFCS) production has increased from three thousand tons in 1967 to 9,227,000 tons in 2005. North Americans consume more calories from HFCS than from any other source. HFCS has been shown to cause resistance to leptin (the hormone that is secreted from our brains to tell our stomachs that we are full).

Artificial Preservatives

Artificial preservatives and colors have been determined to disrupt our endocrine system, inhibit metabolism, and interfere with the ability to lose weight.

Starchy Root Vegetables

Starchy root vegetables should not be consumed in quantities of more than one-half cup one time per day. These calorie-dense vegetables include yams, sweet potatoes, potatoes, carrots, beets, and some squashes. Non-starchy vegetables contain twenty-five calories and five grams of carbohydrates per one-half cup, cooked. Starchy vegetables contain eighty calories and fifteen grams of carbohydrates per one-half cup, cooked.

Tropical Dried and Canned Fruits

Tropical dried and canned fruits are high in sugar and should therefore be avoided or very limited (two to three servings per week). Dried fruits in particular contain sulfites which are highly inflammatory and can cause severe allergic reactions such as hives, nausea, diarrhea, and shortness of breath, and can mimic asthma symptoms.

Alcohol

Excess alcohol releases estrogen into the bloodstream, promotes fat storage, and decreases muscle growth. The average glass of wine contains approximately 150 calories. Consuming two glasses of wine per night will account for a one pound weight gain every twelve days.

Caffeine

Excess caffeine damages the metabolism and causes hormonal imbalance. After the third cup of coffee, the body is set into "fight or flight" mode. The adrenal glands release epinephrine and norepinephrine, which sets off a cascade of weight-inducing hormonal actions. The liver releases blood sugar for quick energy and the pancreas secretes insulin to counter the blood sugar: the result is a drop in blood sugar levels, which causes hunger. The acidity in one cup of coffee will elevate cortisol for up to fourteen hours.

Top Ten High-Glycemic Foods to Avoid:

- Candy
- Cookies
- Juices with added sugar
- White potatoes
- Chips (corn and potato)
- Sweetened cereal
- Sweetened soda
- Sweetened snacks
- White bread and bagels (processed flour)
- White rice

Top Ten Low-Glycemic Foods to Consume:

- Apples
- Berries and cherries
- Barley
- Grapefruit
- Legumes (lentils, beans, and peanuts)
- Nuts (almonds, walnuts, and soy nuts)
- Oatmeal (unsweetened)
- Green peas
- Tomatoes
- Plain yogurt (unsweetened)

Herbal Medicine Indicated for Andropause

Urtica dioica (Nettle root)

Nettle root liberates testosterone that has become bound to serum globulin and thus is not available to cell receptor sites and fails to induce a libido effect. When testosterone binds to sex hormone binding globulin (SHBG), it loses its biological activity and becomes bound testosterone, as opposed to the desirable free testosterone. Some studies show that the decline in sexual interest with advancing age is not always due to the amount of testosterone produced, but rather to the increased binding of testosterone to globulin by SHBG. European researchers have identified constituents of nettle root that bind to SHBG in place of testosterone, thus reducing SHBG's binding of free testosterone.[166]

Lepidium meyenii (Maca)

Also commonly called "Peruvian ginseng," maca is a powerful adaptogen, which by definition is a substance (food or nutritive herb), which brings the body to a heightened state of resistance to disease through physiological and emotional health.

In 1961, Dr. Gloria Chacón de Popovici published research that demonstrated increased fertility in numerous animal species using maca. She discovered and identified the alkaloids present in maca and proved that it was the alkaloids that were responsible for the positive results.

Dr. Chacón suggests that the alkaloids in maca act on the hypothalamus-pituitary axis and the adrenals. She believes that maca has a balancing effect upon the hypothalamus, the master controller of the body, which then regulates the other endocrine glands, including the pituitary, adrenals, ovaries, testes, thyroid, and pancreas.

Maca works differently on the body than estrogenic herbs (e.g., black cohosh). Instead of introducing weak phytoestrogens into the body, maca regulates and balances the entire endocrine system, strengthening and toning the reproductive glands to promote a heightened sense of well-being and prove the body with higher levels of energy and vitality.

---

[166] Hryb DJ, Khan MS, Romas NA, Rosner W. The effect of extracts of the roots of the stinging nettle (Urtica dioica) on the interaction of SHBG with its receptor on human prostatic membranes. Planta Med. 1995 Feb; 61(1):31-2.

Hirano T, Homma M, Oka K. Effects of stinging nettle root extracts and their steroidal components on the Na+,K(+)- ATPase of the benign prostatic hyperplasia. Planta Med. 1994 Feb;60(1):30-3.

Vahlensieck W Jr., Fabricius PG, Hell U. Drug therapy of benign prostatic hyperpla- sia. Fortschr Med. 1996 Nov 10;114(31):407- 11.

Gansser D, Spiteller G. Plant constituents interfering with human sex hormone-binding globulin. Evaluation of a test method and its application to Urtica dioica root extracts. Z Naturforsch. C 1995 Jan-Feb; 50(1-2):98- 104.

Pausinystalia yohimbe (Yohimbe)

The applicable part of yohimbe is the bark. The active constituent for yohimbe's properties is the alkaloid yohimbine. Yohimbine's effect on impotence seems to be mediated through both increased penile blood flow and increased central sympathetic excitatory impulses to the genital tissue.[167] Caution should be exercised with high doses of yohimbe, as symptoms such as high blood pressure, anxiety, palpitations, dizziness, and shortness of breath can occur.

Epimedium (Horny Goat Weed)

Epimedium, known as horny goat weed and yin yang hou, is a pungent herb found in Asia and the Mediterranean. Epimedium is one of the most valued tonics in Chinese herbalism for supporting healthy sexual activity. It causes vasodilation, possibly by blocking calcium channels, and increases testosterone secretion.[168]

Tribulis Terrestris (Puncture Vine)

Tribulis terrestris, also known as puncture vine, contains saponins (diosgenin and protodioscin), avonoids, and alkaloids. Tribulus terrestris has long been used in the traditional Chinese and Indian systems of medicine for the treatment of various ailments and is popularly claimed to improve sexual function in men. The aphrodisiac activity of Tribulis terrestris is attributed to its androgen-increasing properties.[169]

Serona repens (Saw Palmetto)

An excess of sex hormone-binding globulin can bind much of the free testosterone and therefore inactivate it. In this case, one will have low free testosterone, normal or even high total testosterone, and normal estradiol levels. In addition to following the protocol that inhibits aromatase activity, take saw palmetto to block the estrogen receptor sites in the prostate cells and therefore reduce the effects of excess estrogen. Saw palmetto also blocks the conversion of testosterone into a hormone, DHT, which has been directly linked to the development of prostate disease.

Specific Nutrient Therapies Indicated for Andropause

Zinc Citrate

Zinc is essential for maintaining a man's testosterone levels. Zinc is involved in almost every aspect of male reproduction, including testosterone metabolism, sperm formation, and sperm motility. Multiple studies have demonstrated the effectiveness of zinc in treating male infertility due to low testosterone levels.[170] Infertile males have lower seminal plasma zinc with normal or reduced blood zinc. Clinical research suggests that short-term dietary zinc depletion results in reduced serum testosterone concentrations, seminal volume, and total seminal zinc per ejaculate.[171]

Indole-3-Carbinol (I3C)

Indole-3-carbinol (I3C) is a phytonutrient found in cruciferous vegetables such as broccoli, Brussels sprouts, cabbage, and bok choy. Research suggests that I3C is responsible for many of the health benefits of cruciferous vegetables, by supporting a better balance of estrogen metabolite formation.

---

[167] Urology 1997;49:441-4

[168] Alt Med Alert 2001;4:19-22

[169] Life Sci. 2002. Aug 9;71(12):1385-96

[170] Tikkiwal M, Ajmera RL, Mathur NK. Effect of zinc administration on seminal zinc and fertility of oligospermic males. Indian J Physiol Pharmcol. 1987 Jan-Mar;31(1):30-4.

[171] Am J Clin Nutr 1992;56:148-57

DHEA (dehydroepianodrosterone)

DHEA, like other anabolic steroid hormones such as testosterone, begins depleting with age. Reduced levels of DHEA are directly related to decreased libido and impotence in men. Increasing DHEA levels helps men overcome andropause by enhancing the production of testosterone.

Some of the important functions that DHEA helps control in the body include:

- maintaining sex drive or libido and erectile function
- lowering cholesterol reducing fat
- regulating blood pressure

Produced in the adrenal glands, DHEA is responsible for producing chemicals that influence the growth of testosterone in the body. Memory enhancement, stamina build up, and increased levels of libido can restore a man back to his natural state. Dosing with DHEA is dependent upon lab testing to reveal the individual needs. The average dose is 25mg to 50 mg per day. DHEA can be taken orally or applied topically as a bioidentical cream.

Testosterone Boosting Quench

Testro Max for Men™ is formulated with DHEA and a special Boosting Complex Solution, made with the potent herbs tribulus terrestis, tongkat ali, horny goat weed, and mucuna pruriens. Each full press of the Testro Max for Men™ pump provides approximately 75 mg of Boosting Complex Solution and 15 mg of DHEA.

Bioidentical Testosterone

The ability to normalize levels of testosterone, and sustain these levels for a lifetime, is one of the most important anti-aging and health tools a man can have. Sustaining these levels with bioidentical testosterone compounds which are made of exactly the same molecule that a human body produces is superior to utilization of a synthetically created molecule. Most notably, bioidentical testosterone therapy helps improve mood, attitude, cognitive ability, and general outlook on life. In addition, bioidentical testosterone improves muscle mass and strength, rebuilds bone, strengthens the heart and blood vessels, lowers total cholesterol and blood sugar, raises HDL ("good") cholesterol, lowers blood pressure, lessens the chances of blood clots, improves tissue oxygenation, and improves the health of a non-cancerous prostate gland.

In 2002, the *International Journal of Andrology* published a study that examined 207 men, ages forty to eighty-three, who had all been found to have low or low-normal testosterone levels.[172] The researchers looked at multiple parameters, including prostate volume, prostate specific antigen (PSA), and lower urinary tract symptoms, like frequency, urgency, and "dribbling." The researachers measured levels of several other hormones, including di-hydrotestosterone, or DHT, estradiol, and LH, a marker hormone that has an inverse relationship with testosterone levels—the more LH, the less testosterone, and vice versa. Of the 207 men studied, 187 responded favorably to testosterone treatment. These 187 all showed declines in LH production, as well as improvement in every other parameter measured: their prostate glands all decreased in size, their PSA numbers decreased, and frequency, urgency, dribbling, and getting up at night to urinate all improved. This study indicates that, far from causing prostate trouble, testosterone is actually beneficial for the prostate gland in the vast majority of cases.

A portion of testosterone is converted into estrogen. This small amount of estrogen has important functions for men, just as small quantities of testosterone have important functions for women. In younger men, only a minute quantity of testosterone is converted. But in some older men, testosterone-to-estrogen conversion is dramatically accelerated, resulting in levels of estrogen much higher than usual for men. Monitoring hormonal estrogen levels as well as PSA is strongly recommended when using any testosterone replacement therapy.

---

[172] 1.Perchersky AV et al."Androgen administration in middle-aged and aging men: effects of oral testosterone undecanoate on di-hydrotestosterone, oestradiol, and prostate volume." International J Androl 2002; 25(2): 119

Top 5 Strategies for Andropause

1. Complete Hormone testing
2. Stress reduction and management when needed/Adrenal support
3. Consume a nutrient dense, organic, high fiber whole food diet/ Weight reduction when needed
4. Implement exercise program
5. Supplement with Bioidentical testosterone and DHEA when needed, Zinc, B-complex vitamins, MACA, Saw Palmetto, Puncture vine, Horny goat weed, Yohimbe, Nettle root and Vitamin D3

Weight Gain

Obesity is the excess accumulation of body fat in an individual. The Palo Alto Medical Foundation (PAMF) further narrows this definition to individuals who exceed ideal Body Mass Index (BMI) by 20%, in other words, BMI in excess of twenty-five. The BMI is a number calculated from a person's weight relative to their height, measuring, with fairly reliable accuracy, a person's volume of fat, and is used to determine weight categories at risk of health problems.

Obesity is one of the most tragic, costly, and preventable public health problems. The epidemic of obesity drains the economy of billions of dollars annually in direct medical expenses, disability, and lost productivity and, together with a sedentary lifestyle, contributes to over three hundred thousand deaths each year. Next to smoking, obesity is the second leading cause of preventable death in the United States. According to the results of The National Health and Nutrition Examination Survey 111, one in three North American adults is obese. The number of obese children doubled from 1960 to 1991. Obesity in North America has long been considered an issue of cosmetics and poor self-control, much lower on the scale of importance in comparison to the needs of developing countries. This negligence allowed obesity to run rampant in North American society, gorging on our affluence and economic prosperity.

BMI is classified into six categories, each representing a different level of risk:[173]

	BMI range	**Risk of developing health problems**
Underweight	Less than 18.5	Increased
Normal weight	18.5 to 24.9	Least
Overweight	25.0 to 29.9	Increased
Obese Class I	30.0 to 34.9	High
Obese Class II	35.0 to 39.9	Very high
Obese Class III	Greater than or equal to 40.0	Extremely high

[173] http://www.statcan.gc.ca/pub/82-620-m/2005001/article/adults-adultes/4053561-eng.htm

BMI is calculated as follows:

$$BMI = \left(\frac{\text{Weight in Pounds}}{\text{(Height in Inches) x (Height in Inches)}} \right) \times 703$$

$$BMI = \frac{\text{Weight in Kilograms}}{\text{(Height in Meters) x (Height in Meters)}}$$

For example, for someone who is five feet, seven inches (sixty-seven inches) tall and weighs 220 pounds, the calculation would look like this: 220 divided by 4489 (sixty-seven inches times sixty-seven inches) multiplied by 703 equals 34.45 BMI.

The following table illustrates the breakdown of the Body Mass Index:

	NORMAL						OVERWEIGHT					OBESE										EXTREME OBESITY		
BMI	19	20	21	22	23	24	25	26	27	28	29	30	31	32	33	34	35	36	37	38	39	40	41	42
Height (Feet-Inches)	**Weight** (Pounds)																							
4'10"	91	96	100	105	110	115	119	124	129	134	138	143	148	153	158	162	167	172	177	181	186	191	196	201
4'11"	94	99	104	109	114	119	124	128	133	138	143	148	153	158	163	168	173	178	183	188	193	198	203	208
5'00"	97	102	107	112	118	123	128	133	138	143	148	153	158	163	168	174	179	184	189	194	199	204	209	215
5'01"	100	106	111	116	122	127	132	137	143	148	153	158	164	169	174	180	185	190	195	201	206	211	217	222
5'02"	104	109	115	120	126	131	136	142	147	153	158	164	169	175	180	186	191	196	202	207	213	218	224	229
5'03"	107	112	118	124	130	135	141	146	152	158	163	169	174	180	186	191	197	203	208	214	220	225	231	237
5'04"	110	116	122	128	134	140	145	151	157	163	169	175	180	186	191	197	204	209	215	221	227	232	238	244
5'05"	114	120	126	132	138	144	150	156	162	168	174	180	186	192	198	204	210	216	222	228	234	240	246	252
5'06"	118	124	130	136	142	148	155	161	167	173	179	186	192	198	204	210	216	223	229	235	241	247	253	260
5'07"	121	127	134	140	146	153	159	166	172	178	185	191	198	204	211	217	223	230	236	242	249	255	261	268
5'08"	125	131	138	144	151	158	164	171	177	184	190	197	204	210	216	223	230	236	243	249	256	262	269	276
5'09"	128	135	142	149	155	162	169	176	182	189	196	203	210	216	223	230	236	243	250	257	263	270	277	284
5'10"	132	139	146	153	160	167	174	181	188	195	202	209	216	222	229	236	243	250	257	264	271	278	285	292
5'11"	136	143	150	157	165	172	179	186	193	200	208	215	222	229	236	243	250	257	265	272	279	286	293	301
6'00"	140	147	154	162	169	177	184	191	199	206	213	221	228	235	242	250	258	265	272	279	287	294	302	309
6'01"	144	151	159	166	174	182	189	197	204	212	219	227	235	242	250	257	265	275	280	288	295	302	310	318
6'02"	148	155	163	171	179	186	194	202	210	218	225	233	241	249	256	264	272	280	287	295	303	311	319	326
6'03"	152	160	168	176	184	192	200	208	216	224	232	240	248	256	264	272	279	287	295	303	311	319	327	335
6'04"	156	164	172	180	189	197	205	213	221	230	238	246	254	263	271	279	287	295	304	312	320	328	336	344

Adapted from: George Bray, Pennington Biomedical Research Center; *Clinical Guidelines on the Identification, Evaluation, and Treatment of Overweight and Obesity in Adults: The Evidence Report*, National Institutes of Health, National Heart, Lung, and Blood Institute, September 1998.

Obesity often leads to numerous health problems, including heart disease, gallbladder disease, diabetes, hypertension, stroke, and some forms of cancer. Obesity has also been known to shorten life spans.

Causes of Weight Gain

The obvious cause of unwanted weight gain is simple—an excess amount of calories are consumed compared to a decreased amount of calories burned. There are, however, several other underlying factors that may be at work in the cause of unwanted weight gain and the inability to lose it.

Common Nutritional Mistakes That Lead to Unwanted Weight Gain:

- Skipping meals leads to a dramatic slowdown of the body's metabolism, which creates a fat storing environment
- Calorie counting meal plans do not ensure proper weight loss as the specific type of calorie is not always considered
- Low fat diets lead to hormonal disruptions and unwanted weight gain
- A diet with no carbohydrates creates an acidic environment which leads to many health conditions as well as unwanted weight gain
- Skipping breakfast slows the metabolism down by 35% for the rest of the day
- Dehydration leads to a slower metabolism as the muscles of the body are partly responsible for the rate of metabolism and they are made up of two-thirds water
- Consuming foods that a person is unknowingly allergic to can contribute to weight gain

The main cause of weight gain in women is hormonal imbalances. There are numerous hormones that can be part of the underlying cause of the weight gain. The following chart outlines the hormonal imbalances that can cause weight gain:[174]

Specific Hormone or Contributing Factor	**Imbalance that Causes Weight Gain**
Insulin, the hormone that regulates blood sugar. It is the ONLY hormone that is always telling your body to store energy as fat.	Excess insulin (insulin resistance or metabolic syndrome), usually arising as a result of a poor diet, lack of exercise, excess alcohol consumption, stress, or sleep deprivation.
Estrogen, the sex hormone, is dominant in the first half of the menstrual cycle. Excess estrogen is a major cause of weight gain for both men and women.	Excess estrogen—estrogen dominance, which usually arises from estrogen exposure in our environment or because we fail to eliminate estrogen via regular bowel movements and liver detoxification.
Ghrelin, the hormone released from the stomach that increases appetite.	Excess ghrelin released as a result of sleep deprivation or in between meals to trigger hunger.
Inflammation, not a hormone but a definite cause of hormonal imbalance and obesity	When inflammation is too high as a result of poor nutrition, digestion, lack of sleep, or a medical condition.
Cortisol, the hormone released while under chronic stress. It has detrimental effects on the immune system, bones, brain, and muscles and it increases belly fat when present in excess.	Excess cortisol due to any type of chronic stress (emotional, physical, or physiological) can cause weight gain.

174 The Super-Charged Hormone Diet Dr. Natasha Turner ND pg. 6

Thyroid hormones, TSH, free T3, and free T4—thyroid hormones control the metabolism of every single cell in the body.	Deficiency of thyroid hormone, usually as a result of nutrient deficiency, stress, toxin exposure, or an immune system imbalance.
Adrenalin and noradrenalin, the immediate stress response hormones which increase alertness and fat burning.	An excess of both adrenalin and noradrenalin is usually a result of stress.
Glucagon, the hormone that works opposite to insulin to boost blood sugar and encourage fat burning. It is released when our blood sugar drops (e.g., between meals) or during exercise.	Glucagon is too low, usually as a result of not eating enough protein, not exercising regularly, or consuming excess carbohydrates, which spikes insulin and blocks glucagon activity.
Progesterone, the sex hormone dominant in the second half of the menstrual cycle. A deficiency of progesterone is almost always associated with PMS or fertility concerns.	Low progesterone in men and women, normally as a result of stress or aging.
DHEA, the anti-stress, anti-aging, anti-inflammatory, metabolism-enhancing hormone with masculinizing properties.	DHEA is too low, often as a result of stress or aging.
Testosterone, the masculinizing sex hormone that builds and maintains muscle. A deficiency of testosterone can prevent weight loss in both men and women even with dieting and exercise.	Low testosterone in men, often resulting from stress or toxin exposure. Excess testosterone in women causes weight gain, usually as a result of insulin resistance or PCOS.
Growth hormone, the hormone that handles growth and repair, particularly of the bone, muscle, and skin cells while we sleep. It is also released in response to exercise.	Growth hormone deficiency, usually as a result of poor sleep, lack of exercise, low protein intake, or stress.
Melatonin, serotonin, dopamine, acetylcholine, and GABA, the hormones that influence motivation, mood, sleep, and cravings.	Deficiency of all of these hormones; abnormal highs and lows of dopamine are common in individuals with addictions to food, smoking, gambling, alcohol, and drugs. Low serotonin is related to depression, food cravings, eating disorders, sleep disruption, and anxiety.
Vitamin D3 acts like a hormone in the body. Vitamin D supports immunity, protects us from cancer, and aids weight loss. It also reduces inflammation, boosts mood, and can help to reduce pain.	Vitamin D3 deficiency (blood levels less than 125). Low vitamin D3 is common in individuals who live in northern climates, cover up in the sun, or use excessive sunscreen.

Insulin Resistance

Many people with fatigue, depression, hypoglycemia, excess weight, or sugar/starch cravings are suffering from dysglycemia, which is a disruption in blood sugar metabolism caused primarily by diet. Other conditions that can also be linked to this problem include high blood pressure, some types of high cholesterol, metabolic syndrome, prediabetes, adult onset diabetes, and polycystic ovarian syndrome (PCOS).

Insulin is a hormone that is produced by the beta cells, which are cells that are scattered throughout the pancreas. The insulin is released into the bloodstream and travels throughout the body. Most of the actions of insulin are directed at metabolism (control) of carbohydrates (sugars and starches), lipids (fats), and proteins. Insulin is also important in regulating the cells of the body, including their growth.

Insulin resistance (IR) is a condition in which the cells of the body become resistant to the effects of insulin, that is, the normal response to a given amount of insulin is reduced. As a result, higher levels of insulin are needed in order for insulin to have its effects. The resistance is seen with both the body's own insulin (endogenous) and insulin given through injection (exogenous).

People with insulin resistance tend to gain weight and suffer from carbohydrate cravings that in some cases can be quite intense. They may not feel satisfied if they eat a meal that doesn't contain carbohydrates and they may find it difficult to stop eating carbohydrates once they've started, even binging at times. They will also frequently experience elevated cholesterol and triglyceride levels and lowered HDL cholesterol levels. HDL cholesterol is the good type of cholesterol that offers protection against heart disease. Many of these people also suffer from hypoglycemia, which is a condition that can cause fatigue, anxiety, and shakiness if they don't eat frequently enough.

Insulin Resistance is diagnosed when at least three out of the following five findings are present:

1. Blood pressure equal to or higher than 130/85 mmHg
2. Fasting blood sugar (glucose) equal to or higher than 100 mg/dL
3. Large waist circumference (length around the waist):
   Men—forty inches or more
   Women–thirty-five inches or more
4. Low HDL cholesterol:
   Men—under 40 mg/dL
   Women—under 50 mg/dL
5. Triglycerides equal to or higher than 150 mg/dL

Tests that may be done to diagnose metabolic syndrome include:

- Blood pressure measurement
- Glucose test
- HDL cholesterol level
- LDL cholesterol level
- Total cholesterol level
- Triglyceride level

Adrenal Stress Index	The panel utilizes four saliva samples. Salivary cortisol measurement reflects the free (bioactive) fraction of serum cortisol. The test report shows the awake diurnal cortisol rhythm generated in response to real-life stress. The cortisol/DHEA relationship highlights the many facets of stress maladaptation. The cortisol/DHEA ratio helps determine the projected time for recovery and the substances (hormones, supplements, and botanicals) that promote this recovery. The cortisol/DHEA ratio regulates a multitude of functions. The panel measures P17-OH levels in order to evaluate the efficiency of the conversion of adrenal precursors into cortisol. Certain adrenal fatigue patients who are genetically predisposed to low production of cortisol will not benefit from exogenous supplementation of pregnenolone or progesterone.

	The panel includes fasting and non-fasting insulin measurements. The insulin values are used to diagnose insulin resistance-functional insulin deficit (pre-diabetes), as well as to correlate elevated cortisol with insulin to help explain glycemic dysregulation problems.
Complete Female Hormone Panel	Estradiol and progesterone levels and their ratio are an index of estrogen/progesterone balance. An excess of estradiol, relative to progesterone, can explain many symptoms in reproductive age-women. Testosterone levels can also be either too high or too low. Testosterone in excess, often caused by ovarian cysts, leads to conditions such as excessive facial and body hair, acne, and oily skin and hair. Polycystic ovarian syndrome (PCOS) is thought to be caused, in part, by insulin resistance. On the other hand, too little testosterone is often caused by excessive stress, medications, contraceptives, and surgical removal of the ovaries. This leads to symptoms of androgen deficiency including loss of libido, thinning skin, vaginal dryness, loss of bone and muscle mass, depression, and memory lapses. SHBG binds tightly to circulating estradiol and testosterone, preventing their rapid metabolism and clearance and limiting their bioavailability to tissues. SHBG gives a good index of the extent of the body's overall exposure to estrogens.
Thyroid Hormone Testing	A complete thyroid profile includes free T4, free T3, TSH, and TPO and can indicate the presence of an imbalance in thyroid function. Hypothyroidism includes feeling cold all the time, low stamina, fatigue (particularly in the evening), anxiety, depression, low sex drive, weight gain, and high cholesterol. Hyperthyroidism includes heat intolerance, anxiety, palpitations, weight loss, tired but wired feeling, visual disturbances, and insomnia.
Cardiometabolic Profile (hs-CRP), Fasting Insulin, Hemoglobin A1c (HbA1c), Fasting Triglycerides, Total Cholesterol, LDL Cholesterol, VLDL Cholesterol, and HDL Cholesterol	High Sensitivity C-Reactive Protein (hs-CRP) CRP is an established marker of inflammation and has recently been suggested to be an important contributor to pro-inflammatory and prothrombic elements of CVD risk. Increased CRP levels, which correlate inversely with insulin sensitivity, have been found in individuals with polycystic ovarian syndrome and may be a marker of early cardiovascular risk in these patients. Fasting Insulin High fasting insulin levels are a good indicator of insulin resistance, which occurs when the cellular response to the presence of insulin is impaired, resulting in a reduced ability of tissues to take up glucose for energy production. Chronically high insulin levels are seen as the body attempts to normalize blood sugar levels. HbA1c HbA1c levels above 6% can predict CVD and DM2 in high risk individuals. Fasting Triglycerides Hypertriglyceridemia, a triglyceride level greater than 150 mg/dL, is an established indicator of atherogenic dyslipidemia and is often found in untreated DM2 and obesity.

	Total Cholesterol, LDL Cholesterol, VLDL Cholesterol, and HDL Cholesterol Abnormalities in the lipid profile, including high total cholesterol, high LDL cholesterol, high VLDL cholesterol, and low HDL cholesterol, are a significant component of coronary heart disease risk because of their contribution to the development of atherosclerosis.
ELISA/EIA Food Allergy Testing	This is based on the findings that certain subclasses of IgG have been associated with the *in vitro* degranulation of basophils and mast cells, the activation of the complement cascade (both of which are important mechanisms in allergy and anaphylaxis), and the observation that high circulating serum concentrations of some IgG subtypes have been measured in certain atopic individuals. The premise behind this testing is that high circulating levels of IgG antibodies are correlated with clinical food allergy signs and symptoms. The ELISA/EIA test itself involves coating a ninety-six-well plate with food antigens, adding a patient's sera, and looking for a classic antigen/antibody interaction.

Bioelectrical Impedance Analysis (BIA) Testing

What Bioelectrical Impedance Analysis Can Reveal

Bio impedance analysis, or bioelectrical impedance analysis (BIA), is a commonly used, accurate measurement of body composition. BIA can serve as an important assessment of the metabolic status of patients and assist in the recommendation of a lifestyle intervention program, as well as tracking the program's progress for better patient health.

BIA is a simple, rapid, and non-invasive method of measuring body composition (fat-to-lean tissue ratio) that uses imperceptible electric signals at different frequencies. These signals flow through the body via sensor pads placed on one hand and one foot of a patient lying in a prone position on an examination table. The electric signals are impeded variably by body water, fat, and fat-free mass to produce measurements of each. Healthcare practitioners can then utilize these measurements in the assessment of body composition to determine clinical therapies, which is particularly important as people age.[175]

A certain amount of fat is necessary for normal body functioning and a normal balance of body fat in relation to lean muscle tissue is associated with good health (especially in the aging process). Excess fat in relation to lean body mass, a condition known as altered body composition, can greatly increase the risk of a variety of serious health conditions and concerns.

These health concerns include:

- Cardiovascular Disease
- Type II Diabetes
- Arthritis
- Hormonal Imbalance
- Back Pain
- Fatigue

[175] Bere VA, Rousset P, MacCormack C, et al. Reproducibility of body composition and body water spaces measurements in healthy elderly individuals. J Nutr Health Aging 2000; 4(4):243-45.

A higher ratio of muscle to fat increases metabolism because muscle requires a greater amount of caloric fuel for maintenance. As people age, however, their percentage of fat-free mass diminishes.[176] Lifestyle changes such as exercise, diet, and nutritional supplementation can be recommended to help increase the amount of fat-free mass for better health. BIA provides reliable results that are easy to interpret. Research has shown that BIA is capable of reproducible measurements of water compartments. This makes BIA an excellent tool in accurately tracking the progress of fat loss and other health measurements in a therapeutic lifestyle program or body composition program. To establish "normal" values for both men and women, BIA measurements have been collected from a large population of healthy, diseased, obese, and elderly subjects. Using differential equations, these results are used to calculate reference values for age ranges by gender. These reference values are useful in evaluating the health status of patients whose measurements differ from what are considered to be healthy values for men or women.[177]

Nutritional Indications for Weight Loss

The following list of foods should be decreased or avoided at all times as they disrupt hormones and cause weight gain:

Foods that cause allergies

Food sensitivities cause inflammation, faulty digestion, and a compromised immune system and therefore should be detected and then eliminated through food allergy testing.

Refined sugars

Refined white sugar and its products can trigger inflammation by raising blood sugar and insulin. One gram of sugar is equal to four teaspoons of white sugar in any ingredient list and is automatically stored as fat. Each year, the average person consumes forty-five kg (one hundred pounds) of sweetener. The average adult consumes ten to fourteen teaspoons of sugar daily.

Refined grains

White flour, white rice, and other refined grains all spike insulin levels and contribute to insulin resistance. Refined grains are blamed for the obesity epidemic in our nation.

Excess saturated fats

Saturated fats naturally found in meats, shellfish, egg yolks, and dairy products can promote inflammation as they contain arachidonic acid, which contributes to the inflammatory process.

Excess Omega-6 fatty acid.

Omega-6 and omega-3 fatty acids cannot be produced in the body and therefore need to be consumed through the diet. Omega-6 fatty acids are found in abundance in today's diet in foods such as corn, safflower, and sunflower oils, which are used in processed and packaged food items in place of trans fatty acids. Sixty years ago, the average American diet included a one to two ratio of omega-6 to omega-3 and today the ratio is estimated at approximately twenty-five to one. The optimal ratio is one to one.

Trans Fats

Foods that contain trans fats, including margarine and partially hydrogenated oils, greatly contribute to the free radical process in the body and stimulate weight gain.

---

[176] Kyle UG, Genton L, Slosman DO, et al. Fat-free and fat mass percentiles in 5225 healthy subjects aged 15 to 98 years. Nutrition 2001:17(7-8):534-41.

[177] Kyle UG, Genton L, Slosman DO, et al. Fat-free and fat mass percentiles in 5225 healthy subjects aged 15 to 98 years. Nutrition 2001:17(7-8):534-41.

Processed Meats

Processed meats containing nitrates and sulfites, including hot dogs, sausages, and deli meats, are all associated with increased inflammation.

Artificial Sweeteners

Artificial sweeteners such as aspartame have been shown to cause consumers to gain weight. People who consume artificial sweeteners are 65% more likely to gain weight than those who do not consume them.

High Fructose Corn Syrup

High fructose corn syrup (HFCS) production has increased from three thousand tons in 1967 to 9.3 million tons in 2005. North Americans consume more calories from HFCS than from any other source. HFCS has been shown to cause resistance to leptin (the hormone that is secreted from our brains to tell our stomachs that we are full).

Artificial Preservatives

Artificial preservatives and colors have been determined to disrupt our endocrine system, inhibit metabolism, and interfere with the ability to lose weight.

Starchy Root Vegetables

Starchy root vegetables should not be consumed in quantities of more than one-half cup one time per day. These calorie dense vegetables include yams, sweet potatoes, potatoes, carrots, beets and some squashes. Non-starchy vegetables contain twenty-five calories and five grams of carbohydrates per one-half cup, cooked. Starchy vegetables contain eighty calories and fifteen grams of carbohydrates per one-half cup, cooked.

Tropical dried and canned fruits

Tropical dried and canned fruits are high in sugar and should therefore be avoided or very limited (two to three servings per week). Dried fruits in particular contain sulfites, which are highly inflammatory and can cause severe allergic reactions such as hives, nausea, diarrhea, and shortness of breath, and can mimic asthma symptoms.

Alcohol

Excess alcohol releases estrogen into the bloodstream, promotes fat storage, and decreases muscle growth. The average glass of wine contains approximately 150 calories. Consuming two glasses of wine per night will account for a one pound weight gain every twelve days.

Caffeine

Excess caffeine damages the metabolism and causes hormonal imbalance. After the third cup of coffee, the body is set into "fight or flight" mode. The adrenal glands release epinephrine and norepinephrine which sets off a cascade of weight-inducing hormonal actions. The liver releases blood sugar for quick energy and the pancreas secretes insulin to counter the blood sugar: the result is a drop in blood sugar levels, which causes hunger. The acidity in one cup of coffee will elevate cortisol for up to fourteen hours.

Top Ten High-Glycemic Foods to Avoid:

- Candy
- Cookies
- Juices with added sugar
- White potatoes
- Chips (corn and potato)
- Sweetened cereal

- Sweetened soda
- Sweet snacks
- White bread and bagels (processed flour)
- White rice

Top Ten Low-Glycemic Foods

- Apples
- Berries and cherries
- Barley
- Grapefruit
- Legumes (lentils, beans, and peanuts)
- Nuts (almonds, walnuts, and soy nuts)
- Oatmeal (unsweetened)
- Green peas
- Tomatoes
- Plain yogurt (unsweetened)

Specific Guidelines for Nutritional Lifestyle Management

There are several categories of food that need to be consumed each day. The following is a list of categories with the recommended food examples:

Protein

Serving size three to four ounces cooked, or as indicated
(one serving = approximately 150 calories)
Organic chicken, turkey, fish, lamb, buffalo, venison, elk, organic eggs, tofu, tempeh, 1% cottage cheese, ricotta cheese, part skim mozzarella cheese

Legumes

Serving size one-half cup cooked, or as indicated
(one serving = approximately 110 calories)
Beans including garbanzo, pinto, kidney, black, lima, cannellini, navy, mung, fat-free refried, green, soy
Split peas, sweet green peas, lentils

Dairy/Dairy Alternatives

Serving size six ounces, or as indicated
(one serving = approximately eighty calories)
Almond milk—plain, Hemp milk—plain, organic milk—nonfat or 1%, soy milk—plain, organic yogurt—plain and unsweetened, yogurt (goat milk or Greek)—plain and unsweetened, fat-free feta cheese (two ounces)

Nuts

Serving size eight to twelve nuts or one tablespoon of sesame seeds
(one serving = approximately one hundred calories)
Almonds, hazelnuts, pine nuts, pistachios, sunflower, pumpkin, walnut or pecan halves, sesame seeds

Low Glycemic Vegetables

Serving size one-half cup—minimum of three to four servings, unlimited

(one serving = approximately ten to twenty-five calories)
Artichokes, asparagus, bamboo shoots, bean sprouts, bell or other peppers, broccoli, broccoflower, Brussels sprouts, cabbage (all types),cauliflower, celery, chives, cucumber, eggplant, garlic, green beans, greens, bok choy, escarole, Swiss chard, kale, collards, spinach, dandelion, mustard and beet greens, leeks, lettuce/mixed greens, romaine, red and green leaf, endive, spinach, arugula, radicchio, watercress, chicory, mushrooms, okra, onion, radishes, salsa (sugar-free), scallions, sea vegetables (kelp, etc.), snow peas, sprouts, squash, zucchini, yellow, summer, spaghetti, tomatoes or mixed vegetable juice (low sodium), water chestnuts

Medium Glycemic Vegetables

Serving size½ one-half cup
(one serving = approximately forty-five calories)
Beets, winter squash (acorn, butternut), carrots, sweet potatoes or yams, Yukon gold, new, or red potatoes

Fruits

Serving size as indicated
(one serving = approximately eighty calories)
Apple—one medium, apricots—three medium, berries (blackberries and blueberries)—one cup, berries (raspberries and strawberries)—one and one-half cups, cantaloupe—medium, one-half, cherries—fifteen, fresh figs—two, grapefruit—one whole, grapes—fifteen, honeydew melon—small, one-quarter, mango—medium, one-half, nectarines—two small, orange—one large, peaches—two small, pear—one medium, plums—two small, persimmon—one-half, tangerines—two small, watermelon—two cups

Grains

Serving size: one-half cup cooked, or as indicated
(one serving = approximately seventy-five to one hundred calories)
Basmati or other brown rice, wild rice, barley, buckwheat grouts, or millet, bulgur (cracked wheat), quinoa, teff, whole oats, raw—one-third cup, cooked oatmeal-three-quarters cup, whole wheat, spelt, or kamut berries, 100% whole wheat, spelt, or kamut, whole grain rye crackers—two each, bread: mixed whole grain or 100% whole rye-one slice, whole wheat tortilla or pita—one-half, low-carb tortillas—two small or one large, kashi® seven whole grain puffs cereal or equivalent—one cup

Good Fats

Serving size: one teaspoon or as indicated
Oils should be cold pressed
(one serving = approximately forty calories)
Plant oils: avocado (fruit)—one-eighth, coconut milk, light—three tablespoons., coconut milk, regular—one and one-half tablespoon, flaxseed oil, olives—eight to ten medium, olive oil, extra virgin (preferable), coconut oil—-one teaspoon, ghee (clarified butter)—one teaspoon, grapeseed oil—one teaspoon., earth balance® spread or equivalent—one and one-half teaspoon

The following table outlines the recommended allowable number of servings for each category of food depending upon daily caloric requirements:

	1300 calories	1600 calories	1800 calories	2000 calories
Protein Shake *	2	2	2	2
Protein	2	3	3	3

Legumes	1	2	2	2
Dairy	1	1	1	1
Nuts and Seeds	1	1	1	2
Low Glycemic Vegetables	Minimum 3 to 4 servings	Minimum 3 to 4 servings	Minimum 3 to 4 servings	Minimum 3 to 4 servings
Medium Glycemic Vegetables	1	1	1	2
Fruits	2	2	3	3
Whole Grains	1	1	1	1
Oils	4	4	6	6

*Two scoops of protein powder per day provide additional blood sugar and hormone balancing as well as a feeling of being satisfied. Protein choices include rice, hemp, pea, pumpkin and isolated whey (whey is best for men and should be used with caution as it can cause stomach upset).

Herbal Medicine Indicated for Weight Management

Any hepatotropic or hepatoprotective herb will increase the body's ability to detoxify harmful agents that disrupt the hormonal system. Liver detoxification will speed up the metabolism and aid in the elimination of years' worth of fermenting fecal matter stored in the colon.

Milk thistle *(Carduus marianus)*

Silymarin, a flavonolignan, is the main active compound that gives milk thistle its well-researched liver protecting effects. Silymarin protects the liver by inhibiting substances in the liver that cause liver damage. Silymarin has the added ability to increase glutathione, one of the most critical nutrients for liver detoxification in the liver, intestine, and stomach. There are over one hundred studies that involve the ability of milk thistle to protect and regenerate the liver. Milk thistle is proved to be useful in all liver conditions such as hepatitis, cirrhosis, liver damage, cholestasis, and fatty liver. Silymarin's ability to promote the regeneration of damaged hepatocytes renders it as one of the most potent liver detoxifiers.

Turmeric *(Curcuma longa)*

Curcumin, one of the active compounds in turmeric, is a potent liver detoxifier and anti-inflammatory agent. Curcumin is of exponential use in Phase 2 detoxification pathways in the liver as it increases the levels of the enzymes needed to facilitate the action of Phase 2 detoxification. Curcumin also increases the production of bile in the liver which helps to expel toxins and reduce liver inflammation.

Burdock Root *(Arctium lappa)*

Burdock root is one of the foremost cleansing herbs, providing nourishing support for the blood, the liver, and the natural defense system. It is rich in vitamins B-1, B-6, B-12, and E, plus manganese, copper, iron, zinc, and sulfur. Burdock root contains inulin along with bitter compounds and mucilage, which provide its ability to control liver damage and protect from further burdens to the liver. Burdock root also promotes the flow and release of bile, which not only helps cleanse the liver, but also aids the digestive process.

Dandelion Root *(Taraxacum officinalis)*

The *Australian Journal of Medicinal Herbalism* has cited two studies that show the liver-regenerating properties of dandelion in cases of jaundice, liver swelling, hepatitis, and indigestion.

The root of the dandelion plant is effective as a detoxifying agent, acting especially on the liver and gallbladder to remove toxins and waste products. It stimulates and tonifies the digestive system. Its cholagogue, or bile secreting, effect creates a mild laxative effect which allows for expulsion of toxins. Dandelion root is therefore useful in the treatment of liver conditions such as jaundice, metabolic toxicity, hepatitis, and cholelithiasis (gallstones), as well as chronic conditions of the digestive system, conditions of the skin such as acne and eczema, and joint problems such as arthritis.

Globe Artichoke *(Cynara scolymus)*

Globe artichoke contains a powerful compound called cynaropicrin which is a sesquiterpene lactone that stimulates the flow of bile from the liver and makes it a useful liver detoxifier and protector. Due to its ability to promote detoxification and improve bile flow, Globe Artichoke is useful in all cases of insufficient liver production and digestion.

Blue Flag *(Iris Versicolor)*

Blue flag has the ability to detoxify almost all channels of elimination. It stimulates the flow and release of bile from the liver, purges the intestines, and promotes secretions from the pancreas. Blue flag also cleanses the blood of impurities and stimulates the lymphatic system to enhance whole body cleansing effects.

Yellow Dock *(Rumex crispus)*

The major plant chemicals in yellow dock are tannins, oxalates, anthraquinone glycosides (about 3-4%), and nepodin, as well as other chemicals based on chrysophanol, physcion and emodin. These constituents produce alterative, gently purgative, mildly laxative, and mildly astringent tonic effects. The iron content of yellow dock makes it powerful in treating anemia symptoms. Chrysarobin in yellow dock is known to relieve a congested liver.

The anthraquinone glycosides contained in yellow dock have a laxative effect on the bowels, making it useful in all detoxification strategies. The release of toxins from the tissues can create an increasingly symptomatic effect on the body if the channels of elimination are not working efficiently. Yellow dock has the ability to expel toxins from the bowels, as well as from the liver and blood.

Barberry *(Berberis vulgaris)*

Barberry is known for containing berberine, a powerful agent that has numerous actions, including potent anti-microbial, hepato-protectant, bile secreting, and liver detoxifying benefits. Apart from berberine, there are numerous other active substances in the chemical composition of the plant. The bark contains a large number of alkaloids (berberine, berbamine, and oxyacantha) and tannins. Barberry is also effective in reducing nausea and vomiting, toning and strengthening the body, and stimulating bowel action.

Specific Nutrient Therapies Indicated for Weight Management

Hydroxycitric acid

Hydroxycitric acid from standardized garcinia cambogia extract is a natural extract that comes from a tropical fruit grown in several Asian rain forests. Research shows that hydroxycitric acid helps maintain a healthy balance of hepatic lipogenesis and gluconeogenesis, thus preventing excessive conversion of glucose from dietary carbohydrate into body fat. Research also indicates that hydroxycitric acid plays an important role in the regulation of normal appetite. Unlike many commonly used diet ingredients, hydroxycitric acid is not a central nervous stimulant. Dosage: 1000 mg per day

Chromium

Chromium is an essential trace mineral that potentiates insulin's action and thus influences carbohydrate, protein, and fat metabolism. In its biologically active form from brewer's yeast, sometimes called glucose tolerance factor (GTF), chromium is associated with nicotinic acid (vitamin B-3). Chromium polynicotinate closely resembles the brewer's yeast GTF in both biological activity and chemical composition, as it also contains chromium associated with nicotinic acid. Chromium polynicotinate is yeast-free and has documented high bioavailability. Dosage: 200 mcg to 1000 mcg per day

Conjugated Linoleic Acid (CLA)

CLA is a mixture of conjugated dienoic derivatives of linoleic acid from safflower oil. Conjugated linoleic acid is found mainly in meat and dairy and can also be found in certain vegetable oils. Its presence in human tissue comes not only from dietary sources but also from *in vivo* oxidation of linoleic acid. CLA's activity as a potent metabolic modulator was first recognized in metabolic activity studies of its anti-carcinogenic properties in fried hamburgers. Research has now expanded to include its ability to modulate lipid and energy metabolism, body fat and muscle, and atherosclerosis. Research in several animal models has demonstrated that CLA reduces body fat accumulation. Some studies have shown that the reduction in body fat occurs regardless of whether the diet is high or low in fat. It appears that increased energy expenditure is responsible for the decreased fat accumulation. Dosage: 1000 mg to 1500 mg per day

Dietary Fiber

Dietary fiber is defined as complex carbohydrates that are resistant to the action of digestive enzymes, and therefore pass through the intestinal tract, unabsorbed. Dietary fiber includes substances such as cellulose, hemicellulose (xylans, galactans and mannans), pectins, gums, and lignin. Dietary fiber has many nutritional benefits for the health of the gastrointestinal tract. Insoluble dietary fiber, such as cellulose and many hemicelluloses, is not efficiently fermented in the colon. As a result, it provides fecal bulk, binds water, and helps soften stools. Soluble dietary fiber, such as pectin, many gums, and some hemicelluloses, is fermented in the colon to varying degrees. This results in lower colonic pH (acidity) and the production of short chain fatty acids, which are important for the intestinal micro flora and the health of the mucosal cells. Short chain fatty acids also have a role in facilitating colonic water absorption. Many insoluble and soluble fiber types bind dietary cholesterol and bile acids in the intestine and therefore play an important nutritional role in the enterohepatic circulation of cholesterol and cholesterol metabolism in general. Most types of dietary fiber, when hydrated, contribute substantially to the volume of stomach contents and help provide a feeling of fullness. Dosage: 30 g to 45 g per day

Relora®

Relora® is a patent-pending combination of the two herbal extracts magnolia and phellodendron bark. Both herbs have been used in traditional Chinese medicine for several hundred years. Relora reduces cortisol levels caused by excessive stress which in turn helps with weight loss. In a human study, 82% of the participants found that Relora® helped control irritability, emotional ups and downs, restlessness, tense muscles, poor sleep, fatigue, and concentration difficulties. Relora® was found not to cause sedation, although 74% of the patients had more restful sleep. Additionally, no adverse side effects were reported during the trial. A second human trial studied the effects of Relora® on salivary dehydroepiandrosterone (DHEA) and cortisol levels in patients with mild to moderate stress. The effects of stress on the body are sometimes associated with lower levels of DHEA and higher levels of cortisol. Two weeks of Relora® increased salivary DHEA by 227% and decreased total salivary cortisol by 37%. Both hormones were brought into the normal range. Dosage: 500 mg to 1000 mg per day

Garcinia Cambogia

Garcinia Cambogia, also known as Brindall berry, is a native fruit of South India. It is used in Ayurvedic medicine to treat obesity. Garcinia cambogia's high content of the organic acid hydroxycitric acid (HCA) is thought to interfere with the body's ability to produce and store fat, and suppress appetite by promoting glycogen synthesis. Dosage: 500 to 1,000 mg taken three times a day with plenty of water just before meals. The recommended daily allowance for this supplement is 2,500 to 3,000 mg.

Green Tea Extract

Green tea has been attributed to assist in weight loss possibly due to its diuretic and thermogenic effects. Early evidence suggests green tea's epigallocatechin-3-gallate may increase caloric and fat metabolism. Green Tea's active ingredient Conjugated Linoleic acid (CLA) is known to be an effective modulator of metabolism, reducing body fat and increasing muscle mass as well as encouraging healthy glucose homeostasis. Dosage: 500-1,000mg of green tea extract standardized for EGCG two to three times per day.

Acetyl L-Carnitine

Acetyl L-Carnitine can be used in the production of the neurotransmitter acetylcholine that is used in cognitive processing and memory storage. Acetyl L-Carnitine (and other forms of Carnitine) are vital for energy metabolism and help to transport lipids to the cells so that they can be burned to produce ATP. This process whereby fat is converted into energy is known as oxidation. Biomarkers of oxidation have been shown to be increased after taking Acetyl L-Carnitine supplements, resulting in the theory that using this supplement will enhance weight loss. Dosage: 500-3000mg per day

Raspberry Ketones

Raspberry Ketones contain a natural metabolic booster similar to capsaicin known to help the efficiency of the metabolism through thermogenesis (by increasing the body's core temperature and thus increasing the body's fat burning abilities). Raspberry Ketones also increase the level of Adiponectin, the hormone that supports lipolysis, by which fat is stored in the body is broken down into simpler compounds such as free fatty acids and glycerol, and in turn produces energy, rather than being stored as fat. Dosage: 100mg two times per day before meals.

Green Coffee Bean Extract

Green coffee bean extract contains chlorogenic acid (CGA), a biologically active phenol with antioxidant activity that has been shown to aid in weight loss. CGA inhibits the hydrolysis of glucose-6-phosphatase, reducing hepatic glycogenolysis and in turn slowing the release of glucose into the bloodstream. CGA also decreases intestinal absorption of glucose. This slower release of glucose in the bloodstream leads to a reduced insulin response, which minimizes fat deposition. Dosage: 400mg three times per day 30 minutes before meals.

Infrared Sauna and Weight Management

Methods to induce sweating have been used for centuries by many cultures to bring about improved health and relief from disease. Over two thousand years ago, the famous Greek physician Parmenides stated, "Give me a chance to create fever, and I will cure any disease." This traditional wisdom has certainly stood the test of time and is now coupled with the most advanced technology to create the soft heat infrared sauna.

Reducing toxic burdens of the body is a critically important factor in restoring health and vitality to individuals with chronic illness. The main drawback to using saunas in the past has been the discomfort many people experience during a sauna treatment. Traditional saunas use extremely high temperatures to warm the body by intensively heating the surface of the body only. Many people feel claustrophobic and find it hard to breathe. Fortunately, technological advances have resulted in a new type of sauna which is superior in many ways to traditional saunas. The soft heat infrared sauna utilizes infrared light, invisible to the human eye, to warm deeply inside the body tissues without significantly heating the air or external parts of the body. Many people who could not tolerate the traditional saunas will find the soft heat infrared sauna very pleasant and extremely effective at restoring health and well-being.

Health Benefits of Infrared Saunas Include:

- Weight loss (burn 600 calories in one half hour session)
- Pain relief from arthritis, back pain, chronic fatigue syndrome, fibromyalgia, and headaches.
- Eliminates harmful toxins including heavy metals, cholesterol, pesticides, and environmental contaminants.
- Increases circulation and cardiovascular function
- Clears cellulite
- Boosts immune response
- Improves and eliminates skin conditions such as acne, eczema, and psoriasis

Exercise and Weight Management

Exercise influences the hormones in the following ways:

- Improves fat burning and appetite control through leptin sensitivity
- Growth hormone is secreted in higher amounts as skin, bone, and muscle cells are repaired quicker
- Decreases the accumulation of harmful estrogens
- Decreases insulin resistance, resulting in improved fat loss and increased energy levels
- Secretion of serotonin in higher amounts, leading to improved mood, better sleep, and lessened cravings
- TSH, T4, and T3 levels are more balanced and therefore the metabolic rate is increased
- Decreased levels of elevated cortisol, resulting in a balanced nervous system
- Increased dopamine secretion, which improves mood, motivation, and appetite control
- Increased DHEA, which aids in anti-aging effects and improves lean body mass development
- Improved testosterone, which positively influences motivation and muscle building

Types of Exercise

Studies show that even the most inactive people can gain significant health benefits if they accumulate just thirty minutes or more of exercise or other physical activity per day. For the greatest overall health benefits, experts suggest thirty minutes of moderate-intensity aerobic exercise on most days of the week, plus some form of anaerobic exercise such as muscle strengthening and stretching at least two to three times per week.

Aerobic Exercise

Aerobic exercise is any activity involving large muscles, done for an extended period of time, that makes the heart and lungs work harder. Aerobic exercise provides both weight loss and cardiovascular benefits. Examples of aerobic exercise include walking, biking, jogging, running, dancing, boot camp classes, swimming, aerobic classes, and cross-country skiing.

Anaerobic Exercise

Anaerobic exercise usually refers to resistance training, such as lifting weights. Anaerobic exercise is performed primarily for increased muscle mass. Weight training and strength-resistance are examples of anaerobic exercise.

Moderate-Intensity Activities

Moderate-intensity exercise includes normal daily activities such as gardening and housework. These activities are often done in short spurts but the accumulation of thirty minutes of moderate-intensity activities can result in substantial health benefits. To become more active throughout your day, take advantage of any chance to get up and move around.

Some examples of moderate-intensity exercise include:

- Take a short walk around the block.
- Rake leaves.
- Play actively with the kids.
- Walk up the stairs instead of taking the elevator.
- Mow the lawn.
- Take an activity break—get up and stretch or walk around.
- Park your car a little farther away from your destination and walk the extra distance.

Top 5 Strategies for Weight Loss

1. Complete Hormone testing/Cardio Metabolic testing/Food Allergy testing/BIA testing
2. Liver detoxification
3. Consume a nutrient dense, high fiber, organic whole food diet/ Eliminate sugar/Eliminate high glycemic carbs/Limit all grain consumption
4. Implement an exercise program
5. Supplement with Omega 3's, Vitamin D3, B-complex vitamins, Acetyl L-Carnitine, Garcinia Cambogia, Chromium, Green tea extract, Relora, Green Coffee Bean extract and Raspberry Ketones

Nicole's Story - Weight Loss

Nicole is a thirty-one-year-old busy working mom whose main complaint was weight gain. Nicole was five feet two inches and weighed 192 pounds. Nicole had been on a popular weight loss program for about one year and had only lost ten pounds after spending thousands of dollars. Nicole wanted a different approach to weight loss. Nicole complained of severe PMS symptoms. She felt cold all of the time, suffering from Raynaud's syndrome (extremely cold hands/feet) as well as repeated chest infections. Nicole was a pack-a-day smoker who commonly skipped breakfast. At lunch and dinner she ate large amounts of meat and dairy products. She also consumed three to four cups of coffee per day with artificial sweeteners and, at night, consumed lemon gelato with aspartame nearly every night.

Lab testing:

- Low progesterone levels
- Estrogen dominance
- Low Free T3
- Low testosterone levels
- Low daytime cortisol levels
- Low DHEA levels

Management Plan

Nicole was administered the following natural medicine therapies:

- Infrared sauna sessions—thirty minutes three times per week for detoxification and added calorie burning

- Estrogen detoxification: DIM, calcium D-glucarate, SGS (standardized to contain 30 mg glucoraphanin glucosinolate), hops extract (0.12% 8-prenylnaringenin) two capsules with breakfast
- Thyroid support: iodine (as potassium iodide), zinc (as zinc picolinate), copper (as copper chelate), L-tyrosine, thyroid glandular (thyroxine free) two capsules two times per day
- Medical food: a powdered medical food designed to nutritionally support the management of conditions associated with metabolic syndrome (including altered body composition)
- Modified Mediterranean Lifestyle Nutrition Plan to balance hormones (see "Specific Guidelines for Nutritional Lifestyle Plan" in "Weight Gain" section)
- Bioidentical progesterone one pump on days fourteen to twenty-eight of the menstrual cycle
- Vitamin B-complex one capsule two times per day
- Exercise regime including one hour of a mixture of cardiovascular exercise and strength resistance training four times per week
- Smoking cessation

Nicole reported back twelve weeks later as she had previously been away on vacation. She said that she was doing very well with the plan. She had quit smoking "cold turkey" right after our initial appointment twelve weeks ago. She had not had a chest infection since the appointment. She stated that some of her PMS symptoms had improved, such as the breast tenderness and cramping. She added that her mood was much better but had been an issue for two to three days. BIA testing revealed that Nadege had lost a total of twenty-three pounds of fat mass and gained three pounds of lean body mass.

Nicole was recommended to quit drinking coffee altogether and to concentrate on improving water consumption. The remainder of the protocol stayed the same.

Nicole reported back eight weeks later and stated that all of her PMS symptoms were gone. She felt more "grounded" and calm now that she was not relying on caffeine. Nicole had lost a total of thirty-four pounds.

Over the following nine months, Nicole reached her goal weight of 125 pounds. She was thrilled and was strongly counseled on the importance of lifestyle changes versus diets so that she could maintain her weight loss.

Conclusion

Women are experiencing increasing endocrine dysfunction in our society today. There are a plethora of symptoms that are plaguing women of all ages that can be linked to imbalances within the hormonal cascade. Mainstream medicine has limited therapeutic tools to treat the very conditions that comprise most medical visits. The underlying cause is often overlooked or undiscovered and women are recommended masking medications that ultimately offer no cure. Cultural changes have contributed to the accelerated lifestyle to which many women have now become accustomed. It is normal for a woman to have a full-time career and raise children while under the expectation to maintain composure while running ragged.

In the world today, endocrine disruptors have inundated women's bodies and driven hormonal excesses and deficiencies to the extreme. These disruptors invade the body and terrorize the hormonal balance as they lock into the estrogen receptor sites. From the shampoo in the shower to the make-up in the drawer and the pesticides in our morning fruit, the stage is set for xenoestrogen dominance.

Centuries ago, women did not face the same challenges as the modern day woman. Today's woman consumes toxins that were not even thought of or needed by our ancestors. Life was simpler and consumerism was rare; therefore, this driven mentality was not the norm. There was minimal or no exposure to electromagnetic, noise, air and internal stress pollution.

Uncovering the disharmony in the endocrine system is the first step toward healing. A complete holistic approach is needed in order to truly restore balance. Factors such as liver function, nutrition, stress levels, lifestyle, toxin exposure, and stark hormonal imbalances all need to be addressed to bring transformation. Conditions such as depression, anxiety, stress, PCOS, ovarian cysts, adrenal fatigue, PMS, endometriosis, fibroids, weight gain, menopause, and thyroid dysfunction all share common denominators and are intertwined through the hormonal pathways. The body cannot be compartmentalized and separated into self-functioning systems, but rather must be recognized as an interwoven unit that requires all-encompassing consideration.

Bibliography

http://meridianvalleylab.com/bioidentical-hormones-risks-you-should-know-and-how-to-reduce-them/?gclid=CNn3po3x7KQCFQsGbAodI3nz1A

http://www.1-menopause.com/index.htm

http://www.natural-hormones.net/

http://www.cemcor.ubc.ca/

https://www.neurorelief.com/index.php?p=home

http://www.naturalnews.com/024985_cortisol_blood_adrenal_fatigue.html

http://www.estrogendominanceguide.com/

http://www.drlam.com/articles/Estrogen_Dominance.asp

http://www.endotext.org/adrenal/index.htm

http://www.merckmanuals.com/home/sec22/ch241/ch241e.html

http://www.womentowomen.com/healthyweight/naturalweightloss.aspx

http://pcos.insulitelabs.com/PCOS-Elements.php#Anchor-49575

http://www.stopthethyroidmadness.com/adrenal-info/symptoms-low-cortisol/

http://www.alternativehormonesolutions.ca/treatment.htm

http://www.prohealth.com/ME-CFS/library/showArticle.cfm?libid=14383&B1=EM031109C

http://www.diagnostechs.com/Home.aspx

http://www.womensinternational.com/

http://www.zrtlab.com/

http://www.theseventhwoman.org/

http://www.womeninbalance.org/find_help/

http://www.greenmountainhealth.com/news

What Your Doctor May Not Tell You About Perimenopause John R. Lee, MD

What Your Doctor May Not Tell You About Menopause John R. Lee, MD Wellness Central 1996

The Wisdom of Menopause Christine Northrup, MD Bantam Books 2001

The Cortisol Connection Shawn Talbott, PhD Hunter House 2002

Adrenal Fatigue: The 21st Century Stress Syndrome James L. Wilson, ND, DC, PhD Smart 2001

From Hormone Hell to Hormone Well C.W. Randolph, Jr., MD Health Communications Inc. 2009

You've Hit Menopause: Now What? George Gilson, MD Rocky Mountain Analytical Publishing 2004

Are Your Hormones Making You Sick? Eldred B. Taylor, MD Physicians Natural Medicine 2000

Feeling Fat, Fuzzy, or Frazzled? Richard Shames, MD Penguin Books 2005

Fight Fat After Forty Pamela Peeke, MD Penguin Books 2000

Estrogen's Storm Season Jerilynn Prior, MD Centre for Menstrual Cycle and Ovulation Research (CeMCOR) 2005

Hormone Matters for Vital Life- DVD www.theseventhwoman.com

Master Your Metabolism Jillian Michaels Crown Publishers 2009

Ageless Suzanne Somers Three River Press 2006

The Sexy Years Suzanne Somers Crown 2004

The Hormone Diet Natasha Turner, ND Random House Canada 2009

Super Charged Hormone Diet Natasha Turner, ND Random House Canada 2011

Fundamentals of Naturopathic Endocrinology Michael Friedman, MD CCNM Press 2005

Complete Natural Medicine Guide to Women's Health Sat Dharam Kaur, ND Robert Rose Inc. 2005

No More HRT Menopause Treat the Cause Karen Jensen, ND Lorna Vanderhaugue Fitzhenry and Whiteside 2002

The 4-Week Ultimate Body Detox Plan Michelle Schoffro Cook, DNM, DAc, CNC

Medicinal Herbs Quick Reference Guide Julieta Criollo, DNM, CHT 2009

Natural Detoxification A Practical Encyclopedia Jaqueline Krohn MD, Frances Taylor, MA Hartley and Marks 2000

Natural Progesterone-The multiple roles of a remarkable hormone John R. Lee MD Jon Carpenter 1999

Encyclopedia of Natural Medicine Revised 2nd Edition Michael Murray ND Joseph Pizzorno ND Prima Publishing 1998

Natural Medicine Instructions for Patients Elsevier Science Ltd Pizzorno L U, Pizzorno, Jr. J E, Murray M T Pizzorno-5 4/10/02 1:57 PM

The Super-Charged Hormone Diet Dr. Natasha Turner ND

Ultra Metabolism Mark Hyman, MD Atria Books 2006

Nutritional Medicine Alan R. Gaby, MD Fritz Perlberg 2011

Anxiety Orthomolecular Diagnosis and Treatment Dr. Jonathan Prousky CCNM Press, 2006

Treating and Beating Anxiety and Depression with Orthomolecular Medicine Dr. Rodger Muphree Harrison and Hamptom 2005

Healing Depression Integrated Naturopathic and Conventional Treatments Dr. Peter B. Bongiorno CCNM Press 2010

Slow Death by Rubber Duck Rick Smith and Bruce Lourie Counterpoint 2009

Encyclopedia of Nutritional Supplements Michael T. Murray Three Rivers Press 1996

Depression Free, Naturally Joan Mathews Larson Random House 1999

From Fatigued to Fantastic Jacob Teitelbaum Penguin Group 2007

Women's Encyclopedia of Natural Medicine Tori Hudson, ND McGraw Hill 2008

The 4-Week Ultimate Body Detox Plan Michelle Schoffro Cook, DNM, DAc Wiley 2004

Veganist Kathy Freston Weinstein 2011

Writing Your Dissertation in Fifteen Minutes a Day Joan Bolker Henry Holt and Company 1998

A Manual for Writers of Research Papers, Theses, and Dissertations Kate Turabian Chicago Guides 2007

The Craft of Research Wayne C. Booth, Gregory G. Colomb, Joseph M. Williams Chicago Guides 2008

Appendix

Sources Used

Hormonal Lab Testing

ZRT Labs
8605 SW Creekside Place
Beaverton, OR 97008 USA

Diagnos-Techs
19110 66th S, Bldg G
Kent, WA 98032 USA

Food Allergy Testing

Sterochrom Analytical
7825 Edmonds Street
Burnaby, BC V3N 1B9 Canada

Genova Diagnostics
63 Zillicoa Street
Asheville, NC 28801 USA

Supplements:

AOR
3900 – 12 Street NE
Calgary, AB T2E 8H9 Canada
www.aor.ca

Avicenna
North Vancouver, BC Canada
www.avicennanatural.com

Biotics
6801 Biotics Research Dr
Rosenberg, TX 77471
www.bioticsresearch.com

Boiron
1300 René-Descartes
Saint-Bruno-de-Montarville, QC J3V 0B7 Canada
www.boiron.ca

Douglas Labs
552 Newbold Street
London, ON N6E 2S5 Canada
www.douglaslabs.ca

Enzed Nutricorp
2402 Canoe Ave.
Coquitlam BC V3K 6C2
Canada
www.enzednaturals.com

Integrative Therapeutics
825 Challenger Drive
Green Bay, WI 54311 USA
www.integrativepro.com

Metagenics
100 Avenida La Pata
San Clemente, CA 92673 USA
www.metagenics.com

Oona
803 Washington St.
New York, NY 10014 USA
www.oonausa.com

Pascoe
Unit 70-40 Vogell Road
Richmond Hill, Ontario L4B 3N6 Canada
www.pascoecanada.com

Promedics
PO Box 155
2498 W 41st Avenue
Vancouver, BC V6M 2A7 Canada
www.promedics.ca

Restorative Formulations
93 Barre Street, Suite #1
Montpelier, VT 05602
www.restorativeformulations.com

Seroyal (Genestra)
490 Elgin Mills Road East
Richmond Hill, ON L4C 0L8 Canada
www.seroyal.com

Thorne Research, Inc.
P.O. Box 25
Dover, ID 83825 USA
www.thorne.com

Xymogen
6900 Kingspointe Pkwy.
Orlando, FL 32819
www.xymogen.com

100% Pure
2221 Oakland Road
San Jose, California 95131
www.100percentpure.ca

www.ingramcontent.com/pod-product-compliance
Lightning Source LLC
Chambersburg PA
CBHW080328270326
41927CB00014B/3136

* 9 7 8 1 9 9 0 8 3 0 5 4 9 *